Basic Medical Techniques and Patient Care in Imaging Technology

Sixth Edition

Lillian S. Torres, RN, BS, MS, MEd, CNS, NP

Professor Emeritus, Chaffey College
School of Physical, Life and Health Sciences
Rancho Cucamonga, California

TerriAnn Linn-Watson Norcutt, MEd, RT(RM), RDMS

Coordinator, Radiologic Technology Program
Professor, Chaffey College
School of Physical, Life and Health Sciences
Rancho Cucamonga, California

Andrea Guillen Dutton, MEd, RT(RM)

Clinical Coordinator, Radiologic Technology Program
Professor, Chaffey College
School of Physical, Life and Health Sciences
Rancho Cucamonga, California

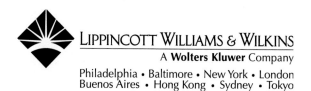

LIPPINCOTT WILLIAMS & WILKINS
A **Wolters Kluwer** Company

Philadelphia • Baltimore • New York • London
Buenos Aires • Hong Kong • Sydney • Tokyo

Editor: *John Goucher*
Managing Editor: *Nancy Peterson*
Marketing Manager: *Mary Martin*
Production Editor: *Jennifer Ajello*
Designer: *Doug Smock*
Compositor: *Techbooks*
Printer: *Courier-Westford*

Library of Congress Cataloging-in-Publication Data is available. ISBN-13 978-0-7817-3191-1
ISBN-10 0-7817-3191-7

06
5 6 7 8 9 10

Basic Medical Techniques
and Patient Care in
Imaging Technology

To Joseph

Foreword

For over 20 years, Lillian Torres has written an outstanding book to facilitate the education of radiography students in patient care. For the first decade, hers was the only book on the subject. Today, with more choices on the subject, Mrs. Torres has refined, yet maintained, the quality and in-depth discussions that have made this book a favorite among educators. *Basic Medical Techniques and Patient Care in Imaging Technology* is used internationally and is published in three different languages making it one of the most widely used tools in radiographic education.

The sixth edition represents the latest contribution to medical skills and techniques. As Mrs. Torres is retiring, she brought her contributors, Andrea Dutton and TerriAnn Linn-Watson Norcutt, on as co-authors. The combined efforts of these individuals have created a work that will be a most valuable resource for radiologic science educators, the students they teach, and their patients.

Stewart C. Bushong, Sc.D., FACR, FACMP
Professor of Radiologic Science
Baylor College of Medicine
Houston, Texas

Preface

The field of radiologic technology has exploded with the technologic advances that have occurred over the past 5 years. When the first edition of this textbook was written and published in 1979, the author and her consultants for the text had no concept of the degree of change that would take place in this discipline. Although each edition of *Basic Medical Techniques and Patient Care in Imaging Technology* has changed and grown to meet the growing professional accountability needs of radiologic technologists, this sixth edition has been expanded significantly.

Hallmarks of the Sixth Edition

Radiologic technology students must understand the responsibilities of membership in their profession. To meet this end, the educational requirements, the necessity of belonging to professional organizations, and the relationship of the radiographer to the other members of the health care team are emphasized. The revised Code of Ethics from The American Society of Radiologic Technologists and the newly adopted rules of ethics are discussed. The subjects of professional ethics and the legal aspects of radiologic technology have been expanded and include a more detailed description of the mandatory consents for imaging procedures.

Individual chapters on each of the following aspects of patient care in imaging technology are included with illustrations to emphasize each technique described.

- Critical thinking (Chapter 1)
- Professional and therapeutic communication (Chapters 1 and 2 and throughout)
- Pediatric and geriatric patient care (Chapter 9)

- Trauma and mobile radiographic techniques (Chapter 8)

The new requirements of health care professionals concerning pain control and the ability to adequately assess patients' safety needs in all aspects of health care is emphasized in the sixth edition (Chapter 4). Infection control in health care continues to be a major concern. With the threat of all forms of hepatitis, HIV and AIDS, tuberculosis, anthrax, and other forms of biologic assault to consider, the techniques of infection control have been updated to protect both the patient and the radiologic technologist (Chapter 3).

Knowledge of pharmacology and safety in drug administration is required in radiology. While chapters on pharmacology and the methods of drug administration were included in the previous edition of this text, the sixth edition has expanded both areas significantly, especially in the area of contrast media administration (Chapters 12 and 13). Patient care in special procedures has been altered to include those areas that are most relevant in imaging at the present time (Chapter 16).

As the scope of radiographers' practice expands and radiographers participate in diagnostic procedures in which continuous cardiac monitoring is required, the need for radiographers to identify ominous cardiac arrhythmias has increased. To meet this need, an entire chapter has been added on interpreting the basic electrocardiogram (ECG) (Chapter 15). Illustrations of normal and abnormal ECG strips with explanations are added for clarification.

It is the hope of the authors that the changes in the sixth edition will assist radiologic technology students to be safe practitioners in every aspect of patient care.

Acknowledgments

When Lillian Torres approached us with the proposal of becoming co-authors of this text, we were both honored and excited at the prospect of being able to work on such an important book. It is to her that we owe the most. She has mentored us over the years, not only in teaching the medical procedures class, but also as a great friend. We did it!

T.A.L.W.N.
A.G.D.

The authors had the valuable cooperation and assistance of the Health Science faculty and Radiologic Technology students at Chaffey College. Sylvia Pompura, RN, MEd, our critic and secretarial assistant; Marcha Talton, RN, MSN; Juanita Mathews, RN, MSN; Sue Herman, RN, MSN; Rene Ketchum, RN, MSN; Kathy Lightner, RN, MSN; Beverly Cox; and all others at Chaffey College who assisted us during the long photo sessions are remembered fondness and gratitude.

Special thanks goes to the following:

Jeffrey A. Jones, our photographer, and his assistant, Pat Amison

James Akamine, MD, for taking time from reading a large stack of radiographic images to assist us with our photographs on a Sunday afternoon

Greg Higgins, RT, Administrative Technologist at San Antonio Community Hospital

Ed Millard, RT, Vice President of Ancillary Services at San Antonio Community Hospital

Michael Segura, RT, Cardiac Catheterization Laboratory Manager at San Antonio Community Hospital, and the catheterization laboratory staff: Larry Seligman, RN, Julie Olney, RN, and Tom Candido, RN

The student models who reported promptly and stayed long hours to pose as directed

C. Davidson, RT, and the radiology staff at Jerry Pettis Veterans Administration Memorial Hospital, Loma Linda, California

We are also indebted to the 2002 and 2003 graduating classes of the Chaffey College Radiography Program for enduring the trial and error chapter revisions put to them. Their candidness and humor were a significant help in redefining the chapter narratives.

Finally, thank you to our gracious editor, Carla Schroeder. Working with her has been a pleasure. She has been patient and understanding to the end.

L.S.T.
T.A.L.W.N.
A.G.D.

Brief Contents

Contents

Professional Issues in Radiologic Technology

Objectives

After studying this chapter, you will be able to:

1. Define the criteria of a profession, and explain how the profession of radiologic technology has evolved to meet these criteria.

2. List the members of the health care team with whom you as a radiographer may frequently interact, and briefly describe the role of each.

3. Discuss the purpose of professional organizations, and list the reasons for you to join organizations in your field.

4. Define ethics and discuss ethics as it applies to radiologic technology.

5. Explain the legal obligations that you as a radiographer have toward your patients, peers, and other members of the health care team.

6. Define *patient rights* and describe the role that you have as a radiographer in protecting these rights.

7. List the responsibilities of the patient who seeks health care.

8. Discuss the legal implications for the radiographer when using immobilization techniques, unusual occurrence reports, informed consent, Good Samaritan Laws, computerized technology, and malpractice insurance.

9. Explain the need for accurate and complete medical records and documentation in health care and the obligations you will have as a radiographer in this aspect of patient care.

10. List and define the four current methods of health care delivery and the levels of health care currently available in the United States.

Glossary

Adhere: To stay fixed or firm

Bias: An inclination or temperament based on personal judgment; prejudice

Common law: Decisions and opinions of courts that are based on local customs and habits of an area within a particular country or state

Continuum: Continuous whole whose parts cannot be separated

Diagnostic imaging: Modern term for radiography, encompassing all specialties devoted to producing a picture of a body part

Euthanasia: Act of deliberately bringing about the death of a person suffering from an incurable disease or condition

Grieving process: An emotional state that a person goes through to maintain sound emotional health when experiencing a loss

Holistic: The view that an organic or integrated whole has a reality independent of and greater than the sum of its parts

Liability: Something that a person is obligated to do or an obligation required to be fulfilled by law; usually an obligation of a financial nature

Litigation: Lawsuit

Malpractice: Professional negligence that is the cause of injury or harm to a patient

Mentor: A teacher, coach, or advisor of conduct

Preceptor: A teacher; directs action or conduct or another individual

Profession: A calling that requires specialized knowledge and intensive academic preparation

Statutory law: Established law that is enacted by a legislative body and punishable by law

Terminal illness: A disease with no known cure that results in death

Therapeutic: Healing

Unethical: Not conforming to the standards of conduct of a particular profession or group

Radiologic technology has evolved to meet the criteria of a profession. As in all professions, the conduct and behavior of radiographers are expected to adhere to the particular ethical and legal standards of the field. Any person who does not adhere to this code may lose his or her license as well as the privileges of that profession.

As a radiographer, you will not work alone in caring for the patient. You will work and interact with members of a health care team whose goal is to improve or restore the patient to good health. The health care team consists of physicians, nurses, therapists, and social workers, all of whom work within their scope of practice and are accountable for performing their professional duties.

As a student who has made the decision to enter the profession of radiologic technology, you must realize that you are committed to accepting the code of ethics of this profession and must work within that scope of practice. You must also understand that you are accountable for your work and may be held legally liable for any errors you make while caring for patients.

Radiologic technology is a profession oriented toward the diagnosis and treatment of trauma and disease. This means that as a radiologic technologist (called radiographer in this text) you will work in intimate contact with people on a daily basis. You must be prepared to work with people of all races, religions, and economic backgrounds and to relate to them in an unbiased, nonjudgmental manner.

If you are contemplating a career in radiologic technology, you need to examine the reasons why you have chosen this profession. It would be helpful to ask yourself the following questions before proceeding:

Am I prepared to accept and practice the profession of radiologic technology and support the ethics of this profession?

Am I prepared to avoid violations of the law in practicing this profession?

Will I be willing and able to learn to relate to my patients in a professional and nonjudgmental manner at all times?

If you cannot answer these questions positively, you should reconsider your career choice.

The Criteria for a Profession

Radiologic technology has evolved from a vocational program into a *profession*. This progression took place over a number of years with the efforts and dedication of the persons who worked in this field. The term profession implies a vocation or occupation that requires extended training and education of its members, who have special skills and serve a specific social need. The criteria for a group of practitioners to identify themselves as a profession were summarized by Chitty (1993) as follows:

1. A vital human service is provided to the society by the profession.

2. Professions possess a special body of knowledge that is continuously enlarged through research.

3. Practitioners are expected to be accountable and responsible.

4. The education of professionals takes place in institutions for higher education.

5. Practitioners have an independent function and control their own practice.

6. Professionals are committed to their work and are motivated by doing good.

7. A code of ethics guides professional decisions and conduct.

8. A professional organization oversees and supports standards of practice.

All professions have a code of ethics and professional organizations that control the educational and practice requirements of its members. The two organizations that assume these roles for radiographers are the American Society of Radiologic Technologists (ASRT) and the American Registry of Radiologic Technologists (ARRT). The professional radiographer is registered by the ARRT and by state licensure, if applicable.

Radiologic technology fulfills the basic requirements of a profession and is becoming increasingly autonomous in professional practice. With the status of a profession come certain responsibility and educational requirements that the person formerly known as an "x-ray technician" did not have. If you are contemplating radiologic technology as a profession, examine the criteria of a profession listed above to make certain that you are willing to uphold the high standards of a professional. These standards include responsibility, accountability, competence, and judgment. As a professional radiographer you are expected to demonstrate all of these qualities.

Standards of Practice and Educational Requirements in Radiography

The ASRT Standards of Practice state, "Radiographers use professional and ethical judgment and critical thinking when performing their duties. Quality improvement and customer service allow the radiographer to be a responsible member of the health care team by continually assessing professional performance. Radiographers embrace continuing education for optimal patient care, public education and enhanced knowledge and technical competence" (ASRT, 2001).

In addition, the radiographer must possess the following qualities: a willingness to become an active member of professional organizations, ethical behavior, an appreciation for the implications that rising health care costs have for patient care, a holistic caregiver perspective, effective oral and written communication skills, problem-solving skills, and a broad computer knowledge base.

The preparatory education for the radiographer has evolved from a hospital-based preceptor training to formal educational programs. Hospital-based programs as well as college or university-based programs of study are now available. To become a registered radiographer, you must complete at least 2 years of formal education in an accredited hospital-based program or a 2-year or 4-year educational program at an academic institution. In addition, you must pass a national certification examination (ASRT, 2001).

Radiography program curriculum includes course work in anatomy, patient positioning, examination techniques, equipment protocols, radiation safety, radiation protection, and basic patient care. As an entry-level radiographer, you will need the skill and ability to perform the following functions:

1. Apply modern principles of radiation exposure, radiation physics, radiation protection, and radiobiology to produce diagnostic images.

2. Use knowledge of medical terminology, pathology, cross-sectional anatomy, topographic anatomy, anatomy and physiology, and positioning procedures to produce diagnostic images.

3. Provide direct patient care such as ECG, contrast media, and other drug administration.

4. Evaluate recognized equipment malfunctions.

5. Evaluate radiographic images.

6. Achieve a level of computer literacy.

7. Teach educational courses at the technical level.

8. Communicate with other members of the health care team.

9. Provide patient and family education.

10. Participate in community affairs.

In addition, as an entry-level radiographer, you should possess the following qualities: an ability to think in a critical manner; a willingness to participate in lifelong learning, including becoming an active member of professional organizations; ethical behavior and an appreciation for the implications that rising health care costs have for patient care; a holistic caregiver perspective; a broad computer knowledge base; problem-solving skills; and the ability to communicate effectively orally and in writing.

As you become more experienced, you will possess all of the qualities and abilities listed above as well as the following:

1. The ability to supervise, evaluate, and counsel staff

2. The ability to plan, organize, and administer professional development activities

3. Superior decision-making and problem-solving skills to assess situations and identify solutions for standard outcomes

4. The ability to promote a positive, collaborative atmosphere in all aspects of radiography

5. Skills as a mentor

6. Knowledge in areas of supervision, in-service and/or continuing education, and regulatory compliance

As a health care professional, you must acquire and maintain current knowledge to preserve a high level of expertise. Continuing education provides you with educational activities to enhance knowledge, skills, performance, and awareness of changes and advances. Continuing education supports professionalism, which fosters quality patient care.

Previously voluntary for radiographers, continuing education became a mandate in 1995 for all who are licensed by the ARRT. Now you are required to earn 24 continuing education credits. These credits must be accepted by the ARRT and are to be earned every 2 years. The licensing body must verify these credits

Chronology of Events in the History of the Radiologic Technology Profession

1895 Wilhelm Conrad Roentgen discovered x-rays in Wurzburg, Germany.

1920 The American Association of Radiological Technicians, the first society for the profession, was created by a group of technologists in Chicago, Illinois. The society was dedicated to the advancement of radiologic technology.

1921 The society's first annual meeting was held. Membership totaled 47.

1922 The American Registry of Radiological Technicians originated.

1930s–1940s Radiographer education was primarily by apprenticeship.

1932 The name of the American Association of Radiological Technicians was formally changed to the American Society of X-ray Technicians (ASXT).

1936 The ASXT was authorized to make appointment to the Registry Board of Trustees.

1952 The ASXT provided a basic minimum curriculum for training schools.

1955 The ASXT created a new membership category— Fellow of AXST—which recognized individual members who have made significant contributions to the profession.

1959 The ASXT membership reached 8600 members.

1960 Registry applicants were required to have at least 2 years of training or experience.

1963 The American Registry of Radiological Technicians changed its name to the American Registry of Radiologic Technologists (ARRT).

1964 The ASXT changed its name to the American Society of Radiologic Technologists.

1966 Registry applicants were required to be graduates of training programs approved by the American Medical Association's Council on Medical Education.

1967 The Association of University Radiologic Technologists was established to stimulate an interest in radiologic technology through the academic environment.

1968 The Society membership reached 14,000.

1970 Registry Certificate No. 1 was awarded to Sister Mary Beatrice by the Registry.

1984 The Association of University Radiologic Technologists changed its name to The Association of Educators in Radiological Sciences (AERS). Currently membership is around 1000 educators from the United States and other countries.

1988 The Summit on Radiologic Sciences and Sonography met in Chicago to develop strategies to alleviate the personnel shortage in the profession.

1995 The American Registry of Radiologic Technologists announced that, beginning in 1995, x-ray technologists would henceforth be obligated to obtain 12 continuing education units per year to maintain their licenses.

1996 The Society membership reached 47,000 members.

1997 ARRT marked 75th anniversary.

1998 ASRT launched an aggressive campaign to protect patients from overexposure to radiation during radiologic procedures and help reduce the costs of health care.

2001 ASRT introduced a bill, known as the Consumer Assurance of Radiologic Excellence (CARE) bill during the 2001 congressional session. It ensures that the people performing radiologic examinations are qualified.

2001 ASRT is the largest of the profession's association membership, with more than 87,000 members.

before your license is renewed. You may achieve the continuing education credits by participating in educational activities that meet the criteria set forth by the ARRT, such as seminars, conferences, lectures, departmental in-service education, directed readings, home study, and college courses. You may earn 24 credits by taking an entry-level exam in another discipline that you did not previously pass, but are eligible to take. The entry-level exams are in radiography, nuclear medicine, or radiation therapy. Another way you can earn 24 credits is by passing an advanced-level examination, after proving eligibility. The advanced-level exams are in mammography, cardiovascular-interventional technology, magnetic resonance, computed tomography, quality management, and sonography. By participating in continuing education activities, you enhance your professional knowledge and professional performance for providing a high standard of quality patient care.

The Evolution of Professional Organizations in Radiologic Technology

Participation in professional organizations is the responsibility of all practicing professionals, regardless of their field. Membership in professional organizations provides you with a pathway to continued successful professional development. It can provide you with comprehensive opportunities to remain current in a constantly changing technological career. Professional organizations provide you with opportunities for technical growth and the development of leadership skills, as well as an arena for professional interaction and problem solving, especially in career issues. Many program and member services are offered by professional organizations, including continuing education, a job bank and career information, events, conferences and seminars, government relations and collective legislative power, group professional liability insurance, and other member benefits and services. In addition, the ASRT works with professional certification bodies and accreditation agencies for radiographers. Ultimately, membership in professional organizations enables you to continue providing quality patient health care and to uphold the standards of your profession.

There are various levels of professional organizations in radiologic technology. Internationally, there is the International Society of Radiographs and Radiologic Technologists. In the United States, the ASRT is the national organization for radiology technology. The ASRT has affiliated societies at state levels, and the state societies have district affiliates. A chronology of the events that stimulated the radiologic technology profession is interesting to review (Display 1-1).

The Health Care Team

As a radiographer, you will interact on a daily basis with your peers in diagnostic imaging and with other members of the health care team. Many of these people will be members of other health care professions, and some will be nonprofessional members in various aspects of the health care delivery system. Recognition of the roles that the other members of the team play in patient care can be helpful to you. Table 1-1 briefly

TABLE 1-1
The Health Care Team

TEAM MEMBER	RESPONSIBILITIES
Physician	Orders treatments, medications, and consultant care as necessary; requires a baccalaureate degree and 4 years of medical education at an accredited medical school to earn a Medical Doctor degree (M.D.). The physician then chooses an area of medical practice and fulfills the requirements to attain certification in that field of specialized medicine.

Nurse	Provides care for the patient that often requires 24 hours a day; also provides home health care, out-patient care, case management, educator, and acts as a patient advocate. Expanded functions in nursing include clinical nurse specialist and nurse practitioner. Nurses administer medications and treatments as ordered by the physician; monitor the patient's health status, coordinate and facilitate all patient care when the patient is hospitalized.
	    Nursing education may be obtained in a university baccalaureate degree or may be achieved in a community college that allows the graduate to take the licensing examination.
	    For the vocational nurse, there is a two-semester certificate program. The vocational nurse works with patients under the supervision of a registered nurse.
	    All nurses must pass a licensing examination to practice in the profession.

Occupational Therapist and Physical Therapists	Members of separate professions who play significant roles in the rehabilitation of patients following illness or injury. Education for these professions is university-based and requires a baccalaureate degree and 1 year of internship. The therapist evaluates the patient's rehabilitation needs, designs, and supervises the program to achieve mobility or perform activities of daily living (ADLs) independently.
Pharmacist	Prepares and dispenses medications and oversees the patient's drug therapy; Requires a baccalaureate degree and 1 or 2 years of internship.
Respiratory Therapist	Is responsible for maintaining or improving the patient's respiratory status; administers various forms of respiratory therapy; monitors ventilatory equipment, and administers drugs that must be given by inhalation. Education may be college-based, and a certificate must be obtained when the course is completed.
Laboratory Technologists	Receive laboratory specimens and analyze them for pathological conditions; requires a baccalaureate degree and an internship of 1 year.
Paraprofessionals	Phlebotomists (draw blood for examination); electrocardiogram technicians; nursing assistants, pharmacy technicians, and many more all must be educated to a lesser degree in the field that they support and work under the supervision of licensed professionals.

DISPLAY 1–2

Practice Standards

Introduction to Radiography

Radiographers must demonstrate an understanding of human anatomy, physiology, pathology, and medical terminology.

Radiographers must maintain a high degree of accuracy in radiographic positioning and exposure technique. He or she must maintain knowledge about radiation protection and safety. Radiographers prepare for and assist the radiologist in the completion of intricate radiographic examinations. They prepare and administer contrast media and medications in accordance with state and federal regulations.

Radiographers are the primary liaison between patients and radiologists and other members of the support team. They must remain sensitive to the physical and emotional needs of the patient through good communication, patient assessment, patient monitoring and patient care skills.

Radiographers use professional and ethical judgment and critical thinking when performing their duties. Quality improvement and customer service allow the radiographer to be a responsible member of the health care team by continually assessing professional performance. Radiographers embrace continuing education for optimal patient care, public education and enhanced knowledge and technical competence.

Professional Performance Standards

Standard One—Quality: The practitioner strives to provide optimal care to all patients.

Standard Two—Self-Assessment: The practitioner evaluates personal performance, knowledge, and skills.

Standard Three—Education: The practitioner acquires and maintains current knowledge in clinical practice.

Standard Four—Collaboration and Collegiality: The practitioner promotes a positive, collaborative practice atmosphere with other members of the health care team.

Standard Five—Ethics: The practitioner adheres to the profession's accepted Code of Ethics.

Standard Six—Exploration and Investigation: The practitioner participates in the acquisition, dissemination, and advancement of the professional knowledge base.

Radiography Clinical Performance Standards/Quality Performance Standards

Standard One—Assessment: The practitioner collects pertinent data about the patient and about the procedure and pertinent information regarding equipment, the procedures, and the work environment.

Standard Two—Analysis/Determination: The practitioner analyzes the information obtained during the assessment phase and develops an action plan for completing the procedure; information collected during the assessment phase and determines whether changes need to be made to equipment, procedures, or the work environment.

Standard Three—Patient Education: The practitioner provides information about the procedure to the patient, significant others and health care providers and informs patients, the public, and other health care providers about procedures, equipment, and facilities.

Standard Four—Implementation: The practitioner implements the action plan and performs quality assurance activities or acquires information on equipment and materials.

Standard Five—Evaluation: The practitioner determines whether the goals of the action plan have been achieved, evaluates quality assurance results, and establishes an appropriate action plan.

Standard Six—Implementation: The practitioner implements the revised action plan and the quality assurance action plan.

Standard Seven—Outcomes Measurement: The practitioner reviews and evaluates the outcome of the procedure and assesses the outcome of the quality assurance action plan in accordance with established guidelines.

Standard Eight—Documentation: The practitioner documents information about patient care, the procedure and the final outcome and also documents quality assurance activities and results.

Source: The American Society of Radiologic Technologists.

outlines many of these professions and the roles they play in health care delivery.

Specialty Areas in Radiography

Radiography has made dramatic progress since its inception in 1895. At present, this profession has practice standards that reflect the increasing responsibilities that you will have as a radiographer (Display 1-2). In addition to radiographic imaging, you may enhance your professional growth by specializing in diagnostic and therapeutic treatment areas that have evolved from the field of basic radiography. Some of the areas for professional advancement include computed tomography (CT), magnetic resonance imaging (MRI), positron emission tomography (PET), mammography, ultrasonography, nuclear medicine, and radiation therapy. These and other areas of specialization are discussed in detail in Chapter 16. The completion of the basic radiologic technology program can be the end of your educational career or merely the beginning.

Professional Ethics

Ethics may be defined as a set of moral principles that govern one's course of action. *Moral principles* are a set of standards that establish what is right or good. All individuals have a personal code of ethics that evolves based on their cultural and environmental background. This same background has taught us to place *values* on behaviors, as well as on objects in our environment; that is, to assign a judgment of either good or bad to an action.

Ethics is a combination of the attributes of honesty, integrity, fairness, caring, respect, fidelity, citizenship, and accountability. As you can quickly see, the terms "ethics," "principles," and "values" are closely linked and may be used interchangeably from time to time.

As a student entering the profession of radiologic technology, you bring your personal code of ethics, your moral principles, and your personal values. All professionals have a set of professional values, and all professionals have a set of ethical principles or a code of ethics that governs professional behavior. This is true of radiologic technology, adopted in July 2001.

The Standard of Ethics is made up of two parts: the Code of Ethics and the Rules of Ethics. The Code of Ethics was developed, revised, and adopted by the ASRT and the ARRT in July 1998. It serves as a guide in maintaining ethical conduct in all aspects of the radiologic sciences. The rules of ethics were added in 2001. Considered to be mandatory and enforced by the ARRT, the 21 Rules of Ethics are designed to promote protection, safety, and comfort of the patient (Display 1-3).

Together, these documents represent the application of moral principles and moral values to the practice of the profession and are considered to be the minimum acceptable standards of conduct. They are concerned with the duties and responsibilities that you have as a radiographer toward yourself, your patients, and your professional peers and associates. Your responsibilities deal with rights and correlated responsibilities and are discussed in the following section.

Unfortunately, as the world of health care becomes increasingly complex and the ability to prolong life expands, there are more difficult choices to be made. This leads to a growing number of ethical conflicts and dilemmas. You will not be immune to these as you perform your professional duties as a radiographer. You must adhere to your professional standard of ethics at all times, even though doing so will, at times, present difficult problems to be resolved.

A set of ethical principles has been derived from the basic ethical philosophies. These are *utilitarianism*, *deontology*, and *virtue*. Utilitarianism is often called *consequentialism* and advocates that actions are morally correct or right when the largest number of persons is benefited by the decision made. An example of this is as follows:

A large accident occurs and a number of persons are critically injured. The triage team assigns a higher priority to the less injured patients and attends last to those who are critically injured, since the chance of survival is less for the most severely injured.

This is an acceptable philosophy if you are not in the minority who does not benefit from the decision. The important element in this example is the result of the action. This is based on the principal known as *teleological theory* (meaning end or completion). In other words, it is based on consequences with the highest good with the greatest happiness for the largest number of people.

Deontology upholds the philosophy that the rules are to be followed at all times by all individuals. Deontology comes from a Greek word meaning "duty"; therefore, you judge action by deciding if it is an obligation. When making decisions using this school of thought, you generally do not take consequences into consideration even if it proves to be beneficial to the patient. Following the rules at all times may be too restrictive, especially when specific circumstances surrounding a situation do not fit a set of rules.

An example of deontology is illustrated by the accident portrayed in a preceding paragraph. Since the health care provider has the duty to "do no harm," then assigning a low priority number to the most critical patients would be wrong. Since deontology and utilitarianism are more or less opposite, the more critically injured patients would get the highest priority, and the most likely to survive would be attended to last because they would survive longest without care.

Virtue is a new philosophical belief that focuses on using wisdom rather than emotional and intellectual problem solving. With holistic medicine gaining popularity in recent years, virtue ethics incorporates certain principles of both utilitarianism and deontology to provide a broader view of issues. Analysis, review of consequences, and societal rules are key in forming decisions using virtue. Again, using the accident example to illustrate, with virtue ethics the triage of the patients would take into account the significance of each individual. How the family and friends of the victims would be affected by the triage decisions would be the deciding factor in who gets first treatment.

Ethical Principles

To resolve ethical dilemmas, you may apply this established set of principles to decision making:

Autonomy: Refers to the right of all persons to make rational decisions free from external pressures.

DISPLAY 1–3

ARRT Standards of Ethics
Effective: July 2002

Preamble

The *Standards of Ethics* of The American Registry of Radiologic Technologists shall apply solely to persons holding certificates from ARRT who either hold current registrations by ARRT or formerly held registrations by ARRT (collectively, "Registered Technologists"), and to persons applying for examination and certification by ARRT in order to become Registered Tehnologists ("Candidates"). The *Standards of Ethics* are intended to be consistent with the Mission Statement of ARRT, and to promote the goals set forth in the Mission Statement.

A. Code of Ethics

The Code of Ethics forms the first part of the *Standards of Ethics*. The Code of Ethics shall serve as a guide by which Registered Technologists and Candidates may evaluate their professional conduct as it relates to patients, health care consumers, employers, colleagues and other members of the health care team. The Code of Ethics is intended to assist Registered Technologists and Candidates in maintaining a high level of ethical conduct and in providing for the protection, safety and comfort of patients. The Code of Ethics is aspirational.

1. The radiologic technologist conducts herself or himself in a professional manner, responds to patient needs and supports colleagues and associates in providing quality patient care.

2. The radiologic technologist acts to advance the principle objective of the profession to provide services to humanity with full respect for the dignity of mankind.

3. The radiologic technologist delivers patient care and service unrestricted by the concerns of personal attributes or the nature of the disease or illness, and without discrimination on the basis of sex, race, creed, religion or socioeconomic status.

4. The radiologic technologist practices technology founded upon theoretical knowledge and concepts, uses equipment and accessories consistent with the purposes for which they were designed, and employs procedures and techniques appropriately.

5. The radiologic technologist assesses situations; exercises care, discretion and judgment; assumes responsibility for professional decisions; and acts in the best interest of the patient.

6. The radiologic technologist acts as an agent through observation and communication to obtain pertinent information for the physician to aid in the diagnosis and treatment of the patient and recognizes that interpretation and diagnosis are outside the scope of practice for the profession.

7. The radiologic technologist uses equipment and accessories, employs techniques and procedures, performs services in accordance with an accepted standard of practice, and demonstrates expertise in minimizing radiation exposure to the patient, self and other members of the health care team.

8. The radiologic technologist practices ethical conduct appropriate to the profession and protects the patient's right to quality radiologic technology care.

9. The radiologic technologist respects confidences entrusted in the course of professional practice, respects the patient's right to privacy and reveals confidential information only as required by law or to protect the welfare of the individual or the community.

10. The radiologic technologist continually strives to improve knowledge and skills by participating in continuing education and professional activities, sharing knowledge with colleagues and investigating new aspects of professional practice.

B. Rules of Ethics

The Rules of Ethics form the second part of the *Standards of Ethics*. They are mandatory and directive-specific standards of minimally acceptable professional conduct for all present Registered Technologists and Candidates. Certification is a method of assuring the medical community and the public that an individual is qualified to practice within the profession. Because the public relies on certificates and registrations issued by ARRT, it is essential that Registered Technologists and Candidates act consistently with these Rules of Ethics. These Rules of Ethics are intended to promote the protection, safety and comfort of patients. The Rules of Ethics are enforceable. Registered Technologists and Candidates engaging in any of the following conduct or activities, or who permit the occurrence of the following conduct or activities with respect to them, have violated the Rules of Ethics and are subject to sanctions as described hereunder:

1. Employing fraud or deceit in procuring or attempting to procure, maintain, renew or obtain reinstatement of certification or registration as issued by ARRT; employment in radiologic technology; or state permit license or registration certificate to practice radiologic technology. This includes altering in any respect any document issued by the ARRT or any state or federal agency, or by indicating in writing certification or registration with the ARRT when that is not the case.

2. Subverting or attempting to subvert ARRT's examination process. Conduct that subverts or attempts to subvert ARRT's examination process includes, but is not limited to:

   (i) conduct that violates the security of ARRT examination materials, such as removing or attempting to remove examination materials from an examination room, or having unauthorized possession of any portion of or information concerning a future, current or previously administered examination of ARRT; or disclosing information concerning any portion of a future, current or previously administered examination of ARRT; or disclosing what purports to be, or under all circumstances is likely

continued on following page

Display 1–3: ARRT Standards of Ethics

to be understood by the recipient as, any portion of or "inside" information concerning any portion of a future, current or previously administered examination of ARRT;

(ii) conduct that in any way compromises ordinary standards of test administration, such as communicating with another Candidate during administration of the examination, copying another Candidate's answers, permitting another Candidate to copy one's answers, or possessing unauthorized materials; or

(iii) impersonating a Candidate or permitting an impersonator to take the examination on one's own behalf.

3. Convictions, criminal proceedings or military court-martials as described below:

(i) Conviction of a crime, including a felony, a gross misdemeanor or a misdemeanor with the sole exception of speeding and parking violations. All alcohol and/or drug related violations must be reported.

(ii) Criminal proceeding where a finding or verdict of guilt is made or returned but the adjudication of guilt is either withheld or not entered, or a criminal proceeding where the individual enters a plea of guilty or nolo contendere.

(iii) Military court-martials that involve substance abuse, any sex-related infractions, or patient-related infractions.

4. Failure to report to the ARRT that:

(i) charges regarding the person's permit, license or registration certificate to practice radiologic technology or any other medical or allied health profession are pending or have been resolved adversely to the individual in any state, territory or country, (including but not limited to, imposed conditions, probation, suspension or revocation); or

(ii) that the individual has been refused a permit, license or registration certificate to practice radiologic technology or any other medical or allied health profession by another state, territory or country.

5. Failure or inability to perform radiologic technology with reasonable skill and safety.

6. Engaging in unprofessional conduct, including, but not limited to:

(i) a departure from or failure to conform to applicable federal, state or local governmental rules regarding radiologic technology practice; or, if no such rule exists, to the minimal standards of acceptable and prevailing radiologic technology practice;

(ii) any radiologic technology practice that may create unnecessary danger to a patient's life, health or safety; or

(iii) any practice that is contrary to the ethical conduct appropriate to the profession that results in the termination from employment.

Actual injury to a patient or the public need not be established under this clause.

7. Delegating or accepting the delegation of a radiologic technology function or any other prescribed health care function when the delegation or acceptance could reasonably be expected to create an unnecessary danger to a patient's life, health or safety. Actual injury to a patient need not be established under this clause.

8. Actual or potential inability to practice radiologic technology with reasonable skill and safety to patients by reason of illness, use of alcohol, drugs, chemicals or any other material; or as a result of any mental or physical condition.

9. Adjudication as mentally incompetent, mentally ill, a chemically dependent person, or a person dangerous to the public, by a court of competent jurisdiction.

10. Engaging in any unethical conduct, including, but not limited to, conduct likely to deceive, defraud or harm the public; or demonstrating a willful or careless disregard for the health, welfare or safety of a patient. Actual injury need not be established under this clause.

11. Engaging in conduct with a patient that is sexual or may reasonably be interpreted by the patient as sexual, or in any verbal behavior that is seductive or sexually demeaning to a patient; or engaging in sexual exploitation of a patient or former patient. This also applies to any unwanted sexual behavior, verbal or otherwise, that results in the termination of employment. This rule does not apply to pre-existing consensual relationships.

12. Revealing a privileged communication from or relating to a former or current patient, except when otherwise required or permitted by law.

13. Knowingly engaging or assisting any person to engage in, or otherwise participating in, abusive or fraudulent billing practices, including violations of federal Medicare and Medicaid laws or state medical assistance laws.

14. Improper management of patient records, including failure to maintain adequate patient records or to furnish a patient record or report required by law; or making, causing or permitting anyone to make false, deceptive or misleading entry in any patient record.

15. Knowingly aiding, assisting, advising or allowing a person without a current and appropriate state permit, license or registration certificate or a current certificate of registration with ARRT to engage in the practice of radiologic technology, in a jurisdiction which requires a person to have such a current and appropriate state permit, license or registration certificate or a current and appropriate certification of registration with ARRT in order to practice radiologic technology in such jurisdiction.

16. Violating a rule adopted by any state board with competent jurisdiction, an order of such board, or state or federal law relating to the practice of

continued on following page

Display 1–3: ARRT Standards of Ethics

radiologic technology, or any other medical or allied health professions, or a state or federal narcotics or controlled substance law.

17. Knowingly providing false or misleading information that is directly related to the care of a former or current patient.

18. Practicing outside the scope of practice authorized by the individual's current state permit, license or registration certificate, or the individual's current certificate of registration with ARRT.

19. Making a false statement or knowingly providing false information to ARRT or failing to cooperate with any investigation of ARRT of the Ethics Committee.

20. Engaging in false, fraudulent, deceptive or misleading communications to any person regarding the individual's education, training, credentials, experience or qualifications, or the status or the individual's state permit, license or registration certificate in radiologic technology or certificate of registration with ARRT.

21. Knowing of a violation or a probable violation of any Rule of Ethics by any Registered Technologist or by a Candidate and failing to promptly report in writing the same to the ARRT.

Patients have the right to make decisions concerning their lives, and you must respect those decisions.

In your practice as a radiographer, you will act as the liaison between the radiologist and the patient. In these circumstances, you must act on behalf of the patient.

Beneficence: Refers to the fact that all acts must be meant to attain a good result or to be beneficial. As a radiographer, you must always plan patient care to ensure safe outcomes and avoid harmful consequences.

Beneficence requires action that either prevents harm or does the greatest good for the patient. This may require you to side with the patient and against his co-workers.

Confidentiality: Refers to the concept of privacy. All patients have the right to have information concerning their state of health or other personal information kept in confidence unless it will benefit him or her or unless there is a direct threat to society if not disclosed. As a radiographer, you must not disclose facts concerning the patient's health or other personal information to anyone not involved with the patient's care.

Double Effect: Refers to the fact that some actions may produce both a good and a bad effect. Four criteria must be fulfilled before this type of action is ethically permissible:

a. The act is good or morally neutral.

b. The intent is good, not evil, although a bad result may be foreseen.

c. The good effect is not achieved by means of evil effects.

d. The good effect must be more important than the evil effect, or at least there is favorable balance between good over bad.

Radiation exposure may be harmful; however, the diagnosis obtained by the exposure will aid in restoring the patient to health.

Fidelity: Refers to the duty to fulfill one's commitments and applies to keeping promises both stated and implied. As a radiographer, you must not promise patients results that you cannot achieve.

Justice: Refers to all persons being treated equally or receiving equal benefits according to need. You must not favor one patient over another or treat one patient differently from another, regardless of personal feelings.

Nonmaleficence: Refers to the duty to abstain from inflicting harm and also the duty to prevent harm. As a radiographer, you are obligated to practice in a safe manner at all times.

Paternalism: Refers to the attitude that sometimes prompts health care workers to make decisions regarding a person's care without consulting the person affected. If you are tempted to make such a unilateral decision, you must consider whether the action is justifiable based on potential outcomes. As a radiographer, you are justified in taking action in instances in which not acting would do more harm than the lack of patient input into the decision.

Sanctity of life: Refers to the belief that life is the highest good and nobody has the right to judge that another person's quality of life is so poor that his or her life is not of value and should be terminated. You cannot make life-and-death decisions for your patients based on your personal values.

Veracity: Refers to honesty in all aspects of one's professional life. You must be honest with your patients, your co-workers, and yourself.

Respect for property: Refers to keeping the belongings of patients safe and taking care not to intentionally damage or waste equipment or supplies with which one works.

Ethical Issues in Radiography

As a radiographer, you are expected to conduct yourself in a professional manner. You must be reliable; that is, you are expected to report for work on time and complete your assigned share of the workload in a timely and efficient manner. You are also expected to work as a cooperative member of the health care team. You must be articulate, and your speech must be free of vulgar expressions or inappropriate slang. You must treat all patients as persons of dignity and worth and not demonstrate preference for one patient over another.

In spite of impeccable behavior on your part as a student radiographer, you may observe behaviors and patient care problems that you may see as ethical concerns as you perform your clinical laboratory practice in health care institutions. Some of the problems that you might encounter are defensive shielding of professional colleagues who are violating the code of professional ethics; unequal medical resource allocation based on the patient's age or socioeconomic status; lack of respect for the patient; breaches of privacy and confidentiality; and overtreatment or undertreatment of patients. In other words, you will observe that what is taught in the classroom often does not match what is seen in the clinical area.

In such cases, as a student radiographer you should observe the issues that you believe to be violations of the ethical code and discuss them with your colleagues and your instructor in a private conference. These issues can become learning experiences for you as you and your colleagues contemplate as a group how they should be resolved.

As the scope of practice and the professional responsibilities of radiologic technology grow, so do the ethical responsibilities of radiographers. Often, an ethical decision involves a choice between two unsatisfactory solutions to a problem. This is often the case with health care. If you conscientiously follow your professional code of ethics and the ethical principles previously listed to make difficult decisions as they arise, you will be able to resolve ethical dilemmas in a manner that allows you peace of mind. Combine this approach with critical thinking and the problem-solving process that will be discussed in Chapter 2 of this text.

For ethical dilemmas of some magnitude, most health care institutions have ethics committees that meet on a regular basis to solve problems and formulate policies that provide guidelines to facilitate decision making. If you encounter an ethical dilemma in your workplace that cannot be readily resolved by following your professional code of ethics, you are obliged to present the problem to such a body.

Legal Issues in Radiologic Technology

While ethics refers to a set of moral principles, law refers to rules of conduct as prescribed by an authority or group of legislators. The *New World Webster's Dictionary* defines *law* as all rules of conduct established and enforced by the authority, legislation, or custom of a given community or group. The group in the case of the radiographer includes the ARRT and the ASRT. The rules of conduct refer to the Practice Standards in Display 1-2. These define the practice and establish general criteria to determine compliance with the law as it applies to radiologic technology.

The standards are general in nature by design to keep pace with the rapidly changing environment in which we live and work. They have been divided into three sections:

1. Professional performance standards—define the activities of the practitioner in the areas of education, interpersonal relationships, personal and professional self-assessment, and ethical behavior.

2. Clinical performance standards—define activities in regard to the care of patients and the delivery of diagnostic or therapeutic procedures and treatments.

3. Quality performance standards—relate to the technical areas of performance such as equipment and material assessment, safety standards, and total quality management.

Patient Rights

As a professional radiographer, you have a legal responsibility to relate to your colleagues, other members of the health care team, and the patient in a manner that is respectful of each person with whom you interact while you adhere to the *Patient's Bill of Rights* (Display 1-4). This bill delineates the rights of the patient as a consumer of health care. Because all health care workers are required to adhere to the provisions of this bill, they must be familiar with it. You must also be aware of the areas of practice in which health care workers may infringe upon the patient's rights and be held legally liable. Some examples of these are as follows:

- Acting in the role of a diagnostician and providing a patient with results, impressions, or diagnoses of diagnostic imaging examinations

DISPLAY 1–4

A Patient's Bill of Rights

Introduction

Effective health care requires collaboration between patients and physicians and other health care professionals. Open and honest communication, respect for personal and professional values, and sensitivity to differences are integral to optimal patient care. As the setting for the provision of health services, hospitals must provide a foundation for understanding and respecting the rights and responsibilities of patients, their families, physicians, and other caregivers. Hospitals must ensure a health care ethic that respects the role of patients in decision making about treatment choices and other aspects of their care. Hospitals must be sensitive to cultural, racial, linguistic, religious, age, gender, and other differences as well as the needs of persons with disabilities.

The American Hospital Association presents A Patient's Bill of Rights with the expectation that it will contribute to more effective patient care and be supported by the hospital on behalf of the institution, its medical staff, employees, and patients. The American Hospital Association encourages health care institutions to tailor this bill of rights to their patient community by translating and/or simplifying the language of this bill of rights as may be necessary to ensure that patients and their families understand their rights and responsibilities.

Bill of Rights

These rights can be exercised on the patient's behalf by a designated surrogate or proxy decision maker if the patient lacks decision-making capacity, is legally incompetent, or is a minor.

1. The patient has the right to considerate and respectful care.

2. The patient has the right to and is encouraged to obtain from physicians and other direct caregivers relevant, current, and understandable information concerning diagnosis, treatment, and prognosis. Except in emergencies when the patient lacks decision-making capacity and the need for treatment is urgent, the patient is entitled to the opportunity to discuss and request information related to the specific procedures and/or treatments, the risks involved, the possible length of recuperation, and the medically reasonable alternatives and their accompanying risks and benefits.

   Patients have the right to know the identity of physicians, nurses, and others involved in their care, as well as when those involved are students, residents, or other trainees. The patient also has the right to know the immediate and long-term financial implications of treatment choices, insofar as they are known.

3. The patient has the right to make decisions about the plan of care prior to and during the course of treatment and to refuse a recommended treatment or plan of care to the extent permitted by law and hospital policy and to be informed of the medical consequences of this action. In case of such refusal, the patient is entitled to other appropriate care and services that the hospital provides or transfer to another hospital. The hospital should notify patients of any policy that might affect patient choice within the institution.

4. The patient has the right to have an advance directive (such as a living will, health care proxy, or durable power of attorney for health care) concerning treatment or designating a surrogate decision maker with the expectation that the hospital will honor the intent of that directive to the extent permitted by law and hospital policy.

   Health care institutions must advise patients of their rights under state law and hospital policy to make informed medical choices, ask if the patient has an advance directive, and include that information in patient records. The patient has the right to timely information about hospital policy that may limit its ability to implement fully a legally valid advance directive.

5. The patient has the right to every consideration of privacy. Case discussion, consultation, examination, and treatment should be conducted so as to protect each patient's privacy.

6. The patient has the right to expect that all communications and records pertaining to his/her care will be treated as confidential by the hospital, except in cases such as suspected abuse and public health hazards when reporting is permitted or required by law. The patient has the right to expect that the hospital will emphasize the confidentiality of this information when it releases it to any other parties entitled to review information in these records.

7. The patient has the right to review the records pertaining to his/her medical care and to have the information explained or interpreted as necessary, except when restricted by law.

8. The patient has the right to expect that, within its capacity and policies, a hospital will make reasonable response to the request of a patient for appropriate and medically indicated care and services. The hospital must provide evaluation, service, and/or referral as indicated by the urgency of the case. When medically appropriate and legally permissible, or when a patient has so requested, a patient may be transferred to another facility. The institution to which the patient is to be transferred must first have accepted the patient for transfer. The patient must also have the benefit of complete information and explanation concerning the need for, risks, benefits, and alternatives to such a transfer.

9. The patient has the right to ask and be informed of the existence of business relationships among the hospital, educational institutions, other health care providers, or payers that may influence the patient's treatment and care.

continued on following page

Display 1–4: A Patient's Bill of Rights, continued from previous page

10. The patient has the right to consent to or decline to participate in proposed research studies or human experimentation affecting care and treatment or requiring direct patient involvement, and to have those studies fully explained prior to consent. A patient who declines to participate in research or experimentation is entitled to the most effective care that the hospital can otherwise provide.

11. The patient has the right to expect reasonable continuity of care when appropriate and to be informed by physicians and other caregivers of available and realistic patient care options when hospital care is no longer appropriate.

12. The patient has the right to be informed of hospital policies and practices that relate to patient care, treatment, and responsibilities. The patient has the right to be informed of available resources for resolving disputes, grievances, and conflicts, such as ethics committees, patient representatives, or other mechanisms available in the institution. The patient has the right to be informed of the hospital's charges for services and available payment methods.

The collaborative nature of health care requires that patients, or their families/surrogates, participate in their care. The effectiveness of care and patient satisfaction with the course of treatment depend, in part, on the patient fulfilling certain responsibilities. Patients are responsible for providing information about past illnesses, hospitalizations, medications, and other matters related to health status. To participate effectively in decision making, patients must be encouraged to take responsibility for requesting additional information or clarification about their health status or treatment when they do not fully understand information and instructions. Patients are also responsible for ensuring that the health care institution has a copy of their written advance directive if they have one. Patients are responsible for informing their physicians and other caregivers if they anticipate problems in following prescribed treatment.

Patients should also be aware of the hospital's obligation to be reasonably efficient and equitable in providing care to other patients and the community. The hospital's rules and regulations are designed to help the hospital meet this obligation. Patients and their families are responsible for making reasonable accommodations to the needs of the hospital, other patients, medical staff, and hospital employees. Patients are responsible for providing necessary information for insurance claims and for working with the hospital to make payment arrangements, when necessary.

A person's health depends on much more than health care services. Patients are responsible for recognizing the impact of their life-style on their personal health.

Conclusion

Hospitals have many functions to perform, including the enhancement of health status, health promotion, and the prevention and treatment of injury and disease; the immediate and ongoing care and rehabilitation of patients; the education of health professionals, patients, and the community; and research. All these activities must be conducted with an overriding concern for the values and dignity of patients.

- Failing to obtain appropriate consent from women of childbearing age before performing a diagnostic imaging procedure

- Failing to obtain a complete history from a patient before administering an iodinated contrast agent

- Failing to correctly identify a patient before performing an examination

- Failing to explain a diagnostic imaging procedure to a patient before the examination

- Failing to document technical factors used to facilitate dose calculations for a procedure

- Failing to maintain a patient's physical privacy during an examination

- Failing to maintain the highest quality of images with the lowest possible radiation dose for the patient

As a radiographer, you must never assume the role of other medical personnel in the department. It is not within your scope of practice to read radiographs or other diagnostic tests or to impart the results of these to the patient or the patient's family. This constitutes medical diagnosis and is the physician's responsibility. If a patient is injured in the diagnostic imaging department in any manner, you must not dismiss the patient from the department until the patient has been examined by a physician and has been deemed safe to be discharged.

Patient Responsibilities

Just as the radiographer has to abide by the *Patient Bill of Rights* and other professional standards, the patient has responsibilities when he or she presents for health care. These responsibilities are as follows (Grieco, 1996):

1. The patient has the responsibility to provide, to the best of his or her knowledge, an accurate and complete health history.

2. The patient is responsible for keeping appointments and for notifying the responsible practitioner or the hospital when unable to do so for any reason.

3. The patient is responsible for his or her actions when refusing treatment or not following the practitioner's instructions.

4. The patient is responsible for fulfilling the financial obligations of his or her health care as promptly as possible.

5. The patient is responsible for following hospital rules and regulations affecting patient care and conduct.

6. The patient is responsible for being considerate of the rights and property of others.

Legal Concerns

Many types of laws affect people in daily life; however, statutory law and common law are the most significant for the radiographer in professional practice. Statutory laws are derived from legislative enactments. Common law usually results from judicial decisions.

Two major classifications of the law are criminal law and civil law. An offense is regarded as criminal behavior, and in the realm of criminal law if it is an offense against society or a member of society. If the accused party is found guilty, he or she is punished.

Criminal law protects the entire community against certain acts. An example of this would be a terrorist bombing that results in the destruction of public property and the death of one or more persons. The crime is a crime against society and is a felony. A felony is a crime of a serious nature punishable by a fine higher than $1000.00 and a prison sentence of more than 1 year, or in extreme cases, by death.

A misdemeanor is a crime of a less serious nature punishable by a fine or imprisonment for less than 1 year. In some instances, driving under the influence of drugs or alcohol may be a misdemeanor provided that no accident or injury has resulted.

Civil law has been broken if another person's private legal rights have been violated. The person who is found guilty of this type of offense is usually expected to pay a sum of money to repair the damage done. An example of a violation of civil law might be a suit by an individual against a physician for a misdiagnosis that results in injury. This injury is to one person and not to the entire society.

Tort law exists to protect the violator of a law from being sued for an act of vengeance, to determine fault, and to compensate the injured party. A tort involves personal injury or damage resulting in civil action or litigation to obtain reparation for damages incurred. A tort may be committed intentionally or unintentionally. An intentional tort is a purposeful deed committed with the intention of producing the consequences of the deed. Defaming a college's character or committing assault or battery are examples of intentional torts. It is possible for a radiographer to be found guilty of a criminal act in professional practice. Generally, in this situation, the radiographer is likely to be legally liable for malpractice in the commitment of a tort. Battery may be charged by a patient to whom the radiographer has administered treatment against the patient's will. Assault and battery are often linked together, meaning that a threat of harm existed before the actual contact; however, assault may be charged without any physical contact if the patient fears that this will occur. Other examples of intentional tort include:

Immobilizing a patient against his or her will (false imprisonment)

Falsely stating that a patient has AIDS (defamation of character)

Causing extreme emotional distress resulting in illness through outrageous or shocking conduct

An unintentional tort may be committed when a radiographer is negligent in the performance of patient care and the patient is injured as a result. The following are examples of unintentional torts:

- Improperly marking radiographic images, such as incorrectly labeling intravenous pyelography images for right and left, which could result in the surgeon removing the healthy kidney, leaving only the diseased kidney

- Omitting to apply gonadal shielding on a female patient with a femur fracture who is subsequently discovered to be pregnant

- Improperly positioning a trauma patient for tibia and fibula projections so that the projections do not adequately demonstrate the entire lower leg, resulting in a fracture being "missed" by the orthopedic physician and the radiologists

- Handing the radiologist the incorrect syringe during a procedure, which results in the injection of Xylocaine (lidocaine) instead of the contrast media

- Leaving an unconscious patient on a gurney while the radiographer leaves the room, thus allowing the patient to jar the siderails and fall off the gurney, since the safety belt was not secure

- Improperly positioning a footboard on an x-ray table, which results in the patient sliding off the table when the table is placed in the upright position during an examination

- Not providing parents of pediatric patients with the proper protective attire when they are aiding in immobilizing their child, especially during fluoroscopic procedures

Radiographers most often have suits brought against them in cases of patient falls. Although the institution where the accident occurs (the employer) may be found liable for the actions of the radiographer (employee) under the principle of *respondent superior* ("let the master answer"), the technologist is responsible for his or her actions if named in a lawsuit.

Ethical and legal issues are frequently combined in the practice of your profession. As a radiographer, you must be aware of this and take precautions to prevent situations that may lead to problems of this nature. Discrimination and bias shown toward a particular person constitute an example of this. You must understand that it is unlawful to discriminate against any patient or co-worker on the basis of race, color, creed, national origin, ancestry, sex, marital status, disability, religious affiliation, political affiliation, age, or sexual orientation. You must practice in a totally nonjudgmental manner and make no decisions or take any action based on these issues.

Use of Immobilization Techniques

Patients may not be immobilized for radiographic imaging procedures simply as a matter of convenience for the radiographer. You must obtain an order from the physician in charge for patient immobilization for a defined period of time to protect the patient's safety. The method of immobilization must be one that is the least restrictive to the patient's movement and freedom. There must be a need to immobilize the patient to achieve the most satisfactory outcome. (The term "restraint" is often substituted for immobilization techniques; the two are used interchangeably in this text.)

Only when you have exhausted all other safe methods of obtaining a radiograph should you consider immobilizing the patient. In most instances, a physician's order is required. If a combative patient threatens you, call security personnel to assist in the immobilization of the patient. All patients who have been immobilized must be carefully monitored.

Immobilizers must be appropriate to the individual needs of the patient. When you feel immobilizers are necessary, you need to document the reasons for use, the type used, and the length of time applied. Immobilizers must be released for specified periods of time when they are in use. You must also document the time and conditions of immobilizer release.

The use of medication as a restraining technique occurs only in extreme circumstances and only as prescribed by the patient's physician. Using immobilization techniques improperly or without a physician's orders can be considered false imprisonment and therefore cause for legal action. An institutional policy for the use of immobilization must be present in all departments, and user instructions must be clearly visible on all immobilizing devices. The technical aspects of application of immobilizers for adults and children are discussed later in this text.

CALL OUT!

Unauthorized use of immobilization techniques can be construed as false imprisonment—a tort.

Unusual Occurrence Reports

An injury to a patient or any error made by personnel in the diagnostic imaging department must be documented in an *incident report* as soon as it is safe to do so. The document may also be called *an unusual occurrence report* or an *accident notification report* (Display 1-5). An injury may seem slight and not worthy of such a report, but all injuries—whether to patient or staff or accidents involving equipment regardless of severity—must be reported. An error in medication administration or any other error in treatment must also be documented in an incident report.

When filing an incident report, write in simple terms what occurred, at what time, on what date, in which room or department, to whom, who was present, and what was done to alleviate the situation at the time. Also report the condition of the patient or person injured. The report is signed by all who participated in the event. All incidents resulting in patient or personnel injury must also be reported by the supervisor of the department to the institution's insurance company. If this is not done, the insurance company may drop the policy.

Good Samaritan Laws

All states in the United States now have Good Samaritan laws. These laws were enacted to protect persons who give medical aid to persons in emergency situations from civil or criminal liability for their actions or omissions under these circumstances. State laws vary, but generally if you stop to render aid at the scene of an accident, you are not held liable for any adverse results of your actions, provided that you act within accepted standards and without gross negligence.

Automatic external defibrillators (AEDs) have been added to emergency medical procedures, and the equipment for this procedure is now available in many areas of public use such as in airplanes and city buildings. "To permit and encourage the use of AEDs by the lay public, nearly all states have enacted facilitating legislation. In addition, the Cardiac Arrest Survival Act provides

DISPLAY 1–5

Unusual Occurrence Reports—Sample form:

Section 1

Name of the individual reporting the incident: _____

Institution where the incident occurred: _____

Date of incident: _____ Time of incident: _____ a.m. _____ p.m. _____

Exact location of incident: _____

Section 2

Incident occurred to: _____

☐ Staff ☐ Student ☐ Patient - ID# _____ ☐ Equipment
☐ Other Explain _____
_____

If staff, student, or patient is checked, see sections 3 & 5.

If equipment is checked, see sections 4 & 5.

Section 3

Occurrence _____ Type of incident _____
☐ Back injury from lifting patients   ☐ Reaction to foreign substances
☐ Miscellaneous back injury   ☐ Contagious disease
☐ Injury from a patient   ☐ Laceration
☐ Needle stick   ☐ Contusion
☐ Unsafe/defective equipment   ☐ Burn
☐ Improper use of equipment   ☐ Fracture
☐ Patient contact   ☐ Sprain/strain
☐ Fall (attended)   ☐ Puncture
☐ Fall (unattended)   ☐ Other
☐ Fire
☐ Other

Did the injury require treatment by a physician? _____

Was the incident reported to the appropriate personnel? _____

Section 4

Type of equipment damaged: _____

How was equipment damaged: _____

Result of damage (e.g., equipment down time for repair) _____

Section 5

Briefly describe the incident: _____
_____
_____

Name(s) of person(s) notified: _____

Name(s) of witness(es): _____

I certify that the above information is correct: _____

Signature of person filling out the form _____ Date _____

Witness Signature _____ Date _____

immunity for lay rescuers who use AEDs and for businesses or other entities or individuals who purchase AEDs for public access defibrillation" (American Heart Association, 2001). You will be instructed to use the AED as part of your Basic Life Support for Healthcare Providers education.

Informed Consent

Many procedures performed in diagnostic imaging departments require special consent forms to be signed by the patient or, in the case of minor children or other special cases, by their parents or legal representative. You must be familiar with the procedures that require special consent and not confuse these with the blanket consent forms that are often signed when the patient enters the hospital, since these are not valid if an informed consent is required.

A consent is a contract wherein the patient voluntarily gives permission to someone (in this case the imaging staff) to perform a service. The legal aspect of obtaining consent deals with the imaging staff's "duty to warn" and the ethic "do no harm." The medical aspect of consent is hoped to establish rapport with the patient through communication to secure a successful outcome.

A consent is not legal if the patient is not informed of all aspects of the procedure to be performed. These include the potential risks, benefits, and suggested alternatives. The patient must also be informed of the consequences if the suggested procedure is not completed. Because a patient usually consents or refuses a procedure based on the information that the health care professional provides, the duty of obtaining the informed consent is the duty of the referring physician or his staff.

Although these special consent forms are usually signed before the patient comes to the diagnostic imaging department, your duty as a radiographer is to recheck the patient's chart to be certain that this has been accomplished. You must also make sure that the patient understands what is going to be done and the essential nature of the choices available to him or her. If the patient, parent, or legal representative denies knowledge of the procedure or withdraws consent, notify the radiologist or the patient's physician. The procedure should be postponed until the matter is satisfactorily resolved. It is not your responsibility to determine whether a procedure should be terminated. It is your responsibility to bring the problem to the physician in charge to resolve.

There are several levels of informed consent:

1. *Simple consent*: is a matter of obtaining a patient's permission to perform a procedure without knowledge of that procedure. Simple consent is divided into express and implied consent.
   a. *Express consent* occurs when the patient does not stop the procedure from taking place. By allowing the procedure to occur, the patient has given his or her express consent to the radiographer; however, legally, silence is not an agreement.
   b. *Implied consent* occurs in emergency situations when it is not possible to obtain consent from the patient, his or her parents, or a legal representative. The health care provider operates under the belief that the patient would give permission if able; it is "implied" that permission would be given.

2. *Inadequate consent* is also known as *ignorant consent*. This occurs when the patient has not been informed adequately to make a responsible decision. The patient can bring charges of negligence (an unintentional tort) when he or she has had inadequate consent, particularly if the patient sustains injury (when consent is not obtained, battery may be charged).

Obtaining informed consent protects you from lawsuits. You must also understand that communicating with the patient is essential to alleviate his or her anxiety as well as to improve outcomes from all procedures.

Malpractice Insurance

In recent years, professional (malpractice) liability protection has become an important kind of insurance, especially for members of the medical profession. All radiographers should carry their own malpractice insurance, even if their employer carries insurance for them. Malpractice is a wrongful act by a physician, lawyer, or other professional, which injures a patient or client. The patient or client may file a civil lawsuit to recover damages (money) to compensate for the injury. As a radiographer, you could be named in a lawsuit in which the legal expenses for defense are not completely covered by your employer. You may still be liable for your own negligence. Without a malpractice insurance policy in your own name, you assume risks. Professional liability insurance provides protection against claims of malpractice. It is not wise to place yourself in professional jeopardy when you can purchase a professional malpractice policy for a reasonable price. With a malpractice liability insurance policy, the insurance company assumes the risk in accordance with the policy contract.

Medical Records and Documentation

A medical record is kept for each patient who seeks medical treatment whether he or she is an outpatient or has been admitted to the hospital for care. This record, called a *chart*, is begun the moment the patient arrives or is admitted for care and is kept until he or she is dismissed or discharged from the hospital. The medical record is kept for a number of reasons:

1. To transmit information about the patient from one health care worker to another

2. To protect the patient from medical errors and duplication of treatments

3. To provide information for medical research

4. To protect the health care worker in cases of litigation

5. To provide information concerning quality of patient care for institutional evaluation teams such as the Joint Commission on Accreditation of Healthcare Organizations

The chart contains the patient's identifying data, documentation of all physician's orders, physician's consultation notes, patient progress notes, medications and treatments received, around-the-clock nurse's notes, all patient visits for outpatient or ambulatory care, laboratory and radiology reports, medical history and physical examination, admitting and discharge diagnosis, results of examinations, surgical reports, consent forms, education received by the patient, discharge planning, health care team planning, nursing care plans, and discharge summaries. All members of the health care team are expected to document the care they have rendered for the patient on this chart.

Certain documentation is specific to radiographic imaging. As a radiographer, you are accountable for the documentation of any radiograph that you take, including the number of films, the exposure factors, and the amount of fluoroscopic time used during a procedure. You must also document any patient preparation for procedures that you make, medications that you administer, and adverse reactions to medications or treatments received.

You must assume responsibility for obtaining a medical history from the patient that is pertinent to the treatment or examination he or she is to receive in the department. This information includes vital signs; female patient's response to questions concerning pregnancy and date of last menstrual period, if pertinent; history of allergies; trauma, if pertinent; contrast media or radionuclide administered; patient education before and after each procedure; names and credentials of the members of the health care team participating in the procedure; and the diagnostic report of the physicians involved following the procedure. Many of these issues are discussed in detail in the chapters that follow.

Nurses and physicians who participate in radiographic imaging examinations or treatments are also responsible for documentation; however, you must review the documentation and bring any omissions to their attention. Any item that has not been documented on the chart is considered to be "not performed" in a court of law. All entries on a medical record must list the time and date of the procedure and be signed by the person who administered it. The credentials of the person must also be listed.

Abbreviations must be approved by the institution in which you are employed. A list of acceptable abbreviations must be on record at that institution and learned by those using them. No others are acceptable.

Charting formats are also made and approved by each institution; however, the contents of the record are reviewed and either approved, disapproved, or changed according to recommendations made by the accreditation bodies inspecting the charts.

If you make an error while writing an entry into a chart, you may draw a single line through the error, write "*mistaken entry*" above the error, and sign your name to the error. You may then write the corrected entry. If documenting by computer, the items listed above must still be included on the chart.

Radiographic images are considered part of the patient's medical record and may be used as legal evidence in the event of a lawsuit. For this reason, clearly mark all radiographic images. Make sure that the patient's name, identification number, the name of the facility where taken, and a marker are correctly placed. A consent written and signed by the patient or legal guardian must be presented before any patient records are released for any reason. Original radiographs should not be released from the department where they are taken; however, there are exceptions to this. Copies are usually made when films are requested.

Computer Technology in Radiographic Imaging

The modern day radiographer has evolved into a multicompetent and multiskilled health care worker. He or she must fit into the new health care environment created by computers and current technology. Computer technology provides methods of quickly storing and retrieving patient information through the use of networks or systems within the radiologic imaging departments, hospitals, health insurance groups, and other nationwide organizations. This is rapidly becoming a major component of diagnostic imaging in health care delivery systems.

One of the most common computer applications in radiologic imaging departments is Picture Archiving and Communication Systems (PACS), or teleradiology systems. The PACS network allows physicians in intensive care units, pediatrics, orthopedics, or any department of medicine to immediately access images. This immediate computer access eliminates problems with lost images that can occur when images are filed or transported as radiographic films to various locations.

Other benefits of this computerized system include improved service to referring physicians and an opportunity for clinicians to work off-site. Such computer systems also allow the patient more flexibility in choosing a health care facility, since the patient records can be accessed immediately by computer. As the use of this new technology expands, however, ethical and legal issues are being raised. Violation of confidentiality, fraud, and illegal access to personal information are of grave concern.

In 1996, Congress recognized the need for national patient record privacy standards, when they enacted the Health Insurance Portability and Accountability Act of 1996 (HIPAA). The law included provisions designed to save money for health care businesses by encouraging electronic transactions, but it also required new safeguards to protect the security and confidentiality of that information.

In November 1999, the Department of Health and Human Services (HHS) published proposed regulations to guarantee patients new rights and protections against the misuse or disclosure of their health records. In December 2000, HHS issued the final rule, which took effect on April 14, 2001. Most covered entities have 2 full years—until April 14, 2003—to comply with the final rule's provisions. All medical records and other individually identifiable health information, whether electronic, on paper, or oral, are covered by the final rule.

As a radiographer, you must abide by the same rules concerning confidentiality, security, and privacy of patient information with computerized records as with previous systems. Written consent by the patient is the only legitimate reason to obtain and pass on confidential material. As a student radiographer, you must familiarize yourself with the potential abuses of the new technology so that you will not unknowingly violate the law.

Health Care Delivery

In the recent past, the rising cost of health care became a major concern of the medical community and of the nation. This gave rise to major changes in the health care delivery system in the United States and has become a major political concern. The belief was that the exorbitant cost of health care and its continued rising cost did not necessarily improve the quality of patient care. Based on this belief, many restraints were placed on the institutions and the practitioners of health care. These changes are complex, and it is not within the scope of this text to discuss them at length. However, a very brief outline of the current methods of health care delivery follows.

Private Insurance Plans: These plans are "private pay" insurance options. They are called third party reimbursement plans because the medical services that the patient receives are paid by the insurer rather than by the patient or the health care agency. The care rendered to the patient is paid either partially or entirely by the insurer and is a costly method of obtaining medical care.

Medicare: This nationwide health insurance program provides health insurance to all persons 65 years of age or older and to persons of any age with permanent kidney failure or with a permanent disabling illness. This insurance is authorized under Title 18 of the Social Security Act. Medicare does not pay the full cost of most diagnostic procedures including imaging procedures. It pays a flat rate and if the health care provider charges more than that cost, the individual receiving the treatment is expected to pay. Health care agencies receive payment for medical services based on what is called diagnosis-related group (DRG). This is a system of major diagnostic categories that is further broken down into 494 divisions depending on the patient's principal medical diagnosis. The health care agency receives payment according to the DRG classification without consideration of the true cost of the patient's care.

Medicaid: This federally funded and state-administered program provides medical care for families with dependent older adults, children, or otherwise disabled persons with incomes below the federal poverty level. It also funds maternal and child care for the poor.

Managed Care Programs: These health care programs are designed to control the cost of health care while meeting the patient's health care needs in a satisfactory manner. All persons enrolled in a particular managed care program are funneled through one party who is called the *case manager*. The enrolled member may not choose any provider of health care but must accept the health care provided by the particular program. Any special care needed must be approved by the case manager. There are a number of managed care programs, but they are too complex to be discussed in this text. At present there is much discontent with many of the aspects of managed care, and legislation is before the U.S. Congress to alter the rights of patients enrolled in these programs.

Levels of Health Care

Health care is no longer rendered only to the person who has an acute illness and comes to the hospital for treatment. There are currently six levels of health care that

TABLE 1-2

Levels of Health Care in the United States

LEVEL OF CARE	EXTENT OF CARE
Preventive Care	Educates healthy people in methods of maintaining their health and preventing illness
Primary Care	Provides early detection of illness and provides routine out-patient care
Secondary Care (also called acute care)	Provides emergency treatment, critical care, complex diagnostic examinations, and treatment
Tertiary Care (also called special care)	Provides largely technical care to persons in a large geographic area
Restorative Care	Provides intermediate follow-up care after medical or surgical treatment; also provides rehabilitative care and home care for those in need
Continuing Care	Provides care either in skilled nursing facilities or in the home for those in need of long-term care, chronic care, hospice care, or personal care

the beginning student radiographer should recognize. Table 1-2 briefly describes these levels of health care.

Summary

Radiologic technology has evolved to meet the criteria of a profession by requiring extended education and clinical practice. It has a theoretical body of knowledge and leads to defined skills, abilities, and action. It also provides a specific service, and its members have a degree of decision-making autonomy when working within their scope of practice.

There are several educational choices for you as you begin your radiologic technology career. Each category has defined educational requirements and responsibilities, and you are expected to fulfill continuing education requirements to renew your license every 2 years.

As a professional radiographer, you are expected to join and participate in professional organizations. Such participation allows you to keep informed of technological changes and alterations in professional standards. You also promote the strength of the profession and prevent infringement from groups that desire to assume parts of the professional responsibilities of the radiographer.

In your work as a radiographer, you interface with members of the health care team on a daily basis. It is advantageous for you to recognize the educational background and duties of these team members so that you may develop a harmonious working relationship with them built on professional knowledge and respect. The health care professionals with whom you will work most frequently are the physician, the nurse, the pharmacist, occupational and physical therapists, and the respiratory therapist.

If you have selected radiologic technology as a profession, you must be aware of and willing to accept the ethical and legal constraints that govern your practice as a member of that profession. You must learn the *Code of Ethics* and understand *The Practice Standards* of your profession and adhere to those principles. You must also understand the rights of the patient and treat each patient as a human being with dignity and worth.

You must work within the scope of your radiography practice at all times. You must understand that to do otherwise is a violation of the law. There are standards of practice in radiographic imaging, as there are in all areas of health care. You must understand and follow these standards as you work. You must follow the policies of the institution or health care facility in which you work concerning unusual occurrence and accident reports. Any patient injured during a procedure must not be discharged from the radiographic imaging department without the consent of the physician.

Documentation and maintenance of medical records constitute an important aspect of health care. It transmits information to other health care workers, protects the patient from errors, provides information for medical research, protects the radiographer and others in cases of litigation, and provides information concerning the quality of patient care for institutional evaluation.

Computer technology is being used in radiographic imaging in most departments. As a radiographer, you must abide by the same rules of confidentiality of patient information that have applied to previous methods and familiarize yourself with other methods of potential abuse when using this new technology. Health care delivery in the United States has been altered considerably in the recent past. It is beneficial for you to recognize the current methods of health care delivery and the levels of health care offered at present.

The radiographer is believed to be a competent professional. As such, you are expected to act in a responsible and safe manner when caring for patients. It is your obligation to communicate effectively with other members of the health care team and document patient care correctly and completely. You are expected to perform in a safe and responsible manner in all areas of patient care including radiation safety; safety in moving patients; infection control; medication administration; knowledge and competency during procedures; and maintenance of patient privacy and confidentiality. You must also respect the patient's right to refuse treatment.

Chapter 1 Test

1. List the criteria of a profession and explain how radiologic technology meets these criteria.

2. The two major professional organizations of radiologic technology are _____ and _____.

3. The document that represents the application of moral principles and moral values for radiologic technology is _____.

4. Match the following:
   a. The right to make decisions concerning one's own life
   b. The intent is good although a bad result may be foreseen
   c. Equal treatment and equal benefits
   d. Honesty to patients
   e. Duty to refrain from inflicting harm

   1. Nonmaleficence
   2. Autonomy
   3. Truthfulness
   4. Justice
   5. Double effect

_____ **5.** The radiographer who mistakenly administers an incorrect drug to a patient may be guilty of a
   a. Tort
   b. Negligence
   c. Crime
   d. Battery

_____ **6.** As a radiographer, you refuse to work with a patient because you do not care for persons of the patient's religion. You are guilty of violating
   a. The law
   b. The ethics of your profession
   c. You own moral values
   d. Both a and b

7. Explain the documentation for which you as a radiographer will be accountable in your department when you participate in a procedure.

_____ **8.** Professional ethics may be defined as
   a. A set of principles that govern a course of action
   b. Standards of any professional person
   c. The same as not violating the law
   d. A set of rules and regulations made up by the department in which you work

_____ **9.** Which of the following is an example of privileged (confidential) information?
   a. Your friend buys a new car and asks you not to tell anyone about it yet.
   b. A colleague discusses his stock market holdings with you.
   c. You assist with a diagnostic study and a large adherent mass is discovered in the colon.
   d. A fellow student is told that he has the highest grades in the class.

_____ **10.** After completing a radiologic technology program, you are employed at the local community hospital in the diagnostic imaging department. You are approached by a colleague who asks you to become a member of the local chapter of your professional organization. You know that you will be expected to pay yearly dues. Which would be your best response to your colleague?
   a. You explain that you have just begun your first job and money is in short supply at this time.
   b. You laugh and say, "No thanks, I've had all of the organization I can take for a while."
   c. You join in 1 or 2 years when your financial status improves.
   d. You join at once because you feel that it is an obligation to be a member of your professional organization.

_____ **11.** You are the radiographer assigned to the special procedures area to assist with an arteriogram this morning. In the room where the examination is to take place, the patient asks you what this examination is for and what the doctor has planned. You check her chart and find that the consent for the procedure has been signed. The next thing you must do is
   a. Explain the procedure to the patient.
   b. Remind the patient that she has signed the consent form and therefore must understand what is going to happen.
   c. Explain the problem to the physician, and ask the physician to review the procedure with the patient.
   d. Tell the patient not to worry because she is in capable hands.

_____ **12.** Information about a patient's condition or prognosis
   a. May be freely discussed with close relatives
   b. Must always remain confidential
   c. Should always be open discussion, since "a well-known fact is no secret"
   d. Should be discussed only on a co-worker-interdepartmental basis

_____ **13.** If you are unable to solve a professional ethical dilemma, you must present the problem to
   a. Your attorney
   b. The ethics committee of the institution for which you work
   c. Your colleagues
   d. Your peers

_____ **14.** As a radiographer you are assigned to a diagnostic imaging procedure for which you have had no education. Your best course of action when this occurs would be
   a. To proceed as best you can
   b. To ask a colleague for directions and then proceed
   c. To explain to your superior that you have never worked with this procedure and do not feel competent to perform the procedure without education
   d. To state that you are ill, and retreat

_____ **15.** If you offer your services at the scene of an accident, you are protected from litigation by the Good Samaritan law.
   a. True
   b. False

_____ **16.** If a patient requests to take his or her radiographic films to another institution for consultation, you must remember
  a. That the patient must present a signed request before the records can be released
  b. That only the original radiographic films can be released
  c. That only copies of the original radiographic films can be released

17. An unconscious child is brought to the emergency suite in your hospital for a diagnostic radiograph. There is no parent or legal guardian with the child. You will proceed with the procedure and will be functioning under the rule of _____ consent.

18. Explain the value of personal malpractice insurance for the radiographer.

19. List and define the levels of health care in the United States.

20. List three areas in which the radiographer may infringe upon patient rights.

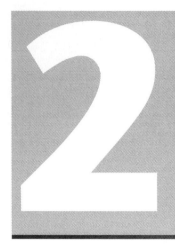

The Patient in Radiographic Imaging

Objectives

After studying this chapter, you will be able to:

1. Explain the basic physical and emotional needs of the patient.
2. Define and explain critical thinking, and describe its place in the profession of radiologic technology.
3. Explain the method used to make an accurate assessment of the patient's needs in the imaging department, and explain the rationale for using this method.
4. List expectations that the patient may have of the radiographer assigned to his or her care.
5. Define therapeutic communication and demonstrate its techniques.
6. Explain the interview process, and list the requirements for its successful completion.
7. Explain the use of the problem-solving process in patient teaching.
8. Describe the special needs of the terminally ill or the grieving patient in terms of radiographic imaging.
9. Define advance directives and differentiate between various types of advance directive documents.

Glossary

Advance directives: Documents (written when client is in good health) granting permission to a responsible person for voicing the desire for medical care for client during times of incapacity

Analytical: The breakdown of a subject into components

Bias: An inclination or temperament based on personal judgment; prejudice

Common law: Decisions and opinions of court that are based on local customs and habits of an area within a particular country or state

Conservator: A person who preserves or protests; a guardian

Despair: A hopeless state; lack of hope or expectation

Infer: To derive by reasoning or implication; conclude from facts

Paralanguage: The sound of speech rather than its content

Personal space: The subjective distance at which one person feels comfortable talking to another

STAT Procedure: A procedure that must be performed at once

Unethical: Not conforming to the standards of conduct of a particular profession or group

As a student radiographer, you are obliged to learn to assess the needs of patients assigned to you for examinations or treatments. After you have made this assessment, you must be able to formulate a plan of care that best fits the individual's needs. The plan is then implemented and, finally, evaluated. To follow these steps in assessment, you must have an understanding of the basic human needs and expectations that a person brings to the diagnostic imaging department when presenting for diagnosis or care.

You need to develop skills in critical thinking and problem solving to accurately assess each patient's unique needs and to effectively plan and implement care. When carefully applied, these skills will enable you to achieve the desired patient care goals.

The ability to communicate effectively and in a therapeutic manner is essential for all health care professionals. This means that you must leave the patient feeling that his or her condition has been improved, not worsened, as a result of the interaction.

Patient education is a part of the radiographer's professional obligation. You must be able to assess the patient's educational needs based on current knowledge and cultural and emotional requirements. When this is done, you can proceed to design an educational plan that adequately informs the patient concerning the procedure to be performed and the preparation for that procedure.

As a radiographer, you will often work with patients who have serious and sometimes terminal, illnesses. The ability to relate to the grieving patient with understanding and sensitivity is a skill no radiographer should be without. The development of this sensitivity is built on an understanding of the phases of the grieving process and an appreciation of your own feelings about loss and death.

Basic Human Needs

Health is often seen as existing on a continuum. At the positive end of the continuum, all body organs are functioning at their best, and one's mental state is positive. The person in this state has a feeling of well-being or health. At the negative end of the continuum, the individual is close to death or is in a state of despair. In the middle are persons at every stage of mental and physical well-being between these two extremes.

Whatever end of the health-illness continuum a person is on, that individual has basic needs that govern his or her life. When basic needs are met, other, higher, needs can emerge. Abraham Maslow, a renowned psychologist, saw humans as governed by a hierarchy of needs, each of which he viewed as a "building block" in a pyramidal structure. At the base of the pyramid are the basic physiological needs; at the top is self-actualization, the end result of all spiritual growth. These and the other needs are defined as follows:

1. *Physiologic needs:* The basic needs are for food, shelter, air, water, sleep, and sexual fulfillment. If these basic needs are not satisfied, a person is unable to pursue other needs.

2. *Safety and security:* After a person has satisfied the most basic needs, he or she begins to seek a place free from harm and can be sure of being able to earn a living.

3. *Love and belongingness:* When primary needs have been met, the person begins to seek someone with whom to share life and seeks a social group in which he or she feels accepted.

4. *Self-esteem and the esteem of others:* Everyone thrives on self-regard and the feeling of being favorably regarded by others beyond their immediate family or circle of significant others.

5. *Self-actualization:* When all the foregoing needs have been met, the person begins to grow spiritually. He or she begins to want to accomplish deeds that will make him or her feel the attainment of the ultimate growth in his or her life.

Persons whose state of mental and physical health is at the most positive end of the health-illness continuum have their basic needs met and are pursuing self-actualization. When illness—whether physical or emotional—overtakes a person, he or she loses the state of well-being and no longer perceives him- or herself as one whose basic needs for food, water, air, love, belonging, and self-esteem are being met. Illness may mean the loss of ability to maintain social and economic status. The individual's place in his or her social group is threatened. As illness progresses, the awareness of unmet basic needs increases, and feelings of great anxiety overwhelm the ill person.

When you as the radiographer meet the patient, he or she is often in this anxiety state. Persons who are in need of diagnostic imaging procedures may present themselves for diagnosis and treatment after a long period of feeling unwell. Others may come to the department immediately after a serious accident has destroyed or threatens to destroy their state of well-being. When one's level of wellness has been compromised and the satisfaction of basic needs is threatened for whatever cause, regressive behavior may result. A person in such a state has difficulty communicating effectively. He or she may resort to aggressive demands or may withdraw in silence and not be able to make his or her needs known at all.

If you are assigned to care for a person, you must be able to determine that person's state of health or illness. Furthermore, you must understand that the fulfillment of the patient's most basic needs may have been interrupted by illness or trauma, thus causing him or her to behave in an unpleasant manner.

Critical Thinking

Each patient care procedure that you encounter requires a different application of your skills and knowledge. The hallmark of an excellent radiographer is the ability to achieve a positive diagnostic or treatment result in a timely, efficient manner while meeting the unique needs of the individual patient. To achieve this goal, you must use your critical thinking skills.

A general definition of critical thinking might be that it is an analytical inquiry into any issue presented. A more specific definition is the one used by Richard Paul, a leader in the critical thinking movement in which critical thinking is described as "the art of thinking about your thinking while you are thinking in order to make your thinking better, more clear, more accurate, or more defensible" (Paul, 1995, p. 6430). If you are not assessing your manner of thought, you are not thinking critically.

Critical thinking requires the ability to interpret, analyze, evaluate, infer, explain, and reflect. This is a lot of work, and it cannot be learned quickly. It must be learned step-by-step fashion. Thinking in this manner requires that you become well acquainted with yourself and well aware of the limits of your knowledge, biases, and prejudices. You must review the life experiences that have created your current thinking methodologies and be willing to expand your thinking methods. You will need to become an inquisitive thinker, become tolerant of the views of others, and be interested in expanding your own thinking to become inquiring and creative in your thought processes.

As you begin to work with patients as a radiographer, you will proceed through levels of thinking. As you mature in your profession, you will grow personally as well as professionally. You must continue to expand your technical abilities as you work with patients, and you must continue to evaluate your thinking methods as they grow from simple to complex.

CALL OUT!

Critical thinking requirements: ability to analyze, evaluate, infer, explain, and reflect.

Modes of Thinking

Thinking comprises several levels: recall, habit, inquiry, and creativity. Recall and habit make up the lower levels, or modes, of thinking. Inquiry and creativity are higher-order thinking skills. Mastering the ability to analyze how you think is another crucial skill of critical thinking. A brief description of the modes of thinking follows:

Recall

As a radiographer, you need to learn a large body of scientific facts that you can recall at a moment's notice as you work with patients. Without the ability to bring these facts to mind quickly, you will not succeed. This is the basic level of critical thinking at which answers are either right or wrong. The beginning radiographer is not qualified to proceed without following the prescribed patterns of those who are experts in the field. For example, let's say that you are called on in the laboratory to make a radiographic exposure of a patient's anterior chest. If you have not learned the basic methodology of this procedure or have learned it but cannot recall it immediately, you cannot proceed.

Habit

As you become more experienced, you will develop habits that make for the efficient practice of learned skills. You will have no need to think deeply about each procedure before performing it, because you will have become habituated to performing a number of procedures. When you engage in habitual thinking, you are neither casual nor careless, but rather quick and efficient in performing habitual procedures.

At this level of critical thinking, you are able to interpret the prescribed patterns of your work assignments as a radiographer and perform with little or no directives in all but the most complex situations. You are able to interpret the work of others and apply it to your own methods of accomplishing each task. You begin to evaluate your own work in a critical manner.

Inquiry

A professional person uses the skills of recall and habit in his or her work, along with a higher mode of thinking called inquiry. To inquire is to process information thoughtfully and to be willing and able to recognize, explore, and challenge assumptions to make sense of complex ideas.

Inquiry is the essence of critical thinking and includes the ability to analyze, infer, explain and reflect upon one's work. As a radiographer, you begin to select options for performing each procedure based on advanced knowledge and an awareness of alternative methods of performing a skill that might be more advantageous for the patient when a problem is present. In other words, you begin to do problem-solving based on your knowledge and skills as a critical thinker. You are able to explain the reasons for your decisions and reflect critically on them. You also become accountable for the decisions you make.

Creativity

Another aspect of higher-level thinking is creativity. Creativity often follows inquiry and is used to solve individual problems and to prevent causing the patient discomfort or pain. If you are able to conceive of an alternative method of performing a task or accomplishing a procedure, particularly one that is more efficient or less traumatic for the patient, you are said to have creatively improved your work.

The creative radiographer does not abandon the standards of practice in the field. "Minds indifferent to standards and disciplined judgment tend to judge inexactly, inaccurately, inappropriately, prejudicially (Paul, 1995, p. 198). Creativity must always work within the standards of safe practice and must be able to be validated within the constraints of ethical and professional standards. Creativity demands accountability.

Knowing How You Think

Your ability to understand how you think may be the most difficult aspect of critical thinking. Once again, you need to be introspective. You must think while thinking. Honesty with yourself is also necessary. Ask yourself the following questions:

1. Am I remaining in the lower-level thinking modes most of the time, using only recall and habit to solve problems?

2. Do I rarely (or never) move beyond these lower levels of thinking into the realm of inquiry by exploring, validating, and analyzing the problems before me?

3. Am I combining (interpreting) thoughts, ideas, and concepts to find better solutions to problems?

4. Am I creating new approaches to solve difficult patient care problems?

5. Am I carefully evaluating my work?

Becoming a critical thinker takes practice and time. The successful radiographer takes the concepts presented above and applies them to each patient care problem. If you have made a habit of higher-level thinking, thinking through each situation in a critical manner to create a successful solution will become second nature. The ability to recall what was learned in the classroom and to perform diagnostic imaging skills from habit are necessary but not sufficient skills for you as a professional radiographer. These lower-level thinking processes must be combined with the higher modes of thinking to care safely for the patient.

Patient Assessment (Problem Solving)

Every patient and every diagnostic procedure presents problems, ranging from simple to complex. When you obtain an assignment, decide how to perform the assignment quickly, efficiently, and as comfortably as possible for the patient. This requires you to go through a problem-solving process before beginning the task. Beginning radiography students should write down the problem-solving process. As you attain proficiency, if becomes a mental process. However the process is conducted, critical thinking is necessary to achieve a satisfactory outcome. The ability to recall the scientific principles of the procedure and the habits cultivated in performing various skills is also needed. Problem solving requires data collection, data analysis, planning, implementation, and evaluation.

Data Collection

There are basically two types of data: subjective and objective. Subjective data include anything that the patient or a significant other who accompanies the patient might say that is pertinent to his or her care. For instance, the patient might say, "The last time I had an x-ray, they gave me some medicine in my vein that made me itch all over," or "When I move it hurts my back." Either of these statements would be significant subjective data and, as such, would need to become part of your database as a radiographer. In other words, anything that the patient or a person accompanying the patient to the radiographic imaging department says that can in some way affect the procedure must be considered important subjective data.

Objective data include anything that you see, hear, smell, feel, or read on the patient's chart; anything reported about the patient by another health care worker that may affect the patient or the procedure to be performed is also considered objective data.

Data Analysis

This part of the assessment process integrates all segments of critical thinking. List all the subjective and objective data and then begin to analyze it. You must then decide what data are relevant to the assignment. This requires the skill of inquiry. You must also recall how the procedure to be done is performed. The relevant data (the problems and potential problems) are then listed in order of priority, beginning with what is most significant to the procedure.

Example

You are assigned to make radiographs of the pelvis of an 84-year-old female who may have a hip fracture. You go to the waiting area to summon the patient and find her on a gurney. You greet her and inquire about her well-being.

The patient says, "I'm very hard of hearing, you'll have to speak louder." You raise your voice and ask the patient again how she is feeling. She responds, "I was very well until last evening when I fell as I was getting into bed. Now I have a lot of pain in my right leg." The patient is then moved to the examining room. During the preceding brief interaction, you have managed to gather the following data:

1. The patient is an elderly female (objective data)

2. The patient is hearing impaired (subjective data)

3. The patient has pain in her right leg (subjective data)

In the examining room, you continue your assessment of the patient. From the data that you gather, you formulate a list of problems and potential problems that you will (or may) encounter as you work with this patient. Remember, considering potential problems initially allows you to anticipate and thus avoid possible difficulties. The problem list might be continued as follows, with problems given in order of priority:

1. Pain and a potential for increasing the patient's pain during your examination (moving the patient may cause further pain)

2. Immobility (the patient is unable to move by herself and requires assistance for safety and to obtain adequate exposures)

3. Potential for impairment of skin integrity (elderly persons have fragile skin that is easily damaged)

4. Potential for further injury (if patient is not moved carefully, the injury may be extended)

5. Hearing impairment (it will be necessary to speak distinctly so the patient can hear directions)

After you have completed your data collection, set a goal and make a plan for achieving the goal. To do this, you must rely on recall of theoretical principles concerning movement restrictions of a patient with a pelvic injury. You must use inquiry and creativity to plan how you are going to be able to obtain the most effective radiographic images of the patient's pelvis without causing her further pain or an extension of her injury.

Patient involvement in goal setting and formulating a plan to achieve the goal is essential. A patient who is not part of the care planning is not able to cooperate to achieve the desired goal. Collaborating with the patient in planning her care instills in her a feeling of responsibility for a successful outcome.

After you complete the assessment and list the problems and potential problems, it is time to establish a goal. Next, formulate objectives or outcome criteria for attaining the goal. The patient outcomes, or objectives, depend on the radiographic exposures needed and the problems identified in the initial patient assessment.

Example

Goal: The radiographs will clearly demonstrate the patient's medical problem.

Example

Objectives

1. The patient will be free of pain during the procedure.

2. The patient's skin integrity will not be impaired.

3. The patient's condition will remain stable during the procedure.

Planning and Implementation

After data analysis, you establish a goal with expected outcomes or objectives for achieving that goal. Write the plan for achieving the goal and then implement it. Planning requires the use of all modes of thinking. You must recall the theoretical concepts learned from classroom and textbook instruction. Any practical experience gained in radiography will have given you the time and opportunity to develop reliable habits for selecting correct exposure factors for each patient assignment. Inquiry is used to analyze the data to assess potential areas in which errors can affect a safe and successful outcome. Creativity is necessary to devise a method of performing the procedure, given the problems listed.

Example

1. Instruct the patient concerning what is to be accomplished.

2. Obtain assistance from as many persons as necessary to move the patient onto the radiographic table to avoid further injury and to prevent pain.

3. Provide adequate radiation protection for the patient and for yourself.

4. Set the correct exposure factors for the radiographs needed.

5. Make the exposures required.

6. Process the radiographs.

7. Return the patient safely to her room.

This plan is then implemented. Implementation of the plan depends on the patient's problems and whether you need to obtain assistance to achieve the desired goal. You will also rely on your creativity to solve problems that you have not anticipated during this phase. The patient's safety during the implementation of the plan must always be the chief priority.

Evaluation

After implementing the plan, it must be evaluated. As a beginning student, you will be expected to perform this phase of care in writing or with an instructor's assistance. You should never cease learning from the patient regardless of how many years of experience you may have. Each patient care situation differs in some ways from all others encountered; therefore, all patient care experiences are learning experiences.

Radiographs are the tangible evidence of your successful attainment of diagnostic goals. However, the condition of the patient after the examination must also be considered. In evaluating the patient care you are giving, ask yourself the following questions:

1. Were the patient's needs met?

2. Was the patient's safety maintained during the procedure?

3. Was the patient's skin intact at the end of the examination?

4. Did the patient complain of pain as the procedure was implemented?

5. What problems arose that I did not anticipate?

6. What can I do differently next time to improve my work or to reduce the patient's discomfort?

7. Did I use higher-level critical thinking skills to successfully complete the procedure?

Make a careful analysis of each patient care situation at the end of each assignment. Radiographic quality is certainly the goal; however, if the patient's safety was jeopardized or if the patient was subjected to a great amount of pain as you implemented your plan, the outcome of the procedure was less than perfect. Honest inquiry is the key to evaluation.

As a radiologic technology student, you will not achieve the optimum level of success with each procedure, but if you have the ability to recognize errors and modify subsequent procedures accordingly, you can achieve your goals most of the time.

Patient Expectations

The patient also has expectations of health care professionals. The patient expects to find an articulate, concerned, clean, and well-groomed professional to care for him or her. While in the diagnostic imaging department, the patient also expects to be the focus of your concern, to the exclusion of any personal concerns that you may have at that moment.

As the world grows smaller, radiologic technology students must expect to find persons from all parts of the world presenting themselves for health care. And with these ethnically diverse patients come a host of expectations concerning health and illness and medical treatment that are affected by different cultural and religious traditions. You must convey understanding and sensitivity for each patient's differences. Otherwise, patients may be left with the feeling that their health care experience was less than therapeutic.

Make sure that you take into consideration the patient's ethnicity and cultural beliefs as the initial assessment and patient care plan are made. You must treat every person whom you are caring for as a person who has dignity and worth, and you should design every care plan with the patient's sociocultural needs in mind. Your care of the patients should be free of any effects of your own feelings of prejudice against particular groups who do not share your beliefs or living habits.

Communication

All members of the health care team must learn to communicate clearly and therapeutically with their patients. They must be able to convey messages in an organized and logical manner. Any problem of communication, whether major or minor, has an impact on the patient's health care. If a patient leaves a health care situation feeling confused or misunderstood, he or she may choose not to continue care that is necessary to that patients' health. On the other hand, the patient who leaves feeling that he or she has been treated with dignity and respect will probably continue needed treatment.

Most patients' feelings about health care, whether positive or negative, are the result of communication between the health worker and the patient. As a radiographer, you receive, interpret, carry out, and give directions in your daily work routine. You also offer consolation and reassurance as you care for your patients. For these reasons, being able to communicate effectively is as important as knowing the correct use of the complex equipment in the department.

To become a successful communicator, you need to develop skills in listening, observing, speaking, and writing. As a student radiographer, you might feel that since you can hear, see, talk, write, and use a computer you are already skilled in the art of communication. However, this is not necessarily the case. Your ability to accept others with an open mind and to interact with people in a perceptive manner is based on learned attitudes and self-understanding.

To communicate effectively, you must first possess a degree of self-knowledge. You must become aware of your own limitations and understand any feelings, values, and attitudes that might lead to bias or discrimination in your interactions with others. Attitudes are a set of beliefs that a person holds toward issues or persons that cause him or her to respond in a predetermined manner. These predetermined behaviors may not be acceptable to another person from a different background.

Human beings are born free of attitudes, beliefs, values, and biases. But, from the first day of life, these begin to develop as a result of exposure to a particular group of people called *significant others*. These significant others may be the mother, father, other relatives in the home, or persons who assume the role of parents. As the child grows and matures, this is the group with whom he or she is in daily contact. Their environment, religious beliefs, morals, food preferences, and preferences for other people become the child's own. As the person grows older, friends and mates are sought from this pool of like-minded individuals. This is done to maintain the balance or harmony essential to a peaceful existence.

This need for harmony eventually affects every aspect of a person's manner of perceiving and reacting to the world, but no two people see the world in exactly the same way. For this reason, a person reacts not to a particular event, but to a personal perception of that event. That perception is the result of learned attitudes. As a radiographer, you must understand this and expect your patients to feel differently from the way you do about many things. For instance, a patient who is experiencing pain may react with a stoicism learned from past experiences. This may at first puzzle you, because you may be used to more open expressions of discomfort.

You must use your newly learned skills of critical thinking to assess how you think about those with whom you relate. You need to make an honest analysis of yourself and your learned beliefs and biases to become a skilled and thoughtful communicator.

Self-Concept and Self-Esteem

How we feel about and would describe ourselves may be defined as *self-concept*. It is made up of attitudes of our significant others toward us as we interact with them over time.

> ## CALL OUT!
>
> Elements of self-concept:
>
> Body image
> Self-esteem
> Role
> Identity

Self-concept evolves over a lifetime and is made up of body image, the roles played throughout your life, self-esteem, and identity. All of the aforementioned are interrelated and yet separate issues that make up who you are and how you see yourself.

Body image plays an important role in how you see yourself. If your body reflects an appearance that is acceptable to the society in which you live, it is a strong beginning for a satisfactory self-concept. If your body does not fit the picture of masculinity or femininity that is expected, if you are too large or too small, or unable to meet society's expectations or norms in any manner, it is a difficult issue to overcome as your self-concept develops. Changes in your body due to injury or illness also affect body image. This type of change is an especially difficult adjustment for the adolescent or the elderly person.

Self-esteem is often confused with self-concept and is directly related to self-concept. Self-esteem is our evaluation of ourselves based on the positive or negative returns we receive from our behaviors as we live our lives. A child who has parents who give praise and approval during his or her childhood has a good start toward having a high self-esteem. The child who is criticized and not valued during childhood will develop negative feelings about him- or herself and will have a low esteem of self.

The roles that a person plays throughout life also affects self-concept. Most persons play many roles as life evolves: that is, the role of student; worker in a profession; an intimacy role with a significant other or spouse; perhaps a parent. A person who identifies as having successfully played his or her roles will have enhanced self-concept and self-esteem.

Identity is the last element of self-concept. This is also the way in which you see yourself; however, your identity rarely changes over time. If you see yourself as a strong, competent person who can accomplish most any task you set out to accomplish, that image will remain with you for a lifetime. If you develop the identity of an incompetent person, it is difficult to alter that identity in your own mind.

Understanding your own feelings and attitudes, their natural evolution, and how you have developed your present self-concept is the beginning of self-acceptance. As a radiologic technology student who enters your chosen profession after having completed a thorough self-evaluation and having the ability to accept yourself as a person of worth, you will have fewer obstacles to overcome when beginning to relate to others in a therapeutic manner.

Nonverbal Communication

There is more to communication than the spoken word. The unspoken, or nonverbal, aspects of communication can be defined as all stimuli other than the spoken word involved in communication. To understand nonverbal communication, you must depend on what you *see* the patient doing as he or she speaks, what you *hear* in speech other than the spoken words, what you *feel* (if you are touching the patient during the communication), and what you *smell* as you come closer to the patient. These unspoken messages can often indicate how the patient feels more quickly than any words can. Nonverbal communication functions in the following ways:

It may repeat or stress the spoken message. In this case, the face or body movements are in agreement with what is said. For instance, a patient who states that he or she is in pain and who is protecting the painful body part and wincing or grimacing while speaking is stressing his or her message.

It may contradict the spoken word. As the patient speaks of the severe pain, he or she may smile and seem to enjoy the experience. The nonverbal behavior is obviously not in agreement with what is being spoken.

It may accent the spoken word. As the patient says "no," he or she slams a fist on the table to make the message clearer or to stress it.

It may regulate the spoken word. If, as a person is speaking, the receiver is nodding his or her head and giving the speaker an interested look, it is an indication to continue. Conversely, if the receiver is looking away and seems uncomfortable or uninterested, the speaker has a cue to stop speaking.

It may totally substitute in some instances for verbal communication, as in the case of a frown or a nod. A person may get his or her message across without saying a word.

The perceptive health care worker can learn a great deal about a patient by other types of nonverbal communication. The manner in which a person moves his or her body and face can say a great deal. The person with a frown and a set jaw is determined or angry about something. The patient who does not look you in the eye may feel insecure or mistrustful. The way in which your patient carries his or her body may tell you about his or her self-concept. The person who walks or sits proudly erect probably has a positive feeling about him- or herself. The person who has a poor self-concept or who is depressed may walk slowly with head down and shoulders slumped. While sitting, he or she will draw the body in and look away from the room.

Nonverbal cues may also suggest social and economic status. Signs may be obvious, such as those indicated by the clothing worn or by posture. Less obvious status cues might be the patient's manner of speech or the manner in which he or she enters a room or addresses those in the environment.

As a radiographer, you must make certain that your verbal and nonverbal message to the patient matches as well. If the patient suspects that you are not sincere in the interaction, his or her anxiety will increase. You may be forced to move into the patient's personal space as you work. This may result in feelings of discomfort for the patient as well as for you. You must be sensitive to the patient's feelings and inform the patient in advance of the need to enter his or her space and to touch the patient before you actually do.

You must understand that the patient who comes to the diagnostic imaging department for a difficult examination may be fearful but does not wish to express this verbally. The sensitive radiographer will be able to detect the patient's nonverbal expression of fear and anxiety. Therefore, by using therapeutic communication techniques, you will be able to establish a trusting relationship with the patient, which allows the patient to express his or her feelings, thereby reducing fear and anxiety.

Cultural Variations

You must be aware of cultural differences in verbal and nonverbal communication so that you will not offend or be offended, misunderstand, or be misunderstood. For instance, in some cultures it is considered courteous to place one's body very close to the body of another person during communication. In the United States, people are very protective of the space close to their bodies and might be offended if a person with whom they are not on very friendly terms invades this "personal space."

Nonverbal symbols such as a nod, meaning "yes," or a shake of the head, meaning "no," do not mean the same thing in all cultures. Symbols also have different meanings to different age groups. People of one age group may not understand the symbols of another. A safe rule when communicating with a patient is to use speech instead of symbols if there is any possibility of being misunderstood. Another common cause of cultural misunderstanding is the use of humor. Although humor is often an effective communication tool, you must use it with care when there are cultural or age differences. Humor can be an effective means of releasing tension or conveying a difficult message, but it should not be used in life-threatening situations, when there is a possibility of legal action, or when there may be a cultural misunderstanding. You must remember, too, that a patient's age may affect a common understanding of humor. In other words, if there is any doubt concerning its appropriateness, do not use humor.

Gender Factors

As a radiographer, you must be aware that the manner of communication will vary depending on the sex of the patient. The male radiographer and the female radiographer may tend to deliver and receive messages in an altered manner based simply on their sex. Men tend to be reticent in their expression of feelings and women often prefer to openly discuss how they feel. Men prefer an activity as a means of interaction, whereas women feel comfortable in discussion rather than in activity as a means of interaction. Whatever the sex of the patient or the radiographer, it is necessary to avoid sexual innuendoes, denigration of, or use of sex as a means of humor.

You must also be sensitive to the issue of gender in your professional interactions with co-workers. A nonbiased and nonjudgmental attitude in manner and speech concerning the differences in sexes and an avoidance of sexual innuendoes and a flirtatious manner will prevent many uncomfortable interpersonal problems in your relationships with co-workers.

Other Factors That Affect Communication

The rate at which you speak along with the volume, fluency, and vocal patterns, is categorized under the term *paralanguage*. Paralanguage has to do with the sound of the speech, rather than the content. The correct pauses and inflections are extremely important if the communication is to be understood. If you speak without proper inflection, a question will not sound like a question, or the words may run together and be difficult to sort out. Poor knowledge of correct grammatical usage may also make it difficult to understand what is being said.

Your first obligation as a radiographer is to thoroughly know the material that you want to communicate so that you can transmit the message correctly. Assess the patient-receiver's age; sex; educational, social, and economic levels; cultural background; and physical ability or disability before beginning, so that you may adapt your communication to the patient. If the patient has difficulty hearing, speak in a normal tone of voice but speak closer to the patient's ear. A patient who is unable to stand comfortably should be placed in a position in which he or she is comfortable enough to listen to the message without the distraction of pain. If the patient is accompanied by another person or group of persons, be certain that the patient hears the message.

Feedback

To be certain that the transmitted message has been correctly received, you should obtain feedback. In interactions between you and the patient, this may mean having the patient repeat the directions that were given or simply observe the patient to be certain that he or she is doing as instructed. If the patient understood the message, he or she will respond in the manner that was anticipated. If the patient does not, it is your responsibility to restate the message in a manner that the patient will understand and will demonstrate understanding by giving the correct feedback.

Developing a Harmonious Working Relationship

The most important responsibility you will have as a communicator is to develop a harmonious working relationship with the patient. Although interactions with a patient are often brief, the patient should be made to feel that he or she is a partner in the examination process. Indeed, the patient *is* the most important member of the health care team. Make the patient feel that he or she is sharing in the process. You

---

TABLE 2–1 _____
Therapeutic Communication Techniques

1. Establishing guidelines
2. Reducing distance
3. Listening
4. Using silence
5. Responding to the underlying message
6. Restating the main idea
7. Reflecting the main idea
8. Seeking and providing clarification
9. Making observations
10. Exploring
11. Validating
12. Focusing

---

create this therapeutic relationship through communication that coveys the message that you are a concerned and caring person. If the patient is made to feel that he or she is an unimportant object being passed through the imaging department in order to get the job done, he or she will leave with a feeling of discontent. This atmosphere of discontent gets created primarily through communication and is called a *nontherapeutic relationship*. There are a series of communication techniques that you should cultivate as a radiography student, which will help you to become a therapeutic member of the health care team. Useful therapeutic communication techniques are listed in Table 2-1.

Establishing Communication Guidelines

Since many of your relationships with patients are brief, to make the best use of the time allowed, you should set guidelines for the interaction as soon as possible. Establishing guidelines includes your introducing yourself to the patient and giving an explanation of the examination or treatment to be performed. Also include in your interaction what is expected of the patient and what he or she can expect of the radiology staff.

Delivering these instructions to the patient in a clear, concise, and nonthreatening manner requires careful thought before the communication. You will not be able to deliver accurate messages until your thinking is organized. If the patient doesn't understand the message, he or she will not be able to comply with the care plan. Successful communication requires critical thought on the part of you, the radiographer.

Reducing Distance

For the communication to be therapeutic, the physical distance between you and the patient should be reduced. This proximity also makes the patient feel included and involved. Avoid physical barriers or a noisy environment. Face the patient and make direct eye contact as you speak and as the patient responds.

If you cross your arms or legs during a communication, this creates a physical barrier that nonverbally conveys a lack of receptiveness. Performing other tasks while attempting to communicate also indicates that you have something more important to do than listen to what the patient is trying to convey. Figure 2-1 shows a good setting for communication.

Listening

To listen in a therapeutic manner, you must be able to overcome your personal biases. We all have biases that we learned as we have grown and developed. Unfortunately, most people see the world and their position in it as the correct and only acceptable way. To be a successful critical thinker, you must know yourself so well that you recognize your biased manner of thinking and of listening to anyone with whom you converse.

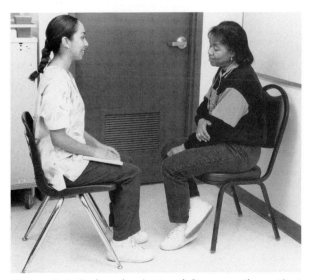

Figure 2–1. Reduce barriers and focus on the patient during radiographer–patient communication.

You can then begin to learn to shut out your own feelings and assume the totally nonjudgmental attitude that is essential to becoming a therapeutic listener.

A therapeutic listener is sympathetic to the patient and attempts to understand the patient's point of view while abandoning his or her own biases. While the patient is speaking, you must not be anticipating your own responses, comparing, or interpreting what the speaker is saying. Your goal must be to gather accurate information. If you are planning your responses instead of listening, you cannot gather the full feeling and meaning of what the patient is telling you.

Using Therapeutic Silence

Related to listening is the therapeutic use of silence. Short periods of silence give the patient a chance to arrange thoughts and consider what he or she wants to say. These periods also give you an opportunity to assess the patient's nonverbal communication as well as your own.

Responding to the Underlying Message

When a patient expresses a feeling of frustration, anger, joy, or relief, it is helpful if you respond in a manner that lets the patient know his or her feelings about the situation have been heard and understood. An example of this type of response follows:

PATIENT: *I'm really discouraged. I'm not sure that being so sick following these treatments is worth it.*

RADIOGRAPHER: *You feel disheartened because you're sick after the treatments, and you aren't certain that they're making you better.*

CALL OUT!

Respond to the feeling and meaning of the patient's verbal expression!

Restating the Main Idea

Restating or repeating the main idea expressed by the patient is a useful communication technique. It validates your interpretation of the message and also informs the patient that he or she is being heard. Consider the following dialogue:

PATIENT: *I am having a lot of pain in my left hip, and I might need help to get up on the examining table.*

RADIOGRAPHER: *You think you'll need help getting up on the table because your left hip is hurting?*

PATIENT: *Yes. Could you please help me?*

Reflecting the Main Idea

Reflecting or directing back to the patient the main idea that he or she has stated is another useful technique. It keeps the patient as the focus of the communication and allows the patient to explore his or her own feelings about the matter. In this instance, you help the patient to make his or her own decision. For example, consider the following dialogue:

PATIENT: *Do you think that I should continue this therapy? It's so expensive, and I'm not sure it's doing me any good.*

RADIOGRAPHER: *Do you think that you should stop the therapy?*

Seeking and Providing Clarification

Seeking clarification is another therapeutic technique that you might use. It indicates to the patient that you are listening to what is being said but are not sure that you have received the message clearly. In such a situation, you simply say, "I'm not sure that I understood you. Will you please repeat that?" or, "I'm not sure that I follow what you've said."

You may clarify directions that you have given to a patient by restating the directions using different terminology.

RADIOGRAPHER: *To prepare for this examination, you will have to take all of this medicine at bedtime tonight.*

PATIENT: *How much of this should I take at bedtime?*

RADIOGRAPHER: *Before you go to bed tonight, take all of the medicine in the bottle at one time.*

Making Observations

Making Observations or verbalizing the perceived feelings of another is a useful communication technique. For example, you might say, "You seem to be very tense, Mr. Smith. Are you concerned about this examination?"

Exploring

A the radiographer, you must direct questions that relate to the problems of the patient. When the patient relates fears or offers information about him- or herself, you may wish to pursue the problem by exploring further. An example of this might be as follows:

PATIENT: *Every time that you give me this medicine, it makes me feel strange.*

RADIOGRAPHER: *Can you tell me what it feels like when you take this medicine?*

TABLE 2–2
Nontherapeutic Communication Techniques

Judgmental statements	Giving advice
Cliché statements	Subjective interpretation
False reassurances	Disagreeing
Defending	Probing
Changing the subject	Demanding explanation

These are a few of the techniques that you may use to communicate with the patient in a therapeutic manner. The guiding principle of therapeutic communication is to keep the communication focused on the patient by asking open-ended questions, questions that allow the patient to expand his or her answers to questions. Avoid "what" and "why" types of questions, or questions that require only a yes-or-no answer. It is important for the conversation to be focused on the patient. Your verbal responses should be kept to a minimum, and the communication should always be redirected to the patient. For example:

PATIENT: *Do you have a family, young lady?*

RADIOGRAPHER: *Yes, I have a husband and two children. And you?*

Validating

When speaking to a patient, you may wish to verify what the patient has told you. This is called validating the message.

RADIOGRAPHER: *Mr. Gleam, you are saying that you have difficulty breathing when you are lying flat.*

PATIENT: *Yes, I must be in a sitting position in order to breathe well.*

Blocks to Therapeutic Communication

Several factors actually block or destroy the possibility of creating a therapeutic atmosphere in communication. Rapid speech, complex medical terminology, and distracting environments, such as a noisy waiting room or a crowded hallway, all are serious barriers to communication. Deliver messages to the patient in a quiet area of the department in a simple and direct manner. Make sure that the patient understands English. If the patient does not understand English, an interpreter should be made available.

Obtaining incomplete answers or failing to explore the patient's description of a problem can also be detrimental to communication. As the radiographer,

you must listen to what the patient tells you; if you are not certain of the message, explore by further questioning until you are certain that you understand. Failure to do this may result in harm to the patient. Some commonly used blocks to therapeutic communication are listed in Table 2-2.

Judgmental statements place the patient in the position of feeling that he or she must gain the approval of the health care worker in order to be cared for. These statements can be simple, such as, "that's good," or "that's bad." Or, they can take the form of clichés such as, "We have to take the bad with the good, you know." Another nontherapeutic communication is falsely reassuring to the client who expresses fear or concern by making a comment such as, "Now don't you worry. Everything will be just fine."

Defending, another block to communication, is an attempt by the health care worker to protect him- or herself, another person, or the institution. This type of communication rejects the patient's opinion and prevents the patient from continuing to communicate. For instance:

PATIENT: *I'm not sure Dr. Jay knows what to do with me.*

RADIOGRAPHER: *Dr. Jay is an experienced physician, and he has taken care of many people with problems just like yours.*

This type of nontherapeutic answer ends the communication with the patient feeling rejected and unworthy. How much better it would have been if the radiographer had simply restated the patient's comments and allowed the patient to complete his or her expression of concern.

Changing the subject while the patient is speaking is a nonverbal means of informing the patient that what he or she is saying is unimportant.

Also, avoid giving advice, offering subjective interpretations of a patient's statements, disagreeing, probing, and demanding explanations, all of which interfere with communication.

The Patient Interview

The goal of an interview is to unearth information concerning the patient's current and past health status for the purpose of providing a safe examination or treatment. An interview may be structured or unstructured. A *structured* interview consists of a list of written questions that require direct responses; it is conducted before a particular treatment or examination. An *unstructured* interview is informal and is based on questions asked by the health care worker that depend on patient responses to previous requests for information.

As an interviewer, you will be asking direct, personal questions of a relative stranger. During an interview, you must convey a professional image to ensure the patient's confidence as he or she relates confidential information.

Establishing rapport with the patient and providing an atmosphere that is private and as quiet as possible is the first priority during the patient interview. Because many people are offended if a stranger addresses them by their first name, you may want to ask the patient how he or she wishes to be addressed, or simply use the formal address.

Next, the patient is informed of the purpose of the interview; he is also advised that the information will be shared only with the medical personnel for whom it is necessary. It is appropriate for you as a radiologic technology student to inform the patient of your student status and that the information elicited will be shared with your supervisor or instructor.

An interview is composed of open-ended and closed-ended questions. *Closed-ended questions* are designed to elicit information quickly, as in an emergency situation or in situations that require only a one- or two-word answer. For example:

RADIOGRAPHER: *What is your age, Mr. Gleam?*

PATIENT: *I'm 24 years old.*

There are many situations in which a closed-ended question is inappropriate because the patient is not allowed to expand on the information requested with these brief responses. When this is the case, an open-ended question is appropriate. An *open-ended* question is used to assess the patient's feelings about a health care problem or to acquire information from the patient's point of view. For example:

RADIOGRAPHER: *Can you tell me what makes your pain worse, Mr. Smith?*

PATIENT: *In hurts all of the time. If I turn on my left side, the pain stops for awhile, but when I'm on my back, it is much worse.*

The therapeutic communication techniques described earlier in this chapter may be used during an interview when seeking information concerning a patient's feelings, as well as to extend or to validate information.

To conduct an effective interview, you must listen, observe, reply, and question in an organized and analytical manner, which requires critical thought

preceding action. While the interview is in progress, you should also be analyzing your patient's strengths and weaknesses so that you can use this information in your plan of care. After a structured interview, it is appropriate for you as the radiographer to summarize with the patient the information gathered. You can then inform the patient that the interview is concluded and thank him or her for cooperating.

The information that you seek in an interview is of great importance and is often of a highly personal nature. The patient's diagnosis is often part of the record that you receive when you obtain the requisition for the diagnostic image. The interview provides additional information required for the radiologist. Information obtained during the interview that is of great importance is as follows:

1. The matter of pregnancy or the possibility of pregnancy for the female patient of childbearing age. This information must be obtained before any radiologic procedure to protect the fetus.

2. The confirmation with the patient of the diagnostic imaging examination to be performed. Performance of an incorrect diagnostic imaging examination is a threat to the patient's health as well as a threat to the integrity of the department.

3. The information gathered during the patient interview provides vital information for the physician. This is particularly true when there is a need for a "STAT" procedure and the radiologist has little previous information concerning the patient on which to base his or her diagnosis.

Samples of structured interview questions are presented in each chapter that deals with a particular body system.

Patient Education

A patient who comes to the radiographic imaging department for treatment or diagnosis has a right to expect that he or she will be instructed in the procedure to be received. It is you, the radiographer, who provides the instruction, which should include the following:

1. A detailed description of the preparation necessary for the procedure

2. A description of the purpose of the test, the mechanics of the procedure, and what will be expected of the patient, for instance, frequent position changes, medications to be taken or injected, and contrast agents to be used

3. The approximate amount of time that the procedure will take

4. An explanation of any unusual equipment that will be used during the examination

5. The follow-up care necessary when the procedure is complete

The patient who is hospitalized before radiographic imaging procedures receives pre-examination preparation from the nurse assigned to his or her care. The radiographer's obligation as a member of the health care team is to communicate the preparation needs for radiographic imaging procedures in his or her department to other members of the health care team who will be preparing the patient. The member of the health care team who usually prepares hospitalized patients for radiographic imaging examinations is a member of the nursing staff.

You must be certain that the nurses who prepare the patient have explicit and current preparation instructions for each procedure to be performed. You must also plan the scheduling of imaging procedures with other members of the health care team so that the examinations are performed in a logical sequence that meets the patient's health care needs and accomplishes the diagnostic goals in the most time- and cost-efficient manner.

The possible adverse effects of a procedure should be addressed by the patient's physician before the patient is left in your care. Your job as radiographer is to determine the extent of the patient's knowledge of the procedure and his or her understanding of what is to occur. The techniques of therapeutic communication can be used to do this effectively. If the patient's understanding is not satisfactory or if he or she continues to be concerned about what is to occur, you should not begin the examination until the patient's concerns have been addressed by the physician. You must also be certain that procedures requiring special informed consent are signed by the patient and are in order.

CALL OUT!

If the patient questions the examination, do not begin until the problem is resolved by the patient and the physician!

You must understand that there are three aspects of learning that may be involved in each patient teaching situation: cognitive, affective, and psychomotor. If the patient must learn why he or she needs a particular imaging examination, the cognitive domain will be called on; therefore, the patient must be able to understand what is taught. If the patient must accept an examination that he or she finds distasteful, the affective domain will be involved, and the patient's response will be based on his or her emotions, opinions, and values. If the patient must learn a procedure necessary for preparation for a diagnostic imaging examination, the psychomotor domain will be affected, and he or she will need to call on muscular activity as well as mental processes.

The problem-solving process is an effective guideline for patient teaching. It can be used to:

1. Establish your teaching goal or expected outcome.

2. Assess the patient's need for teaching and ability to understand instruction. Include:
   a. *Previous experience with the procedure to be performed.* A patient who has had a particular procedure previously does not need as much education as a person who has no idea of what is involved in a complex examination.
   b. *Knowledge of the preparation needed for the procedure.* A person who understands how to administer an enema does not need instruction about the procedure.
   c. *The patient's age, culture, ethnicity, and educational level.* The child as well as the parent need to be instructed, depending on age; an elderly person or caregiver may need additional instruction. Persons from foreign countries or whose cultures prohibit particular medical treatments or examination need additional instruction and demonstration of equipment.
   d. *The patient's health status.* A very ill person may not be receptive to teaching. You may need to enlist the help of a family member to facilitate patient teaching.
   e. *The patient's anxiety level and ability to assimilate the instruction.* A highly anxious individual cannot retain information and may need an alternative method of instruction.

3. Use your critical thinking skills to plan how to instruct the patient based on your assessment. Everyone has a different learning style. The styles are as follows:
   a. *Global versus linear:* some persons look at an entire picture and then the details (global); some look at each component of the material before looking at the whole (linear).
   b. *Visual:* material must be presented as a graphic design or in pictures.
   c. *Auditory:* learning is by verbal explanation alone.
   d. *Kinesthetic:* learning is by demonstration and followed by return demonstration.

4. Plan your method of evaluation to be certain that the patient has understood your instruction. This can be done in several ways:
   a. Obtaining verbal feedback

b. Having the patient perform a return demonstration
c. Obtaining written feedback
5. Implement your plan.
6. Evaluate your plan.

Immediate verbal feedback is usually the best method of evaluating a teaching plan in radiography because of the brief time allowed for teaching. If the patient or caregiver is able to repeat the instructions accurately, you can proceed with the examination. If it seems that the patient does not understand or agree with the examination, postpone the examination until you can successfully convey the information. This requires reformulation of the educational plan. Another member of the health care team might be able to assist you in this regard. If English is not the patient's native language and you cannot communicate in the patient's language, you may need to call an interpreter. This is necessary because if you work with a patient who is poorly instructed, it is sure to result in frustration for you and for the patient, and the examination may not be successful.

When an examination is completed, you must reinforce what you initially taught the patient concerning follow-up treatment or care. Keep in mind that the anxiety caused by the procedure may cause the patient to be somewhat forgetful. Give written follow-up instructions to the patient along with verbal instruction.

Loss and Grief

Grief is a normal emotional response to the loss of a loved one, a prized possession, social status, or a bodily function or body part. It is also to be expected when a person is faced with the possibility of imminent death. Unfortunately, the process of grieving is a long and difficult one.

How a person manages the process of grieving depends largely on cultural, religious, and economic factors, as well as on the value placed on the loss. Grief reactions are often more severe for children and the elderly, especially if they have lost a person on whom they have depended.

In all health care professions, exposure to the loss and grief of others is common. Radiologic technology is no exception. Before exposure to persons who are in various stages of the grieving process, as a student you must examine your own feelings and attitudes concerning death and loss. It is not unusual for a health care worker to be filled with emotion when caring for a person who has suffered a tremendous loss; however, these emotions must not prevent you from caring for the grieving patient. If you feel that you may have

difficulty in this aspect of patient care, seek counseling or discuss these fears with a respected colleague.

Scholars have presented many concepts and theories that may be used to facilitate understanding of persons who are grieving. Each theory identifies phases in the process of grieving. Remember that grieving is a human process and, as such, does not follow an orderly sequence. The grieving person may go from one phase of grief to another and then return to a previous phase; he or she may even be in more than one phase of grief at a time.

I have selected the theory of grieving proposed by Dr. Elisabeth Kubler-Ross to summarize the phases of the grieving process in a concise manner. Remember that the picture of the grieving person presented here is general and varies with each individual. Your ability to care for the grieving patient is enhanced by assessing the patient before beginning care to determine which phase of the grieving process he or she may be going through.

Phase I: Denial

When a human being has an illness that will ultimately lead to death, he or she usually senses this before being informed of this fact by the physician. It is the physician who informs the patient of approaching death, and no other member of the health care team should assume this responsibility. Often a sensitive physician waits for the patient to bring up the matter. When the physician has verified impending death, the patient's initial response is usually one of shock and denial. The patient uses this first response as a defense until he or she can become accustomed to the idea.

The idea of one's own death is difficult to face. Death happens to other people, "not me." If you are questioned about the possibility of death or permanent disability, respond with reflective answers and give support without being unrealistic. For example:

PATIENT: *Do you think my disease is incurable?*

RADIOGRAPHER: *You feel that you have an incurable disease?*

Phase II: Anger

If the illness preceding death is lengthy, or as the recognition of disfigurement and handicap is verified, the patient moves into the second phase of the grieving process. In this phase, the client becomes angry. He may hurl criticism and abuse at family members or at health care workers. He feels that he has been done a serious injustice, and hopeless rage is his only defense. If you are insulted or verbally abused, you should not take the abuse personally. You should be matter-of-fact and understanding in your responses. Releasing anger is therapeutic to these patients and should be permitted.

Phase III: Bargaining

The third phase in the grieving process is a period of bargaining. The patient becomes a "good patient." He or she tries to follow all medical advice and becomes submissive. He or she may feel guilty about outbursts of anger. The patient has hopes that being "good" will spare him or her. Perhaps there will be a miraculous cure or, at least, less pain and suffering.

During this phase, the person who has a terminal illness may seek alternative modes of treatment, some of which may seem unusual or even nontherapeutic.

Phase IV: Depression

The fourth phase of the grieving process is a period of depression. The patient accepts the reality of impending death, permanent disability, or disfigurement. The patient begins to mourn for his or her past life and all that was lost or is being lost He or she is often silent and retiring at this time. Quiet support is the best response of the health care worker during this period.

Phase V: Acceptance

The fifth phase in the grieving process is a period of acceptance. If the patient is dying, he or she will lose interest in the outside world and become interested only in the immediate surroundings and the support of persons near him or her. The patient deals with the pain and illness and begins to disengage from life. The health care workers should be quietly supportive during this time. Communication should be reflective, and the client should be allowed to discuss whatever he or she desires.

If the patient is facing a permanent disability or disfigurement and not death, this is the time when he or she makes the first attempts at rehabilitation. He or she faces the reality of the necessity of making the most of life. This does not mean that the disability is forgotten or totally accepted. The disabled person may have a longer grieving period than the person who suffers the loss of a loved one because of being constantly reminded that he or she is no longer the same person as before. You must remember this and use consideration and understanding. The rehabilitating patient must be allowed to direct his or her own care as much as possible. You should stand by to assist, rather than take the lead. You should also be matter-of-fact as you care for the disabled patient and comply with requests for assistance.

Some persons who are going through the process of grieving may not wish to avoid the subject of their grief. When confronted with a grieving person, many people avoid the grief issue because of their own discomfort with the topic. However, many grieving persons have a desire to discuss their problem. If you are an astute radiographer and a sensitive communicator, you will be able to differentiate those who wish to discuss their grief from those who do not. If the patient refers to the grief issue, a simple reflective statement will allow the patient to proceed if he or she wishes to do so. For example:

PATIENT: *It's been 6 months since I lost my leg, but I still feel that it is not true.*

RADIOGRAPHER: *You sometimes find it hard to believe that this has happened to you?*

When you are caring for a person who is dying or has suffered a serious loss, always be supportive and allow the patient to retain hope for attaining his or her short-term or long-term goals. Perhaps the person can be assisted in making short-term goals that can be realistically attained. All patients have the right to be treated as persons of dignity and worth until they have taken their last breath. Depriving patients of hope or treating them as if their reason for living is no longer valid is a violation of patient rights.

Grief is a normal human reaction to loss. If the person or object of loss was of vital importance in the individual's life, the process of grieving is often not complete for 1 or 2 years. However, in some situations the grieving process becomes maladaptive. This may happen when a person cannot adequately express grief or has a feeling of guilt concerning the relationship of the survivor with the deceased. When the loss results in social dysfunction and mental illness, the grieving person must seek or be taken to a counselor or psychiatrist for assistance in resolving the grief.

Patient Rights Related to Death, Dying, and Medical Treatment

The science of medical care has advanced to the point at which life can be maintained by mechanical means almost indefinitely, or at least long after the quality of life has deteriorated. This may not be in the patient's best interest. Indeed, if the patient were able to make the decision, he or she would likely refuse this type of treatment.

To keep their families from being caught up in the potential legal and ethical issues associated with decisions concerning prolonged medical treatment, many people are choosing to draw up, well in advance of need, legal documents for use by significant others in the event these decisions must be made.

DISPLAY 2–1

Advance Health Care Directive

PART 1

1. *Power of Attorney for Health Care:* A designated person who is instructed to make health care decisions for someone unable to do so. This designated person may be a friend or relative who has been instructed in an individual's wishes concerning the prolonging of life in case of an illness or injury from which his or her chances of recovering are highly questionable. An alternate designee should also be named.

2. *Agent's Authority:* The appointed agent who is authorized to make all health care decisions for an individual. These decisions might include the decision to provide, withhold, or withdraw artificial nutrition and hydration and all other forms of health care to keep the person alive. Exceptions should be stated.

3. *Time Agent's Authority Becomes Effective:* When the physician in charge of a patient's care determines that the patient cannot make his or her own health care decisions or cannot do so immediately, if so written.

4. *The Agent's Obligations:* Health care decisions shall be made by the agent according to the instructions as written in Parts 1 and 2 of the document and any other wishes known by the agent. If the person's wishes are unknown, the agent will make decisions deemed to be in the best interests of that person as he or she considers the personal values of that individual.

5. *Agent's Postdeath Authority:* The agent may be authorized to make anatomical gifts, authorize an autopsy, and direct disposition of the person's remains with exceptions as stated.

6. *Nomination of a Conservator:* A conservator is chosen with an alternative also chosen in case the chosen conservator is unable or unwilling to act in that capacity.

PART 2

Includes or omits any of the following:

End-of-Life Decisions: Directs health care providers and anyone involved in an individual's care to withhold or withdraw treatment in accordance with the choices made. They may be as follows:
Do not prolong my life if I have an incurable and irreversible condition that will result in death or if I will (with a degree of certainty) not regain consciousness or if the most likely risks and burdens of treatment will outweigh the benefits.
Choice to Prolong Life: The individual in question may wish to have his or her life prolonged as long as possible within the limits of generally accepted health care standards.
Pain Relief: The individual may direct that any pain relief methods be provided even if the method may hasten death.
Other Wishes: Any alternative wishes the person desires must be listed.

This document is called an *Advance Health Care Directive*. All persons have the right to give instruction concerning their own health care. These directives must be written, signed, witnessed, and made available to anyone who may be in charge of the person concerned if he or she is not able to make decisions so that these directives may be followed. The Advance Health Care Directive should include the information in Display 2-1.

Organ or tissue donations to be made at time of death may be listed and to whom they should be donated. A primary physician may be selected along with an alternative. The document must be signed by the individual for whom it is made and must be witnessed by two persons who are not relatives of the designator or who are not any of the person's health care providers. These rules may be different in each state, and the person making the designation must be certain that the person is following the rules of the state in which he or she lives. Persons living in a skilled nursing facility may need a patient advocate or an ombudsman to also be a witness.

When this document is complete, copies should be made available to all who may be involved in end-of-life issues with this individual. A copy of this document should be placed in the person's medical file and on his or her chart when admitted to the hospital.

The U. S. Congress passed a Patient Self-Determination Act in 1990, which requires that all health care institutions that receive federal funding ask patients if they have advance health care directives. The patient's response must be a part of their health record.

As the radiographer, you must become familiar with this type of legal document since it is frequently a part of the patient's chart and you must be able to understand the patient's wishes. You must also be familiar with other forms of advance directives. They are as follows:

Living Will: A document that lists the patient's wishes if terminally ill.

Durable Power of Attorney for Health Care: Designates a person who will make health care decisions for the patient if he or she is unable to do so.

DNR: Instructions on a patient's chart that direct health care workers not to resuscitate the patient if he or she stops breathing and the heart stops beating.

DNI: Instructs health care workers not to intubate the patient if a question of such a need arises.

Full Code: Instructs health care workers to initiate a full cardiopulmonary resuscitation if the patient stops breathing and the heart stop beating. This type of emergency is usually referred to as a *Code Blue.*

Summary

All human beings have basic needs. The patient who seeks medical care does so because his or her basic needs are no longer being met owing to illness. An ill person's behavior often regresses because of an inability to have his or her needs satisfied. The patient who comes to the diagnostic imaging department for diagnosis or treatment may be unable to relate to the health care worker in a pleasant manner. You, as the radiographer, must be able to recognize that the patient is behaving in a regressive manner because of unmet basic human needs. If this is understood, you will be able to care for the patient in a sensitive and caring manner, regardless of how the patient behaves.

The successful radiographer has learned the skills of critical thinking. This skill requires a great deal of practice and introspection. To think in a critical manner you need to be able to interpret, analyze, evaluate, infer, explain, and reflect. These are all parts of the higher levels of thinking and are required in your daily professional life.

To learn these critical skills, you must understand how you yourself think. This requires introspection and honesty. As a student, you must become aware of the limits of your current knowledge and understand the reasons for your limitations, which are often the result of personal biases. You can then begin to improve your ability to think in a critical manner.

Each patient care assignment involves problem solving that requires both lower and higher modes of thinking. The steps in the problem-solving process are data collection, analysis of data, planning, implementation, and evaluation. The patient's racial and cultural differences must be considered when planning care.

When a patient enters the diagnostic imaging department for care, he or she expects to encounter a professional health care worker who is articulate, clean, well groomed, and caring. The patient also expects to be treated as a person of dignity and worth.

Communication is central to all health care situations. As a radiographer, you must be able to communicate in a therapeutic manner with your patients. This begins with self-understanding. You must understand your own biases and attitudes. You need to recognize how you feel about yourself and develop a positive self-concept before you can be an effective communicator.

In general, the radiologic technology student must learn to use the techniques of therapeutic communication and recognize potential blocks to therapeutic communication. When these techniques are applied correctly, the patient will leave the imaging department feeling positive about the treatment received.

The interview is another form of communication used frequently in health care. You must use your critical thinking skills to determine when it is appropriate to use open-ended or closed-ended questions in conducting a successful interview.

Patient education before procedures is an obligation that you have as a radiographer. You must assess your patient's level of knowledge and cultural differences before making an instructional plan. Then design your teaching based on each individual's need. Assessment of the teaching plan can be done by obtaining a return demonstration or by requesting verbal or written feedback from the patient.

A patient who is suffering from loss of a body part or body function or who is grieving from another type of personal loss must have special consideration. You must be able to assess the needs of your patient and communicate with him or her in a manner that conveys understanding and sensitivity.

You must also respect the patient's right to make choices concerning his or her own health care. As a student radiographer, you must familiarize yourself with the Advance Health Care Directive, the various alternatives available, and the terminology used in these documents.

Chapter 2 Test

1. All persons have basic needs that must be met. Match the situations listed below with the basic need that is not being satisfied:

    a. A patient is waiting alone on a gurney in a corridor. Everyone rushes by without offering explanations or communicating.

        1. Physiologic need

    b. No food was allowed before this examination after dinner the previous evening. The examination is late; it is now 11:00 AM.

        2. Safety and security need

c. A middle-aged patient who is having a lower gastrointestinal (GI) series has an involuntary evacuation of the barium on the examination table.

d. A young mother is studying music in her leisure time.

e. A child is taken from her parents into the diagnostic imaging department for examination. The parents wait outside.

3. Love and belonging need

4. Self-esteem need

5. Self-actualization need

2. Define *critical thinking*, and list and define the modes of thinking.

_____ **3.** You are preparing for an anatomy examination. You are certain that the instructor will ask you to identify the bones of the skull. What type of answer will this question demand?
   a. Synthesis
   b. Analysis
   c. Recall
   d. Inquiry
   e. Habit

4. You have just completed your first barium enema with your instructor's supervision. Your next step is to complete a written evaluation of your work. What questions will your ask yourself as your write this evaluation?

_____ **5.** How a patient feels about his health care experience is most often the result of
   a. The expense of the procedure
   b. The time of the visit
   c. The knowledge level of the technologists
   d. The communication skills of the health care persons caring for him
   e. The diagnosis

_____ **6.** Miss Myrtle Mulberry has just been informed that she has been accepted into the radiologic technology program at Glucose State University. She is very happy about this; however, she begins to worry about her ability to succeed in this program. She is concerned about her manner of speaking, her ability to help other people, and her appearance. One might say that Ms. Mulberry has
   a. Low self-esteem
   b. A negative self-concept
   c. Depression
   d. A grief reaction
   e. Poor critical thinking skills

7. List the elements of self-concept and explain how a person develops his or her own self-concept.

8. Explain the goal of therapeutic listening.

9. A patient who speaks little English is assigned to you for care. You are not able to communicate in the patient's language. In this situation, if no interpreter is available, how will you plan your communication with this patient?

_____ **10.** Merry Mae is an 83-year-old white female. She has been admitted to the hospital to which you are assigned for your clinical education. Ms. Mae must have a computed tomography scan of the abdomen, and you have been asked to assist with preparing her for this. You approach the patient and greet her. She is silent for a moment and then begins to cry. Your best response to this situation might be
   a. To ignore the fact that she is crying and begin to explain the procedure

b. To take her hand and after a moment say, "You seem to be upset, Ms. Mae. Can you tell me about it?"

c. Approach her and say, "Don't worry, Ms. Mae. Everything will be all right."

d. Leave the patient alone for a few minutes

e. Call for help

_____ **11.** You are interviewing a male patient before placing him on the examining table. He tells you that it is difficult for him to move from a sitting to a standing position. You say, "You feel that you need help to stand?" This therapeutic communication technique is called

a. Exploring

b. Silence

c. Making observations

d. Proving

e. Validating

_____ **12.** The concerns of the radiographer preparing to interview a patient must include

a. Privacy and a quiet environment

b. Ensuring confidentiality

c. Your own personal appearance and professional demeanor

d. Establishment of rapport with the patient

e. All of the above

_____ **13.** As a specialist in your area of health care, radiologic technology, you have patient-teaching responsibilities. These responsibilities include

a. A description of the preparation, purpose, time involved, and equipment used for examinations

b. A description of the adverse reactions possible and the diagnosis made during the examination

c. The toxic effects of the barium and the amount of work involved for the radiographer

d. The risk to the patient, family, and health care team

_____ **14.** The process of grieving, though painful and difficult, is normal and cannot be avoided in the case of a significant personal loss.

a. True

b. False

_____ **15.** Mr. Nathan Nilhouse was diagnosed with cancer 6 weeks ago and told that the disease is incurable. He has decided to seek treatment in another country that promises instant cure with natural herbs. One might conclude that Mr. Nilhouse is in the _____ stage of grieving.

a. Denial

b. Anger

c. Bargaining

d. Acceptance

e. Depression

16. Explain the patient's rights concerning his health care and define Advance Health Care Directive.

_____ **17.** You are the student assisting with the treatment of Mr. George Watson, a patient who has been diagnosed with a terminal illness. During the treatment, he stops breathing. You recall that you saw a note on the front of the Mr. Watson's chart that said DNR. You realize that this means

a. That the emergency resuscitation team must be called

b. That the patient has specified that he does not wish to have cardiopulmonary resuscitation if the question should arise

c. That you should begin cardiopulmonary resuscitation

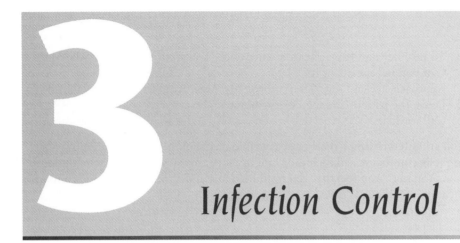

Infection Control

Objectives

After studying this chapter, you will be able to:

1. Define the basic terminology used in the practice of infection control.
2. List and describe the four known microorganisms that may cause infection.
3. List and define the factors that contribute to the process of infection.
4. Describe and demonstrate the methods of controlling infection in health care settings.
5. Discuss the modes of transmission of HIV, hepatitis, and tuberculosis and the methods of preventing their spread in health care settings.
6. List the regulatory agencies that set and maintain the guidelines for safety in health care settings.
7. Define the two tiers of isolation precautions as outlined by the Centers for Disease Control and Prevention (CDC), and describe the precautions required in each tier.
8. Demonstrate the isolation precautions used in each tier of isolation precautions, as required by the CDC.
9. Explain the action you should take if you are exposed to blood or body substances or have a needle-stick injury in the course of your work.

Glossary

Antimicrobial: A type of agent that kills or inhibits the growth or replication of microorganisms

Carrier: A person or animal that harbors and spreads a disease-causing organism without becoming ill

Capsid: The complete virus particle that is structurally intact and infectious

Capsomeres: A subunit of the protein coat or capsid of a virus particle

Ciliate: Of or having cilia; a cell having hairlike projections on its surface

Enteric: Pertaining to the intestines

Exudate: Type of cell fluid or other substance with a high content of cellular material from blood vessels

The AIDS epidemic and the rising threat of tuberculosis and various forms of hepatitis in the United States and throughout the world have forced all health care workers to be more vigilant in the practice of infection control in order to protect themselves and others from acquiring fatal diseases. This makes the practice of infection control measures a necessity for all who are working in, being treated in, or visiting health care settings.

As a radiographer, you must at all times understand the methods of isolating body substances (called Standard Precautions) and correctly perform the required isolation techniques. Correct cleaning of equipment, proper hand washing, and proper disposal of contaminated waste must be part of every procedure in diagnostic imaging to guard against the spread of infection.

Nosocomial Infections

In spite of increasing use of infection control measures, infections in patients while they are receiving health care has increased. Infections acquired in the course of medical care are called *nosocomial infections.* This term is most often applied to infections contracted in an acute care hospital; however, it also applies to infections patients receive while in extended care facilities, outpatient clinics, and behavioral health institutions. Infections contracted at birth by infants of infected mothers are also classified as nosocomial. A nosocomial infection that results from a particular treatment or therapeutic procedure is called an *iatrogenic infection.* Although a patient acquires a particular infection while in a health care unit, he or she

may not develop symptoms of the illness until leaving the health care environment. This is still considered to be a nosocomial infection. A person who enters a health care facility with an infection is said to have a *community-acquired infection.*

Everyone has microorganisms in their bodies at all times. These microorganisms are called normal flora. An infection that is caused by microorganisms that are not normal flora are called *exogenous* nosocomial infections. When a person acquires an infection in the health care setting as a result of an overgrowth of normal flora, it is called an *endogenous* nosocomial infection.

Endogenous infections are often the result of the alteration in the number of normal flora present in the body or the alteration in placement of normal flora into another body cavity. Endogenous infections may also be the result of treatment with a broad-spectrum antimicrobial drug that alters the number of normal flora. Many factors in health care facilities encourage nosocomial infections. Table 3-1 lists these factors.

Factors That Increase the Patient's Potential for Nosocomial Infection

People who present themselves for health care come from many social and economic environments. A variety of factors in the social and economic environment may render a person more susceptible to acquiring a nosocomial infection. Table 3-2 describes some of these factors.

The urinary tract is the most common site of nosocomial infection and is associated with the use of indwelling catheters. Infections in wounds after surgical procedures and respiratory tract infections also occur frequently. Early removal of urinary catheters,

---

TABLE 3-1
Factors That Encourage Nosocomial Infections

FACTOR	REASONS FOR INCREASED INCIDENCE
Environment	Air contaminated with infectious agents; other patients who have infectious diseases; visitors; contaminated food; contaminated instruments; hospital personnel
Therapeutic regimen	Immunosuppressive and cytotoxic drugs used to treat malignant or chronic diseases, which decrease the patient's resistance to infection; antimicrobial therapy, which may alter the normal flora of the body and encourage growth of resistant strains of microbes sometimes called hospital bacteria
Equipment	Instruments such as catheters, intravenous tubing, cannulas, respiratory therapy equipment, and gastrointestinal tubes that have not been adequately cleaned and sterilized
Contamination during medical procedures	Microbes transmitted during dressing changes, catheter insertion, or any invasive procedure may introduce infective microbes if correct technique is not used.

TABLE 3-2 _____

Factors That Increase the Potential for Nosocomial Infection

FACTOR	REASONS FOR SUSCEPTIBILITY
Age	The very young have immature immune systems and are more susceptible to nosocomial infections. Also, as one ages, the immune system becomes less efficient and organ function declines making infections more difficult to resist.
Heredity	Congenital and genetic factors passed on from birth make individuals more or less resistant to disease.
Nutritional status	Inadequate nutritional intake, obesity, or malnourishment as a result of illness render one increasingly susceptible to nosocomial infections.
Stress	Work-related or other stress factors increase potential for infection as levels of cortisone in the body increase related to constant tension.
Inadequate rest and exercise	Efficient elimination and circulation decline as a result of inadequate rest or exercise.
Personal habits	Smoking, excessive use of drugs and alcohol and/or dangerous sexual practices contribute to lowering the body's defenses against nosocomial infections.
Health history	Persons with a history of poor health such as diabetes, heart disease, or chronic lung disease, or children who have not been immunized against diseases of childhood are at increased risk for acquiring a nosocomial infection.
Inadequate defenses	Broken skin; burns or trauma; or immunocompromised persons related to a medical regimen are at increased risk of acquiring a nosocomial infection.

---

intravenous catheters, and other types of invasive treatment devices is recommended whenever possible to reduce the incidence of nosocomial infections.

Microorganisms

Microorganisms do not fit into the plant or animal kingdom; therefore, a third kingdom was formulated by Haickel, named the Protista kingdom. This kingdom includes algae, protozoa, fungi, and bacteria. Algae, fungi, and protozoa have cells with a true nucleus as do all higher animals. These cells are called *eukaryotic or eukaryotes*. Bacteria have a much simpler cell structure and do not have a true nucleus within the cell. They are called *prokaryotes*.

Four major groups of microorganisms are known to produce diseases: bacteria, fungi, viruses, and parasites. If a microorganism is known to produce disease, it is called a *pathogenic microorganism*, or a *pathogen*. There are also believed to be unidentified pathogens that produce newly recognized diseases. Within the known groups of microorganisms, many different species may produce infections in humans, and many are useful or, at least, not harmful. Microorganisms are used in a variety of ways: in food and drug processing to destroy waste and, frequently, as a means of effecting a positive change in the environment.

Some microorganisms that are natural flora in one area of the body produce infection if they are accidentally relocated to a site other than their natural habitat. For example, *Escherichia coli*, which normally inhabits the human intestinal tract, does not cause disease

there; however, if it gains entrance to the urinary bladder, it can cause a urinary tract infection. Often, it is the quantity of microorganisms in an area that produces infection. A small number of a particular bacterium in the body may be harmless; however, if the number increases, it may produce an infection.

Another factor that determines the pathogenicity of a microorganism is its ability to find susceptible body tissue to invade. For example, the skin is a normal habitat for staphylococci; however, if this microorganism enters the lungs, it can cause an infection. Some microorganisms are more virulent than others. This means that some microbes are more certain than others to cause disease if they enter the human body.

The human body houses *resident flora*. This means that there are microbes that live in the body at all times in a quantity that is usually stable. When the quantity of resident flora increases, these flora may become pathogenic. Staphylococci are resident flora on the superficial layers of the skin that in large numbers may cause a serious infection. Resident flora require firm friction and an effective soap and quantities of water to remove from the skin.

Flora that are acquired by contact with an object on which they are present are called *transient flora*. Transient flora are more easily removed from the dermal layers of the skin because they are not firmly adherent. For an infection to occur, the microorganism must be able to survive and multiply in the body of the host, whether the host is human, plant, or animal. Moreover, the microorganism must be able to produce a disease, and the host must be unable to mobilize its defenses against the infectious microbes.

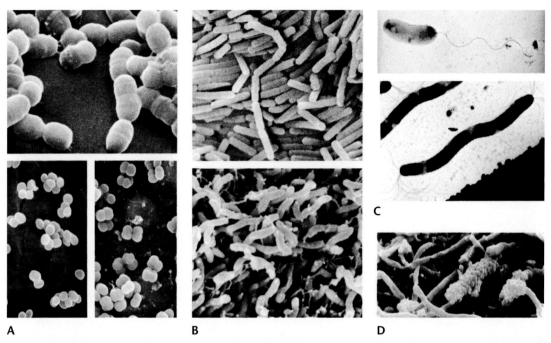

Figure 3–1. Forms of bacteria **(A)** Cocci, *Top: Streptococcus mutans,* demonstrating pairs and short chains. (×9400). *Bottom left:* Single cells and small clusters of Staphylococcus epidermis (×3000). *Bottom right:* Pairs, tetrads, and regular clusters of *Micrococcus luteus* (×3000). **(B)** Bacilli. *Top:* Single cells and short chains of Bacillus cereus (×1700). Bottom: Flagellated bacilli (unnamed) associated with periodontitis (×3700). **(C)** *Top:* A cell of *Vibrio cholerae;* note curved cell and single flagellum (×8470). *Bottom:* The spirillum, *Aquaspirillum bengal;* note polar tufts of flagella (×2870). **(D)** Variety of organisms in dental plaque after 3 days without brushing (×1360). (Volk WA, Benjamin DC, Kadner RJ et al.: *Essentials of Medical Microbiology,* 5th ed. Philadelphia: Lippincott-Raven, 1996)

Bacteria

Bacteria are colorless, minute, one-celled organisms with a typical nucleus. They contain both deoxyribonucleic acid (DNA) and ribonucleic acid (RNA). DNA carries the inherited characteristics of a cell, and RNA constructs cell protein in response to the direction of DNA.

Bacteria are classified according to their shape, which may be spherical (cocci), oblong (bacilli), spiral (spirilla), or pleomorphic (lacking a definitive shape). Short rods are called *coccobacilli.* They may also be classified according to their divisional grouping as diplococci (groups of two), streptococci (chains), or staphylococci (grapelike bunches) (Fig. 3–1).

Bacteria must be stained to be seen under a microscope and are classified according to their reaction to various staining processes in the laboratory. They may be gram-positive, which means that they take the stain; gram-negative, which means that they do not take the stain; or acid-fast, which means that the bacteria are resistant to colorization by acid alcohol. Bacteria may also be classified according to their immunologic or genetic characteristics (Gladwin and Tattler, 2000).

Rickettsias, chlamydias, and mycoplasmas are gramnegative bacteria that are smaller than other bacteria and do not have all of the characteristics of other bacteria. They used to considered viruses because they are too small to be seen under normal microscopic conditions. Rickettsias and chlamydias usually live as parasites inside another cell. Rickettsias are transmitted from animal to animal by the bite of an infected arthropod vector, such as a tick or flea. Typhus and Rocky Mountain spotted fever are caused by rickettsias. Chlamydias are transferred by direct contact between hosts often during sexual contact. They cause infections of the urethra, bladder, or sexual organs of the host. Mycoplasmas may be parasitic or free-living and cause pneumonia and genitourinary infections in humans (Fig. 3–2).

Some forms of bacteria are able to form a protective coat or *spore* when conditions are unfavorable for survival. Bacterial spores are called *endospores.* Endospores encase the genetic material in the cell and may protect it for many years. When conditions for survival are again favorable, the endospore germinates and the bacterial cell again grows and replicates. Endospores are more difficult to destroy than are vegetating bacteria; therefore, many methods of destroying pathogenic bacteria do not affect their endospores (Fig. 3–3).

There are bacteria that survive and thrive only in an oxygen environment. These are called *aerobes.* Others are unable to live in the presence of oxygen and are

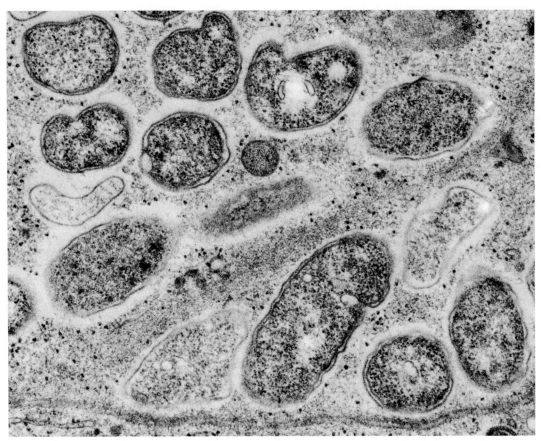

Figure 3–2. *Rickettsia prowazekil* in experimentally infected tick tissue. (Volk WA, Benjamin DC, Kadner RJ et al: *Essentials of Medical Microbiology*, 5th ed. Philadelphia: Lippincott-Raven, 1996.)

called *anaerobes*. Many bacteria are opportunists and learn to adapt or thrive in any condition. They may also learn to live in the presence of antimicrobial drugs or disinfectants.

Diseases caused by bacteria include tuberculosis, streptococcal infections of the throat, staphylococcal infections of many parts of the body, salmonella poisoning, Lyme disease, gonorrhea, syphilis, and tetanus.

Fungi

Fungi are eukaryotic cells that require an aerobic environment to live and reproduce. Fungi exist in two forms—yeasts and molds. Yeasts are one-celled forms of fungi that reproduce by budding. Molds (also called mycelia) form multicellular colonies and reproduce by spore formation.

There is a form of fungi that can grow as either a yeast or a mold, depending on temperature and environment. It is called a *dimorphic fungus*. Another variety of fungi that lives in and utilizes organic matter such as rotting vegetation as a source of its energy is called *saprophytes*.

Yeasts and molds can be harmful and cause a number of infectious diseases. On the other hand, molds are often extremely useful. They are a primary source of material for the production of antibiotic drugs;

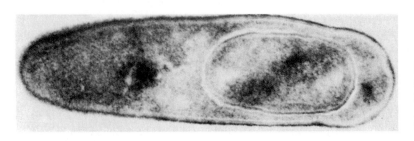

Figure 3–3. A bacillus with a well-defined endospore. (Burton, GW, Englekirk, P: *Microbiology for the Health Sciences,* 6th ed. Baltimore: Lippincott Williams & Wilkins, 2000.)

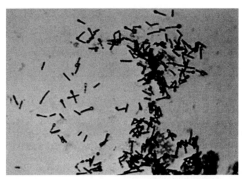

Figure 3–4. Colonies of the yeast, *Candida albicans*, on a blood agar plate. The footlike extensions from the margins of the colonies are typical of this species. (Burton, GW, Englekirk, P: *Microbiology for the Health Sciences*, 6th ed. Baltimore: Lippincott Williams & Wilkins, 2000:6.)

they produce enzymes for medical use and are used in the production of foods to flavor various cheeses. Yeasts are used commercially to produce beer and wine and to leaven bread. They are also a source of vitamins and minerals; however, some yeasts are pathogens that produce diseases in humans and animals. Some commonly seen diseases caused by yeast infection are thrush and meningitis. Diseases caused by dimorphic fungi are blastomycosis and coccidioidomycosis (Fig. 3–4).

Parasites

Parasites are organisms that live on or in other organisms at the expense of the host organ. Parasites may be plant or animal, but animal parasites are those that are pathogenic to humans. A large number of parasites produce disease, and they are roughly classified as *protozoas* and *helminths*.

Protozoa

Protozoa are more complex one-celled microorganisms than those described in the preceding paragraphs. They are often parasitic and are able to move from place to place by pseudopod formation, by the action of flagella, or by cilia.

Pseudopod movement is an amoeboid action in which a part of the cell is pressed forward and the rest of the cell rapidly follows. Flagella are whiplike projections on the protozoa, which move the cell by their swift movements. Cilia are smaller and more delicate hairlike projections on the exterior of the cell wall, which move swiftly and in a synchronous manner to propel the microorganism (Fig. 3–5). Many protozoa are able to form themselves into cysts, which are

protected by a cyst wall in adverse conditions to prolong their existence.

Many of the diseases in humans caused by protozoa affect the gastrointestinal tract, genitourinary tract, and circulatory system. Some of the common protozoal diseases are amebiasis, giardiasis, trichomoniasis, malaria, and toxoplasmosis.

Helminths

Helminths can be simply described as parasitic worms classified as either *Platyhelminthes* (flatworms) or *Aschelminthes* (roundworms). Many of these worms can live in the human intestinal tract for long periods of time if they are not treated.

Some of the more pathogenic types of helminths migrate to the body organs, where they cause serious illness. Although some can be seen with the naked eye, an examination of their eggs is necessary to make a positive identification before initiating treatment. Common diseases caused by helminths are enterobiasis (pinworm), trichinosis, and infection with *Diphyllobothrium latum* (tapeworm) (Fig. 3–6).

Viruses

Viruses are minute microorganisms that cannot be visualized under an ordinary microscope (Fig. 3–7). They are the smallest microorganisms known to produce disease in humans. The genetic material of a virus is either DNA or RNA, but never both. A *virion* is a complete infectious particle with a central nucleoid. The genetic material is protected by a capsid or protein coat that is composed of minute protein units called *capsomeres*. The complete nucleocapsid with a nucleic acid core constitutes a complete virus. Some viruses are surrounded by an envelope that is composed of a lipoprotein. Viruses must invade a host cell in order to survive and reproduce.

Whatever its structure, the virus is transported by way of its capsid to a host cell that has receptor sites on its surface that are suitable to a particular virus, which it invades. A virus does not invade a cell at will. It must attach itself at a membrane receptor site for which it has a specificity; that is, specific for that particular type of host cell and no others.

Once in the cell, production of new viral particles does not take place with certainty. Other factors in the cell environment must be favorable for the multiplication to take place. There are various theories concerning what makes the environment favorable. These include, but are not limited to, poor nutritional status of the host, increased life stress for the host, or excessive use of drugs and alcohol.

To reproduce, the virus uses the genetic machinery of the host cell. When reproduction is complete, new

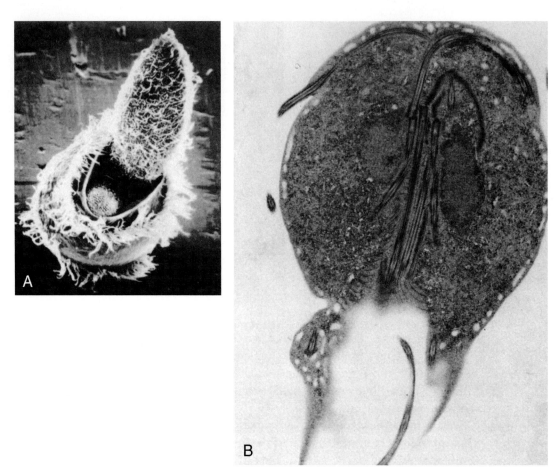

Figure 3–5. Protozoa. (**A**) *Didinium nasutum* with partially ingested prey. (**B**) Longitudinal section of *Giardia lamblia* by transmission electron microscopy. (Burton, GW, Englekirk, P: *Microbiology for the Health Sciences,* 6th ed. Baltimore: Lippincott Williams & Wilkins, 2000.)

viruses leave the original host cell. As some types of viruses leave the host cell, they destroy the cell by the rapid release of new viruses. This is called *lysis*. The second type of viral replication produces viruses that lie dormant, but very much alive and destructive, within the host cell.

Some viruses have the capacity to invade nerve ganglia and leave their genetic material in the ganglia in a

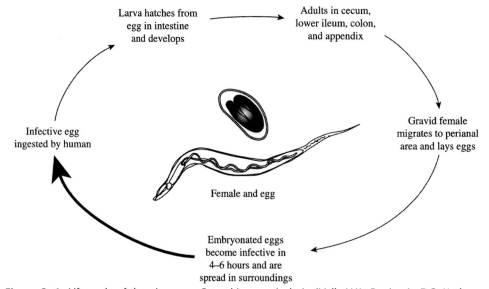

Figure 3–6. Life cycle of the pinworm, *Enterobius vermicularis*. (Volk, WA, Benjamin DC, Kadner RJ et al.: *Essentials of Medical Microbiology,* 5th ed. Philadelphia: Lippincott-Raven, 1996:45.)

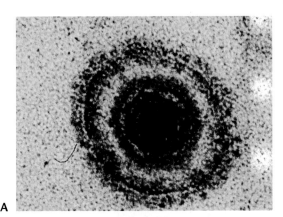 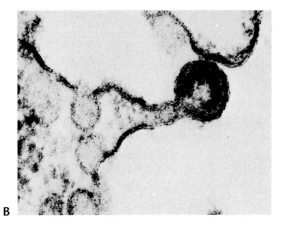

A   B

Figure 3–7. (A) *R*Section through a herpes virus (×330,000) (Rolzman B, Committee on Virology, University of Chicago.) **(B)** A C-type RNA virus budding from an infected cell (×168,000). (Cardamone JJ Jr., and Youngner JS, Department of Microbiology, University of Pittsburgh School of Medicine. In Volk WA, Benjamin DC, Kadner RJ et al.: *Essentials of Medical Microbiology,* 5th ed. Philadelphia: Lippincott-Raven, 1996:45.)

latent phase after an acute infective period. The virus remains there until the body is under some type of stress such as an emotional life event or illness or until it is exposed to sunlight for a period of time. This will often induce the virus to take over nearby cells and produce more viruses, as in the case of herpes simplex (fever blisters). Such viral infections may occur repeatedly.

A virus may be classified on the basis of its genetic composition; the shape or size of the capsid; the number of capsomeres or the absence of an envelope; the host it infects; the type of disease it produces; or its target cell and immune properties.

Viruses are capable of infecting plants, animals, and humans. Some common viral diseases that affect humans are influenza, the common cold, mumps, measles, and hepatitis A, B, C, D, and E. Other increasingly common viral diseases are varicella-zoster and AIDS.

Elements Needed to Transmit Infection

Infection cannot be transmitted unless the following elements are present (Table 3-3):

1. *An infectious agent, which may be a bacterium, a fungus, a virus, or a parasite.* Infectious agents vary in their ability to cause disease. These characteristics are pathogenicity, virulence, invasiveness, and specificity.

   Pathogenicity refers to the causative organism's ability to cause disease.

   Virulence refers to the causative organism's ability to grow and multiply with speed.

   Invasiveness is the term used to describe the organism's ability to enter tissues.

   Specificity characterizes the organism's attraction to a particular host.

2. *A reservoir or an environment in which the pathogenic microbes can live and multiply.* The reservoir can be a human being, an animal, a plant, water, food, earth, or any combination of organic materials that support the life of a particular pathogen.

3. *A portal from which to exit the reservoir.* In the case of a human reservoir, the portals of exit might be the nose, mouth, urinary tract, intestines, or an open wound from which blood or purulent exudate can escape. There can be more than one portal of exit.

4. *A means of transmission.* Infection is transmitted by direct or indirect contact, by droplet, by vehicle,

---

TABLE 3-3

Elements Needed to Transmit Infection

1. An infectious agent
2. An environment in which the pathogenic microbes can live and multiply
3. A portal of exit from the reservoir
4. A means of transmission
5. A portal of entry into a new host

by vector, or by airborne route. Contact is direct when a person or an animal with a disease or his blood or body fluids are touched. This contact can be by touching with the hands, by kissing, or by sexual intercourse.

Indirect contact is defined as the transfer of pathogenic microbes by touching objects (called *fomites*) that have been contaminated by an infected person. These objects include dressings, instruments, clothing, dishes, or anything containing live infectious microorganisms.

Droplet contact involves contact with infectious secretions that come from the conjunctiva, nose, or mouth of a host or disease carrier as the person coughs, sneezes, or talks. Droplets can travel from approximately 3 to 5 feet and should not be equated with the airborne route of transmission, which is described later.

Vehicles may also transport infection. Vehicle route of transmission includes food, water, drugs, or blood contaminated with infectious microorganisms.

The *airborne route* of transmission indicates that residue from evaporated droplets of diseased microorganisms are suspended in air for long periods of time. This residue is infectious if inhaled by a susceptible host.

Vectors are insect or animal carriers of disease. They deposit the diseased microbes by stinging or biting the human host.

5. *A portal of entry into a new host.* Entry of a pathogenic microorganisms into a new host can be by ingestion, by inhalation, by injection, across mucous membranes, or, in the case of a pregnant woman, across the placenta.

A human host can be any susceptible person. Persons particularly susceptible to infection are those who are poorly nourished or are fatigued. Those at greater risk are persons with chronic diseases such as diabetes mellitus or cancer.

Socioeconomic status and culture also play a role in host susceptibility. Persons living in poor environments are more likely to contact some diseases owing to poor hygienic conditions and the poor diets that they are forced to endure. Some diseases have a strong hereditary aspect, which makes them more likely to occur in particular races or families who are genetic carriers of the disease.

The Body's Defense Against Disease

The human body has both specific and nonspecific methods of warding off contamination and infection. As a radiographer, you must be aware of these defenses because this knowledge will play a role in your professional work and your personal life. These defenses may be divided into three categories or lines of defense.

The First Line of Defense

The first line of defense against disease is nonspecific and not selective when dealing with foreign material that enters the body. It is usually a protein or a microbe that attempts to invade the body through a break in the skin or by penetrating a vulnerable body organ.

The skin, hair, ciliated mucous membranes in the upper respiratory tract, and the acidic mucoid linings of body organs all react to any foreign substance or microbe to prevent infection from beginning. The composition and flowing action of urine prevents urinary tract infections. Lysosome in human tears protects the eyes against infection.

In the gastrointestinal tract, the acidic condition of the stomach and intestines, pancreatic enzymes, bile, and normal bacterial flora inhibit infection. Peristaltic action mechanically empties pathogenic microorganisms from the intestines.

There are also inborn traits in humans that protect us from diseases. Some of these are specific to particular races and are called *species resistant*. An example might be human resistance to diseases that affect animals in some regions of the world.

There are microorganisms that live on and in all parts of the human body. These are called indigenous microflora, which prevent colonization of a particular site by foreign flora. These microbes utilize the various nutrients at their site of residence and also produce substances called *bacteriocins*, which discourage foreign invaders.

When a person has had excessive or prolonged use of broad-spectrum antimicrobial drugs, the indigenous flora are reduced in number, and pathogenic microorganisms are free to replicate indiscriminately. An overgrowth of pathogenic microorganisms is called a *superinfection. Candida albicans* in the vagina or *Clostridium difficile* in the colon are examples of superinfections.

The Second Line of Defense

If the body is unable to ward off invading microbes initially, the second line of defense—an inflammatory reaction—begins at the site of injury. This process includes cellular secretion of interferon, prostaglandins, and histamine. It is followed by the activation of serum proteins, chemical changes, and phagocytosis. Phagocytosis is a process in which invading particles are surrounded and ingested by particular white blood cells. The toxic particles are then neutralized, debris is disposed of, and the damage to the cell is repaired.

If the invasion becomes systemic (involving the entire body), the body reacts by producing a fever to assist in destroying the invading microbe; the number of white cells increases (leukocytosis); the infected person develops generalized malaise, enlarged lymph nodes, and often nausea and vomiting.

When the infection is viral, a substance called interferon is produced. Interferons are specific to one host species. That is, interferon produced by one species is not effective in another; however, it is not specific to a particular virus in the infected host. When a virus infects a cell, interferon in secreted in small amounts and leads to the formation of enzymes that produce antiviral activity.

Interferon can now be produced in laboratories for clinical use. Its clinical uses are still in the experimental phase, but interferon is known to be effective against some herpes infections and chronic hepatitis B. Its use in the treatment of cancer and AIDS is still in the trial phase but shows promise as a chemotherapeutic agent.

The Third Line of Defense

The human body has a highly complex immune system that reacts to specific invaders that are able to bypass the nonspecific body defenses by forming antigens. Antigens are foreign or unrecognizable organic substances that invade the body and induce it to produce antibodies. An antibody is a protein substance produced by a particular white blood cell, the lymphocyte or, more specifically, the B cell. B cells work with other lymphocytes called T cells, macrophages, and neutrophils. Together, the components of this highly complex system attempt to destroy invading antigens. All antibodies are immunoglobulins (Ig), but not all immunoglobulins are antibodies. Antibodies in the bloodstream and in other body systems react against specific antigens to produce an immunity to further infection by that particular antigen.

Antibodies are also found in human tears, saliva, and colostrum. Colostrum is the fluid initially secreted by the mammary glands of a new mother. If given to the infant during breast feeding, it protects the infant, because the infant's body is not capable of producing antibodies for itself.

There are several types of immunity and various methods of acquiring immunity, as described in Table 3-4.

Vaccines are administered to produce artificial immunity to a number of diseases that have been extremely pathogenic in times past. These may be made from living or dead (inactivated) microorganisms. If made from living microbes, the pathogenic microbe is rendered less pathogenic and is called an attenuated vaccine. A third type of vaccine called a toxoid is made from inactivated, nontoxic exotoxin of a pathogenic microbe. Diphtheria and tetanus are immunized against with a toxoid.

TABLE 3-4
Methods of Acquiring Immunity

TYPE OF IMMUNITY	HOW ACQUIRED
Acquired immunity	Results from active production or receipt of antibodies.
Active acquired immunity	Antibodies actually produced within a person's body; usually a long-term immunity.
Passive acquired immunity	Antibodies are received from another person or an animal; usually short-term immunity.
Natural active acquired immunity	Antibodies acquired by actually having a particular disease; re-infection may be short or long-term.
Artificial active acquired immunity	Antibodies formed by vaccination that enable one to form antibodies against that particular pathogen.
Passive acquired immunity	Antibodies formed in one individual are transferred to another to protect against infection.
Natural acquired immunity	Antibodies present in a mother's blood or colostrum are passed on to the infant to protect him temporarily from some infections.
Artificial passive acquired immunity	Antibodies are transferred from an immune individual to a susceptible individual to give temporary immunity. This is usually done by administering hyperimmune serum globulin or immune serum globulin (ISG) from the blood of many immune persons.

TABLE 3-5
The Process of Infection

STAGE	PROCESS
Incubation stage	The pathogen enters the body and may lie dormant for a short period, then begins to produce nonspecific symptoms of disease.
Prodromal stage	More specific symptoms of the particular disease are exhibited. The microorganisms increase, and the disease becomes highly infectious.
Full disease stage	The disease reaches its fullest extent or, in some cases, produces only vague, subclinical symptoms; however, the disease continues to be highly infectious.
Convalescent stage	The symptoms diminish and eventually disappear. Some diseases disappear, but the microbe that caused the disease goes into a latent phase. Examples of these diseases are malaria, tuberculosis, and herpes infections.

Occasionally, antibodies function as antigens and produce diseases called *autoimmune diseases*. This occurs when substances identical with one's own tissues stimulate antibody production, and these substances react with the host's tissues in an adverse manner. In other words, one's own antibodies destroy healthy tissue. Some diseases believed to be autoimmune diseases are rheumatoid arthritis, systemic lupus erythematosus, and multiple sclerosis.

The Process of Infection

Infection invades the body in a progressive manner, that is, "in stages." Although some diseases are considered to be infectious (contagious or communicable) during only one or two of their stages, in your practice you should deal with all diseases as if they are highly infectious at all stages, since it is difficult to be certain of the period of infectivity. Table 3-5 outlines the process of infection.

Hereditary Diseases

Some diseases are the result of alterations in a person's genetic makeup, which are inherited from his or her parents or grandparents. The environment may also play a role in influencing the course of these diseases. They may result from aberrations in chromosomal makeup, monogenic (Mendelian) alterations, or other multifactorial errors as the fetus develops. Monogenic disorders are defined as a mutation of one gene that produces disease. It is not possible in this text to fully discuss these problems; however, you must be aware that such problems are seen relatively often and are diagnosed as hemophilia, rheumatoid arthritis, diabetes mellitus, and congenital heart anomalies.

Immune Deficiency

A person whose body does not adequately defend itself against disease is said to be *immunodepressed* or *immunocompromised*. This condition may be present at birth, may be the result of malnutrition, or may be the result of medical treatment, disease, injury, or an unknown cause later in life. An immunocompromised person is unable to neutralize, destroy, or eliminate invading antigens from his or her body systems. These conditions are often chronic and untreatable. Immune deficiency results in frequent, sometimes life-threatening infections. HIV, which causes AIDS, is an example of an infection that can have disastrous consequences for the body's immune system.

HIV *and* AIDS

Because HIV and AIDS are critical health conditions that have a huge impact on health care workers, it is necessary you as a radiographer to understand the underlying disease process. HIV usually results in AIDS, a disease that is currently incurable and has a high mortality rate. Before it was understood how the spread of HIV could be controlled, health care workers were insecure and, in some cases, frightened when caring for persons known to be infected with HIV or who had symptoms of AIDS. They were also concerned when caring for potential HIV-positive carriers who had not yet been identified as being infected with this virus.

HIV is a retrovirus. This means that it converts its viral material from RNA to DNA after it penetrates the host cell. Retroviruses have an enzyme complex called *reverse transcriptinase*, which boosts their ability to replicate and destroy the host cell. After the host cell has been destroyed, the viruses leave and infect other cells. As retroviruses in the bloodstream increase in number, they begin to destroy the cells of the immune system. The infected cells (T4 cells) malfunction and cause the entire immune system to lose its ability to protect the body from infection.

There are two subtypes of HIV: HIV-1 and HIV-2. HIV-2 is related to the HIV virus and causes a disease similar, but slightly less virulent, than AIDS. HIV-2 is found in western Africa.

Phases of HIV Infection

HIV enters the body after exposure through contact with the blood or body fluids of an HIV-positive person and begins an assault on the human immune system. The process of infection is divided into five phases and not until the fifth phase is the person diagnosed as having AIDS. The Centers for Disease Control and Prevention (CDC) has established criteria for reporting persons with AIDS based on a uniformity of symptoms. The five phases are as follows:

Phase 1: HIV enters the body and replicates in the bloodstream. No signs of infection are physically present or present in the laboratory tests; however, HIV can be transmitted during this phase.

Phase 2: There is a period of illness with flu-like symptoms; lymph nodes may enlarge, and fever, a skin rash and malaise may be present. Symptoms may be somewhat more severe with a stiff neck and seizures present. HIV diagnosis may be possible at this time, but the symptoms may be mild and ignored. The infected person may continue to transmit HIV during this time.

Phase 3: No external symptoms of HIV infection are present on an average of 1 to 10 years. The immune function of the body is declining during this phase, and the T lymphocytes (also called CD4 cells) are decreasing in number.

Phase 4: The HIV-infected person develops persistently enlarged lymph nodes; has low-grade fevers, night sweats, mouth lesions, weight loss, and rashes; fatigues easily; and develops changes in cognition and develops peripheral neuropathy.

Phase 5: The infected person becomes immunosuppressed and meets the criteria for the diagnosis of AIDS as established by the CDC. These criteria include all persons who have a CD4 T-lymphocyte count of less than 200 cells per mm. The infected person suffers from multiple opportunistic viral, protozoal, and bacterial infections and possibly cancer. Eighty to 90 percent of persons with this diagnosis die within 3 years.

An infectious disease commonly seen in persons with AIDS is *Pneumocystis carinii*, a type of pneumonia. Also seen are cytomegalovirus infections, *Candida*, herpes simplex, Kaposi's sarcoma (a malignant tumor of the endothelium), AIDS dementia complex (in which it is believed that nerve cells are directly attacked resulting in dementia), tuberculosis, and many other diseases. Death is usually the result of recurrent opportunistic infections. Malignant diseases may also be the cause of death.

Diagnosis and Treatment of HIV-Infected Persons

Confirmation of the presence of HIV is most often made by analyzing the blood for HIV antibodies. The initial test for HIV infection is done to screen for enzyme-linked immunosorbent assay (ELISA). If ELISA is positive, it is repeated on the same blood sample because there are a significant number of false-positive results from this examination. If ELISA is positive a second time, a test called the Western blot test is performed on the same blood sample to confirm the diagnosis and determine the severity of immunosuppression present. Measuring the number of CD4 lymphocytes in the blood is a much more rapid means of making the diagnosis of HIV presence, according to the CDC. A report of fewer than 300 CD4 lymphocytes increases a person's risk of opportunistic infections, and a count of 200 or less confirms an AIDS diagnosis.

Treatment of HIV-infected persons has changed and improved over the past few years; however, a vaccine for prevention of infection or a cure for AIDS has not been found. Antiretroviral drugs used in several combinations greatly slows the progression of infection and prolongs an HIV-infected person's life. Protease-inhibiting antiviral drugs are also effective in delaying symptoms. CD4 count and viral burdens in the blood determine when treatment should begin. Some of the current drugs being used in various combinations are zidovudine (ZDV) and lamivudine (3TC) in combination; and zidovudine, lamivudine, and protease inhibitor in combination. Many other combinations are being used or tested for use. The goal of treatment remains the same at present—decreasing the viral load in the bloodstream. The cost of drug therapy for the HIV-infected person is great, and, because of this, persons in developing countries are often deprived of treatment.

A new problem is the increasing laxity of persons in danger of being exposed to HIV because of the success of drug therapy. This has resulted in a new increase in the number of persons acquiring HIV infection. Education in the methods of prevention of the populations throughout the world who are not infected with HIV and the education of the already infected constitute the greatest defense. Those infected with HIV must be instructed regarding the slow progression of the disease, the potential for infecting others, and the need to be treated to retard the disease progression. Education must include the following for all populations:

1. Avoid sexual contact with high-risk persons (prostitutes, persons who have multiple sex partners, and IV drug users).

2. Follow safe sex practices such as use of condoms.

3. Health care workers must always practice Standard Precautions and be cautious in handling needles and other items that may puncture their skin in the workplace.

4. Maintain good nutritional practices.

5. Get adequate amounts of rest and sleep.

Remember that the patient with HIV infection or with AIDS has a right to confidentiality in regard to his or her diagnosis. Maintenance of strict confidentiality is mandatory when caring for persons with a known AIDS diagnosis or with a patient who is known to have an HIV-positive blood test. In some areas of the United States, violation of the patient's right to confidentiality concerning this issue is punishable by fine and, in some cases, imprisonment. The chart of a patient containing information concerning an AIDS diagnosis or HIV-positive test must be kept in a place where it cannot be inspected by anyone other than the persons directly caring for that patient. You must not discuss the diagnosis with anyone other than the patient's immediate caregivers. Patients who are HIV-positive and are not ill feel that their livelihood or status in their family or community are threatened if this confidentiality is violated.

If you or any health care worker is accidentally exposed to HIV while working with a patient diagnosed with HIV or AIDS, you must report the incident to a superior immediately. If you receive a needle-stick or other penetrating injury while working, report the incident and follow the policy of your institution and of the state in which you reside concerning testing to determine the HIV status of the person to whose blood you were exposed.

CALL OUT!

Immediately report to your superior any accidental exposure to HIV or AIDS sustained while working with an infected person!

Viral Hepatitis

Viral hepatitis is an inflammation of the cells of the liver that is initially acute, but, in some cases may render its victims chronic carriers of the disease. It may be caused by five separate RNA viruses: hepatitis A virus (HVA), hepatitis B virus (HVB), hepatitis C virus (HVC), hepatitis D virus (HVD), hepatitis E virus (HVE), and hepatitis G virus (HVG). Other hepatitis viruses may exist, but this has not been proved at this time.

Both hepatitis A and hepatitis E are transmitted by the fecal-oral route; the others are transmitted by blood or body fluid contacts. Hepatitis F and G are still in the research phase, as are GB-A and GB-B, and GB-C. Health care workers most often contract hepatitis B from needle-stick injuries. Persons who share contaminated needles or have multiple sex partners and hemophiliacs are most susceptible to blood-to-blood methods of contracting HVB and HVC.

The onset of viral hepatitis is most often sudden with symptoms ranging from mild to severe. The resolution is most often complete. However, it may have a prolonged course that eventually becomes chronic, or the victim may become a silent carrier of the disease. HVB, HVC, and HVD can cause chronic hepatitis.

The onset of acute viral hepatitis demonstrates flu-like symptoms with a low-grade fever, muscle aches, and fatigue. After 1 or 2 weeks, the patient becomes jaundiced and as the disease progresses, the liver becomes enlarged, and the liver cells die. If the disease does not progress, the inflammation subsides and the liver regenerates. If the inflammatory process continues, the disease may become chronic. Cirrhosis of the liver, a spontaneous relapse, or a severe fulminating hepatitis resulting in rapid cell destruction, no regeneration, and encephalopathy may result. If this occurs, the outcome may be fatal. The disease is communicable during the incubation period and throughout the course of the illness.

Tuberculosis

Tuberculosis is a recurrent, chronic disease caused by the spore-forming *Mycobacterium tuberculosis* bacterium. The disease most commonly affects the lungs, but is capable of infecting any part of the body. With the increasing immigrant population from third-world countries into the United States and the increase of HIV, tuberculosis is increasing in incidence in the United States. It is a communicable disease and must be treated as such by all health care workers.

Pulmonary tuberculosis may be asymptomatic and most often the onset and early states of the disease go unnoticed. Early symptoms of the disease are fatigue, loss of appetite, weight loss, and fever that occurs late in the day. A shallow cough and hemoptysis (coughing up bloody sputum) occur later in the course of the disease. As the disease advances, wheezes, rales, tracheal deviation, and pleuritic chest pain develop. The initial infection may subside as the bacteria are walled off and lie dormant for an indefinite period of time. If the host organism becomes weakened, the disease process may reappear.

Pulmonary tuberculosis is a treatable disease if it is diagnosed and treatment is begun early its course. If left untreated, massive destruction of lung tissue and respiratory failure may result. A number of anti-infective drugs are used to treat pulmonary tuberculosis; unfortunately, there is an increased incidence of drug-resistant bacilli.

You must recognize that tuberculosis consists of infectious, airborne bacilli to which you may be exposed. There are several methods of preventing this disease. Tuberculin testing is required of all health care workers on a yearly basis to detect possible exposure to infected persons. This is a skin test called a PPD test. If there is a positive tuberculin reaction, a chest x-ray is done. If there is an indication of need, a 1-year course of isoniazid is instituted as prophylaxis.

Anthrax

There is an emerging crisis focusing around the disease, anthrax. This disease is caused by *Bacillus anthracis*, a gram-positive bacterium. "Anthrax is usually a disease of domestic and wild plant-eating animals such as cattle, goats, sheep, swine, buffalo, and deer" (Ingram and Ingram, 2000). It can be contracted by humans and once systemic clinical symptoms appear, it is often fatal. The bacteria that cause anthrax produce endospores that are extremely difficult to eradicate and may last in the soil for as long as 40 years. The disease demonstrates in three clinical forms in humans.

The most common form is cutaneous anthrax (Fig. 3–8). The bacteria enter through a break in the skin, which begins with a blister that later develops into a blackened ulcer. If the bacteria do not invade the bloodstream, the ulcer heals and the infection ends; however, if the infection becomes systemic, it is difficult to control and is often fatal.

The second form of anthrax contracted by humans results from inhaled anthrax spores and demonstrates initially as a mild respiratory infection. It rapidly escalates into a generalized septicemia and is often fatal.

The third and most rare human form of this disease results from eating the flesh of infected animals. This is a gastrointestinal infection and is also often fatal.

Control of anthrax is accomplished by immunizing animals for the disease or destroying infected animals. It is currently being spread in the United States and other countries by terrorists who are sending anthrax spores through the mail to unsuspecting persons. If exposure to anthrax or its spores is recognized, it can usually be controlled by a lengthy course of prophylactic anti-infective drugs. Once symptoms of the disease demonstrate, it is difficult to cure. Anthrax cannot be transmitted from person to person. It is contracted only by direct exposure to the spores.

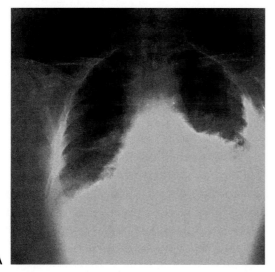

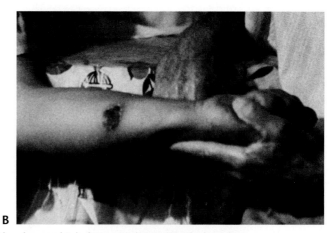

A B

Figure 3–8. (A) Chest X-ray of patient with advanced inhalation anthrax. **(B)** Black eschar on forearm of patient with cutaneous anthrax. (From Coleman, Elizabeth Ann, coordinated by Kearney, K. from *American Journal of Nursing,* December 101[12]: 48-49, 2001.)

DISPLAY 3–1

Institutions that Control Safety of Patients, Workers, and the General Public

The Joint Commission on Accreditation of Health Care Organizations (JCAHO): Sets requirements for hospital safety, infection-control practices and patient care standards (Quality Assurance, QA) that must be met *if the institution or agency is to receive accreditation*

The Occupational Safety and Health Administration (OSHA): A federal agency that protects workers and students from work-related injuries and illnesses; inspects work sites; makes and enforces regulations concerning workplace safety

Centers for Disease Control and Prevention (CDC): Performs research and compiles statistical data concerning infectious diseases; develops immunization guidelines and administers OSHA and OSHA's research institute, the National Institute of Occupational Safety Health (NIOSH)

United States Public Health Service: Investigates and controls communicable diseases and controls carriers of communicable diseases from foreign countries;

prevents spread of endemic diseases; and controls manufacture and sale of biologic products

Food and Drug Administration (FDA): The United States Public Health Service branch responsible for protecting the public from false drug claims and regulates the manufacture and sale of medications. Requires pre-clinical tests for toxicity of new drugs on animals and the testing of medications clinically on humans in three phases before marketing

World Health Organization (WHO): Works under the auspices of the United Nations to reduce famine and disease throughout the world. Compiles information concerning infectious diseases from all countries and compiles this information into reports for every country

United Nations Children's Fund (UNICEF): Helps children, especially children in developing countries to avoid malnutrition and disease; also assists with educational programs for deprived children

---

Agencies Controlling Institutional, Patient, and Workplace Safety

There are international, federal, state, and local agencies that control safe practices for the general public and for all accredited health care institutions, including the various extended care facilities. As health care in the United States changes, more emphasis is being placed on transferring patients from acute care institutions to extended care facilities and into their own homes for care as soon as it is safe to do so. This increases the burden of overseeing the safety of both the patient and the health care worker. Agencies now being overseen by some or all of the regulatory agencies are acute care hospitals; skilled and intermediate care nursing facilities; inpatient rehabilitation centers; inpatient chemical dependency centers; inpatient mental health; and home health agencies. Display 3-1 lists the agencies that control institutional, patient, and workplace safety in the United States and throughout the world.

Infection Control Practices in Health Care Settings

Controlling infection or breaking the cycle of infection is the duty of all health care workers. Medical aseptic practices and use of universal blood and body

fluid precautions must become routine for the radiographer.

People who are ill are particularly susceptible to infection. It is your duty as a radiographer to practice strict medical asepsis at all times in your work. There is a difference between medical asepsis and surgical asepsis. *Medical asepsis* means that insofar as possible, microorganisms have been eliminated through the use of soap, water, friction, and various chemical disinfectants. *Surgical asepsis* means that microorganisms and their spores have been completely destroyed by means of heat or by a chemical process. It is not practical or necessary to practice surgical asepsis at all times, but you must always adhere to the practice of strict medical asepsis.

Most health care institutions now require all students and staff involved in patient care to be immunized or to show proof of immunization—to hepatitis B, rubella, rubeola, poliomyelitis, diphtheria, and tuberculosis. Some institutions require varicella titers for health care workers.

Dress in the Workplace

Fingernails must be short. Shoes must have closed, hard toes. Jewelry, such as rings with stones, and cracked or chipped nail polish harbor microorganisms that are difficult to remove. You should not be wearing these items when involved in patient care. A plain wedding band and a wristwatch are the only pieces of jewelry that are acceptable for the health care worker to wear in the patient care setting.

CALL OUT!

Acrylic fingernails must not be worn in the workplace. They often harbor infectious microorganisms!

Always wear freshly laundered, washable clothing when working with patients. Uniforms are recommended because they will not be worn for other purposes. Short sleeves are recommended because cuffs of uniforms are easily contaminated. If you wear a laboratory coat to protect your clothing, button or zip it closed and remove it when you are not in the work area.

Laboratory coats and uniforms must be washed daily with hot water and detergent. A chlorine bleach is recommended for clothes that have become heavily contaminated.

You should wear a protective gown when working with any patient who may soil your clothing or if it is possible that blood or body fluids will contaminate clothing. On some occasions, you may need to wear a moisture-proof apron along with a gown. (Gowns for isolation patients are discussed later in this chapter.)

Hair

Hair follicles and filaments also harbor microorganisms. Hair is a major source of staphylococcal contamination. For these reasons, wear your hair short or in a style that keeps it up and away from your clothing and the patient. Hair should be shampooed frequently.

Hand Washing

Microbes are most commonly spread from one person to another by human hands. It follows that the best means of preventing the spread of microorganisms is hand washing. Correct hand-washing procedure before and after handling supplies used for patient care and before and after each patient contact is required, even if gloves have been worn for the procedure. Treat all blood and body substances as if they contain disease-producing microorganisms and dispose of them correctly. Then wash your hands. Cover any exposed break in your skin with a waterproof protective covering. If you have an open or weeping wound, you must not work with patients until it has healed.

You should follow a specific hand-washing technique that is accepted as medically aseptic when working with patients (Fig. 3–9). This technique must not be confused with the surgical scrub procedure described later in this text. The medically aseptic hand-washing procedure is as follows:

1. Approach the sink. Do not lean against the sink or allow your clothing to touch the sink because it is considered to be contaminated. Remove any jewelry except for a wedding band.

2. Turn on the tap. A sink with foot or knee control is most desirable but is not always available. If the faucet is turned on by hand, use a paper towel to touch the handles, then discard the towel.

3. Regulate the water to a comfortable warm temperature.

4. Regulate the flow of water so that it does not splash from the sink to your clothing.

5. During the entire procedure, keep hands and forearms lower than your elbows. The water will drain by gravity from the area of least contamination to the area of greatest contamination.

6. Wet your hands and soap them well. An antibacterial liquid soap is the most convenient. If you use a bar of soap, hold it during the entire procedure and rinse it before replacing it in the soap dish. If you replace the soap bar during the procedure and then reuse it, you will contaminate your hands.

7. With a firm, circular, scrubbing motion, wash your palms, the backs of your hands, each finger, between the fingers, and finally your knuckles. Fifteen seconds should be the minimum time allotted for this.

8. Rinse hands well under running water. If your hands have been heavily contaminated, repeat steps 6, 7, and 8.

9. Clean fingernails with a brush or an orange stick carefully once each day before beginning work and again if your hands become heavily contaminated. Scrubbing heavily contaminated nails with a brush is recommended.

10. Rinse your fingers well under running water.

11. Repeat washing procedure as described above after cleaning nails.

12. If you use a bar of soap, rinse the soap well and replace it in the dish. Do not touch the sink or the soap dish.

13. Turn off the water. If the handles are hand-operated, use a paper towel to turn them off to avoid contaminating your hands.

14. Dry your arms and hands using as many paper towels as necessary to do the job well.

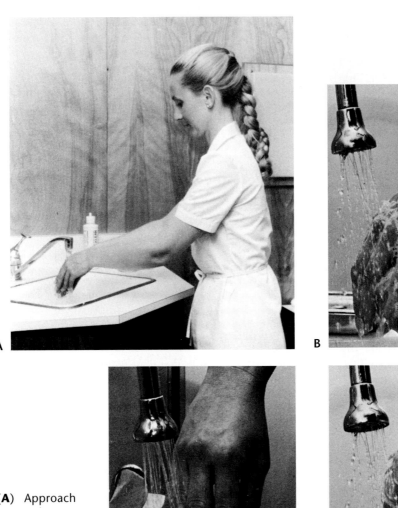

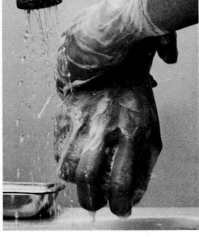

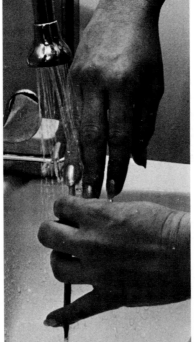

Figure 3–9. (**A**) Approach the sink and turn on the tap. Do not allow your uniform to touch the sink. (**B**) Clean your hands and knuckles and the areas between your fingers with a firm, rubbing motion. Continue to hold the soap while doing this. (**C**) Clean your fingernails with running water to flush away dirt and microorganisms. (**D**) Clean your wrists and forearms with a firm, circular motion, then drop the soap into the soap dish.

15. Use lotion on your hands and forearms frequently. It helps to keep the skin from cracking and thereby prevents infection.

Perform the foregoing procedure at the beginning of each workday, when in contact with a patient's blood or body substances, when preparing for invasive procedures, before touching patients at greatest risk for infection, and after caring for patients with known communicable diseases. This is the case even if gloves are worn. A 15-second hand washing should precede and follow each patient contact.

Standard Precautions (Tier 1)

In 1996, the CDC published revised guidelines for infection control for all persons working in health care settings. A two-tier system was established to be applied as prescribed for patients with particular diagnoses. The first tier is called Standard Precautions and is to be used at all times when you or any health care worker is caring for a patient. The second tier is to be used when called for (see next section).

The threat of infection with HIV, hepatitis B, C, D, E, or tuberculosis was the impetus for establishing these guidelines. Use of Standard Precautions in all patient care relieves the health care worker of the unnecessary burden and the unreliable result of trying to differentiate persons infected with an infectious disease from those who are not. Standard Precautions are effective because they are based on the assumption that every patient has the potential for having an infectious disease. Strict adherence to these principles greatly reduces the threat of infection.

The Occupational & Health Safety Administration (OSHA) amended federal regulations concerning infection control in the workplace. OSHA states that all workplaces in which employees may be exposed to human blood or body substances shall formulate a plan to control employee exposure to pathogenic microorganisms borne by these substances. This plan was to be implemented in all affected workplaces by Spring of 1992. These precautions must be followed at all times. The regulations required of all employers are as follows.

1. An infection control policy conforming to OSHA guidelines must be developed. This policy must specify when personal protective equipment (PPE) is required and how to clean spills of blood or body substances, how to transport specimens to the laboratory, and how to dispose of infectious waste.

2. All staff must be instructed in the application of these policies.

3. Hepatitis B immunizations are to be provided to staff who might be exposed to blood or body substances free of charge.

4. Follow-up care must be provided to any staff member accidentally exposed to splashes of blood or body fluids or to needle-stick injuries.

5. Personal protective equipment must be readily accessible to any staff member who needs it.

6. Impermeable, puncture-proof containers that are disposable must be provided for all used needles, syringes, and other sharps; they must be changed frequently or when full (Fig. 3–10).

7. All health care workers without exception are obliged to follow Standard Precautions and Tier

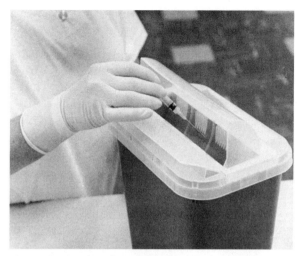

Figure 3–10. Placed used needle uncapped into a puncture-resistant container.

2 precautions as indicated. If an employee or the institution in which he or she is employed is remiss in this practice, legal action should be taken to enforce these rules.

8. Body substance isolation procedures define body fluids and substances as infectious (National Safety Council, 1993). Body substances and fluids that may be infectious include vaginal secretions, breast milk, cerebrospinal fluid, synovial fluid, pleural fluid, peritoneal fluid, pericardial fluid, and amniotic fluid. Urine, feces, nasal secretions, tears, saliva, sputum, and any purulent or nonpurulent drainage from wounds are also considered potentially infectious.

CALL OUT!

If a needle-stick or sharps injury occurs, report the incident immediately and follow the procedure dictated to repair the injury according to institutional policy as quickly as possible.

Additional Infection Control Considerations

Items to be reused must be placed in designated puncture-resistant containers for transport to the area designated for cleaning and disinfecting. Mouthpieces and resuscitation bags must be kept in all diagnostic imaging examination and treatment rooms so that mouth-to-mouth contact with the patient can be

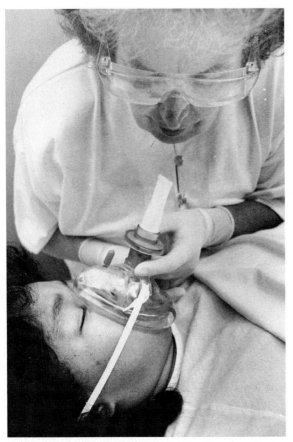

Figure 3–11. Use a protective mask with a mouthpiece to perform cardiopulmonary resuscitation.

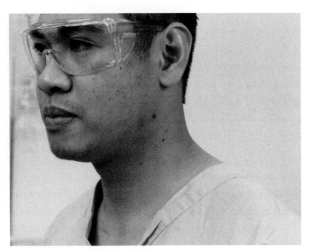

Figure 3–12. Wear goggles to protect your eyes.

avoided in the event of cardiopulmonary resuscitation (Fig. 3–11).

The patient may not be familiar with the requirements dictated for infection control and may feel that you or any other health care worker may be questioning his or her sanitation practices when seeing you wearing gloves and other protective items. Tell the patient about these required precautions, and make the patient understand that these precautions also protect him or her from infection by the health care worker.

Eye Protection

If you are in a patient care situation in which a spattering of blood or body fluids is possible, you must wear goggles to protect your eyes from becoming contaminated. These goggles must have side protectors. If you wear eyeglasses for enhancement of vision, the goggles must fit over the glasses (Fig. 3–12). Keep hands away from your eyes during the course of work so that infection is not introduced into them.

Gloves

Wear disposable, single-use gloves any time you feel that you might touch a patient's blood or body substances in the course of your work. These gloves should be readily available in containers in each treatment room. Since these gloves are to be used for medical aseptic purposes and not for surgically aseptic purposes, you may simply pull them on after hand washing. When they are no longer needed, remove the gloves by use of the following technique to prevent contamination of the radiographer's hands or clothing (Fig. 3–13).

1. With the gloved right hand, take hold of the upper, outside portion of the left glove and pull it off, turning it inside out as you do so (see Fig. 3–13A).

2. Hold the glove that you have just removed in the palm of the remaining gloved hand (see Fig. 3–13B).

3. With the clean, bare index and middle fingers, reach inside the top of the soiled glove and pull it off, turning it inside out and folding the first glove inside it as you do so. Be careful to touch only the inside of the glove (see Fig. 3–13C and D).

4. Drop the soiled gloves into a receptacle for contaminated waste (see Fig. 3–13E).

5. Wash your hands.

CALL OUT!

If exposure to blood or body fluids is possible, wear gloves!

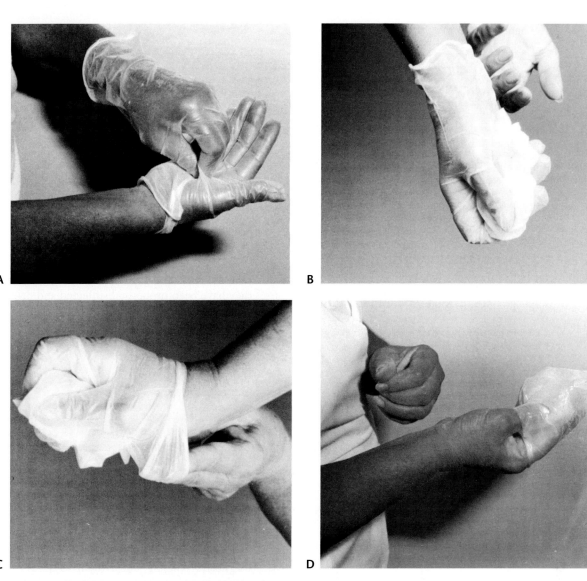

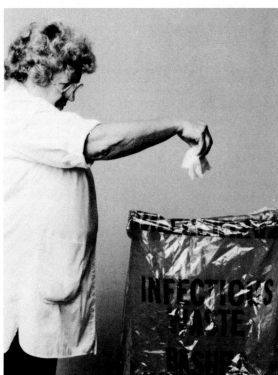

Figure 3–13. (**A**) Pull the first glove off by grasping it on the outside with the other gloved hand. (**B**) Hold the glove that has been removed in the remaining gloved hand. (**C**) With the bare fingers, reach inside the top of the remaining soiled glove and pull it off. (**D**) Turn the glove inside out and encase the other glove inside it. (**E**) Drop the soiled gloves into a designated waste receptacle.

Cleaning and Proper Waste Disposal

Not all disinfectants are equally effective. Before a disinfectant is chosen for the diagnostic imaging department, it should be thoroughly studied by an infection-control consultant. Microorganisms begin to grow in disinfectant solutions left standing day after day. This is also true in liquid-soap containers. If such items are used, they should be changed and cleaned every 24 hours. A more detailed description of disinfection and sterilization methods is presented in Chapter 5. The following are guidelines for the disposal of waste or the cleaning of equipment after each patient use in the diagnostic imaging department.

1. Wear a fresh uniform each day. Do not place your uniform with other clothing in your personal closet. Shoes should be cleaned and stockings should be fresh each day.

2. Pillow coverings should be changed after each use by a patient. Linens used for drapes or blankets for patients should be handled in such a way that they do not raise dust. Dispose of linens after each use by a patient.

3. Flush away the contents of bedpans and urinals promptly unless they are being saved for a diagnostic specimen.

4. Rinse bedpans and urinals and send them to the proper place (usually a central supply area) for resterilization if they are not to be reused by the same patient.

5. Use equipment and supplies for one patient only. After the patient leaves the area, supplies must be destroyed or resterilized before being used again.

6. Keep water and supplies clean and fresh. In the diagnostic imaging department, use paper cups and dispose of them after a single use.

7. Floors are heavily contaminated. If an item to be used for patient care falls to the floor, discard it or send it to the proper department to be recleaned.

8. Avoid raising dust because it carries microorganisms. When cleaning, use a cloth thoroughly moistened with a disinfectant.

9. The radiographic table or other imaging or treatment equipment should be cleaned with a disposable disinfectant towelette or sprayed with disinfectant and wiped clean and dried from top to bottom with paper towels after each patient use.

10. When cleaning an article such as a radiographic table, start with the least soiled area and progress to the most soiled area. This prevents the cleaner areas from becoming more heavily contaminated. Use a good disinfectant cleaning agent and disposable paper cloths.

11. Place dampened or wet items such as dressings and bandages into waterproof bags, and close the bags tightly before discarding them to prevent workers from handling these materials from coming in contact with bodily discharges. Place in contaminated waste containers.

12. Do not reuse rags or mops for cleaning until they have been properly disinfected and dried.

13. Pour liquids to be discarded directly into drains or toilets. Avoid splashing or spilling them on clothing.

14. If in doubt about the cleanliness or sterility of an item, do not use it.

15. When an article that is known to be contaminated with virulent microorganisms is to be sent to a central supply area for cleaning and resterilizing, place it in a sealed, impermeable bag marked "contaminated." If the outside of the bag becomes contaminated while the article is being placed in the bag, place a second bag over it (Fig. 3–14).

16. Always treat needles and syringes used in the diagnostic imaging department as if they are contaminated with virulent microbes. Do not recap needles or touch them after use. Place them immediately (needle first) in a puncture-proof container labeled for this purpose. Do not attempt to bend or break used needles because they may stick or spray you in the process.

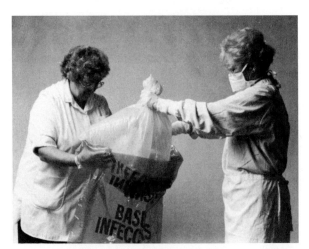

Figure 3–14. Place contaminated bag into a second bag that is not contaminated.

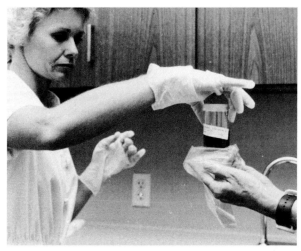

Figure 3–15. Specimens must be sent to the laboratory in a clean container and then encased in an outer bag.

17. Place specimens to be sent to the laboratory in solid containers with secure caps. If the specimen is from a patient with a known communicable disease, label the outside of the container as such. Avoid contaminating the outside of the container, and place the container in a clean bag. If a container becomes contaminated, clean it with a disinfectant before placing it in the bag. Specimens must be sent to the laboratory after collection for examination (Fig. 3–15).

18. Medical charts that accompany patients to the diagnostic imaging department must be kept away from patient care areas to prevent contamination. Keep charts in an area where only those directly involved in patient care may read them.

Disinfection

Disinfection is a term used to describe the removal, by mechanical and chemical processes, of pathogenic microorganisms, but frequently not their spores, from objects or body surfaces. Usually in reference to body surfaces, the term *antisepsis* or *antiseptic* is used rather than disinfect or disinfectant. Items are disinfected when they cannot withstand the process necessary to sterilize them or when it is not practical to sterilize. This is often the case with objects leaving an isolation unit. If an object leaving an examining room or isolation unit has been contaminated, it is cleaned first by vigorous scrubbing (mechanical means) and then disinfected by wiping it with, or soaking it in, a chemical selected by the institution for this purpose.

When a patient enters the diagnostic imaging department and you know or suspect that this patient has a contagious disease, it is your responsibility to prevent the spread of infection. If the patient is coughing and sneezing, you must provide the patient with tissues and a place to dispose of them. Instruct the patient to cough and sneeze into the tissues and then discard them safely. The patient should be removed from a crowded waiting room to prevent infecting other persons. You should put on a gown to protect your uniform. Put on a mask and goggles, if necessary. The patient should be cared for and returned to his or her room or discharged as quickly as possible.

After the patient has been cared for and leaves the imaging department, wash your hands thoroughly and then disinfect the radiographic table and anything in the room that the patient has touched. This can be accomplished with a disinfectant solution. Then remove your gown, goggles, and gloves and scrub your hands again.

Transmission-Based Precautions (Tier 2)

Standard precautions to prevent spread of infection are used daily for all persons cared for in all health care settings. There are particular diseases, or the suspicion of a communicable disease, which require you to take additional precautions to prevent infection of other health care workers, patients, other persons in the health care setting, and yourself. These precautions are presently called *transmission-based precautions* and are designed to place a barrier to the spread of highly infectious diseases between persons with such diseases and the persons caring for them.

It is believed that there are three specific routes or modes of disease transmission, which may differ with each disease. These routes are by air, by droplet, and by contact. Isolation precautions are meant to separate the patient who has a contagious illness from other hospitalized patients and from the health care workers. This separation may be accomplished in a hospital ward or in a private hospital room. The method chosen depends on how the pathogenic microorganism is transmitted and on the reliability of the patient with the disease. If the patient is very young or cannot be relied on to use necessary hygienic practices to control infection, he or she must be placed in a private room. In some institutions, Tier 2 guidelines continue to be referred to as *category-specific* guidelines. If this is the case, there may be a card posted on the patient's door with instructions informing the staff and visitors of the isolation requirements to be observed (Fig. 3–16).

If a disease can be transmitted only by direct contact, the reliable thing may be for the patient to remain in a ward or a room with another patient. If the disease is spread by airborne route, a private room is necessary; however, two patients who have the same disease may share a room. Some diseases may be spread by more than one route, and so more than one method of isolation is required. Following are the transmission-based precautions for the three modes of preventing transmission of infectious diseases.

Airborne Precautions

This method of transmission occurs when microbes are spread on evaporated droplets that remain suspended in air or are carried on dust particles in the air and may be inhaled by persons in that room or air space. In some instances, air currents carry microorganisms, and special air handling and ventilation are required to prevent infectious microbes from circulating. Diseases that are spread by airborne route are tuberculosis, chicken pox, and measles. When diseases require this type of isolation, the following precautions are required.

- A private room, negative air-pressure ventilation, and a mask for most airborne pathogens
- For tuberculosis, a particulate air filter respirator (Fig. 3–17)
- Standard Precautions
- A mask for a patient to be transferred within the hospital

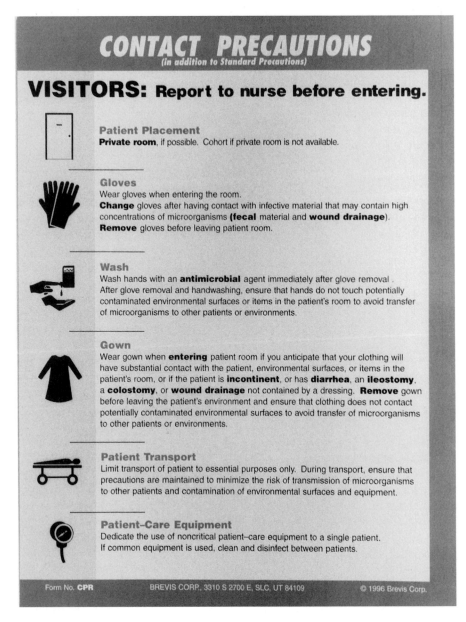

Figure 3–16. Category-specific card.

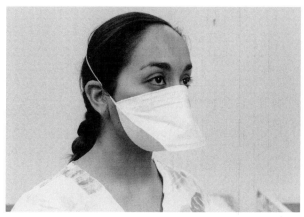

Figure 3–17 Particulate mask is worn for tuberculosis isolation.

Droplet Precautions

Transmission by droplets occurs when droplets contaminated with pathogenic microorganisms are placed in the air from a person infected with a droplet-borne infection. This happens when a patient sneezes, coughs, talks, or deposits infection from his or her eyes, nose, or mouth in other ways, and these droplets are inhaled or internalized in other ways to an uninfected person. Usually, droplets are not spread for more than 3 feet by coughing, sneezing, or talking. Diseases spread by this route are influenza, rubella, most pneumonias, and meningococcal meningitis. The following are requirements for precautions for disease spread by droplet transmission:

- A private room or a room with another person infected with the same disease or a room where the bed of another person is at least 3 feet away from the infected person
- A mask for any procedure that requires less than 3 feet in proximity to the infected patient
- Standard Precautions

Contact Precautions

There are two types of contact spread of infection, *direct contact* and *indirect contact*. Direct contact occurs when a susceptible person actually touches an infected or colonized person's body surface in an area where infectious microbes are present. *Colonization* is defined as the presence of microorganisms on the skin or body surface of an individual who has no symptoms of the disease.

Indirect contact occurs when a susceptible person touches or comes into contact with an object that has been contaminated with infectious microorganisms. These contaminated objects are called *fomites*. A fomite can be a soiled instrument, a used syringe, or

contaminated hands. Diseases transmitted by contact are drug-resistant wound infections; *Shigella* and other gastrointestinal infectious diseases; hepatitis A; herpes simplex; impetigo; scabies; drug-resistant gastrointestinal, respiratory, and skin diseases; and draining abscesses. The following are precautions to prevent disease spread by contact:

- A private room or a room with another person infected with the same disease if the patient cannot be relied on to maintain adequate precautions or is too young to do so
- Gloves to be worn by health care workers before entering the patient's room and removed before leaving it
- Wearing a gown if there is a possibility of touching the patient or items in the room or if the patient is incontinent or has diarrhea, an ileostomy, a colostomy, or a draining wound that does not have a barrier dressing in place
- Standard Precautions
- *Precautions* to minimize disease transmission if the patient is to be transported within the hospital

Protective or Reverse Isolation

Standard Precautions are used for all patients; however, if a patient has a disease that can be transmitted by airborne contact, a private room is recommended. There are specific diseases that also require what is called negative-pressure air flow. This prevents pathogenic microorganisms from flowing out of the isolation room.

In some situations, a patient who is highly susceptible to becoming infected because of a particular treatment or condition, isolation precautions are used to protect the patient from becoming infected. In this case and in some cases in which diseases may be contracted by direct or airborne contact, you must adhere to a strict method of entering and leaving the isolation unit, which encompasses airborne, droplet, and contact precautions. This type of isolation is called *strict isolation* in some institutions and is referred to as such in this section. The procedure for strict isolation techniques follows:

1. Wash hands using the procedure prescribed earlier in this chapter.

2. All items used for patient care are sterilized, disinfected, or disposed of to prevent spread of infection.

3. Bag and label as contaminated all items from isolation rooms before being sending for disinfection.

4. Place all hypodermic needles in labeled, puncture-resistant receptacles used only for this purpose. Do not bend or recap needles after use.

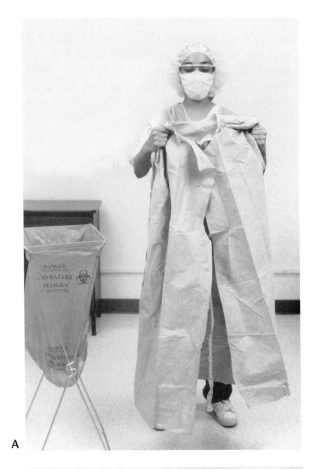

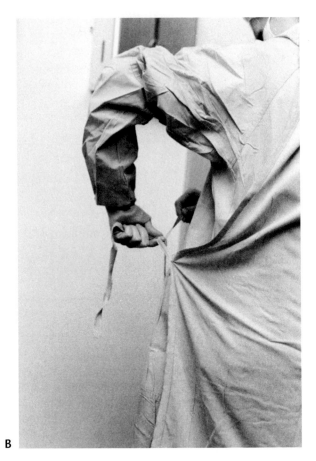

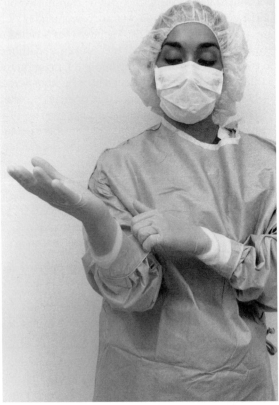

Figure 3–18. (A) Cap must cover hair that touches collar. Goggles and mask and lead apron follow. Then take the gown from the stack and let it unfold in front of you. **(B)** Tie the gown in back and make certain that the back of your uniform is completely covered. **(C)** Make certain that the cuffs of the gloves cover the cuffs of the gown.

To enter and leave a strict isolation unit, you will need the assistance of another radiographer or member of the nursing team who is caring for the patient in the unit. Remember that the patient who is in a strict isolation unit may feel alone and rejected. Such patients are forced to remain in solitude for long periods of time and are often treated by visitors and hospital personnel as if they are undesirable. It is possible to carry out strict isolation procedures and at the same time treat the patient as a human being with dignity and worth. Before beginning your work with the patient, spend a few moments explaining the radiologic procedure. When the procedure is complete, allow a few moments for discussion, and respond in a therapeutic manner to any questions that the patient may have.

When a patient is placed in a strict isolation unit in the hospital setting, a special room is set aside for this purpose. At the entrance to the room there is a sink for hand washing, a stack of paper or cloth gowns, a container for masks and caps, and a box filled with clean, disposable gloves. Many items in the isolation unit that are used for patient care remain in the unit until the patient leaves.

Before entering the isolation room, you must have the portable radiographic machine prepared with as many cassettes on hand as are needed. Make sure the cassettes are covered with protective plastic cases to keep them from becoming contaminated. Also, place extra pairs of clean gloves on the machine before placing it in the patient's room. Have an assistant available and then use the following procedure (Fig. 3–18):

1. Assemble the supplies and equipment you need.

Rationale: Prevents loss of time and reduces risk of breaking isolation procedure.

2. Stop in area where you will put on your protective clothing. Remove any jewelry that you are wearing and pin it into your uniform pocket so it will not be lost.

3. Wash your hands as for medical aseptic practice.

Rationale for steps 2 and 3: Prevent transmission of microorganisms.

4. If your hair touches your collar, you must wear a cap.

Rationale: Hair collects and transmits microorganisms.

5. Remove a mask from the container and put it on, making certain that it your covers mouth and nose tightly. Put on a lead apron (see Fig. 3–18A).

6. Take a gown from the stack. Hold it in front of you and let it unfold. Place your arms into the sleeves and pull it on at the shoulders.

7. Tie the back of the gown, making certain that the gown covers all of your clothing (see Fig. 3–18B).

8. Put gloves on, making certain that the cuffs of the gloves cover the cuffs of the gown (see Fig. 3–18C).

9. Push machine into the room; introduce yourself to the patient, and explain the procedure. Make necessary adjustments to the machine at this time.

Rationale: That patient will have less anxiety if he or she understands what is to occur. It also gives the patient the opportunity to refuse the procedure. Once you have touched the patient, change gloves before touching the machine again.

10. Place the cassette for the exposure (Fig. 3–19).

11. Remove contaminated gloves as described earlier in this chapter, and discard them in a waste receptacle.

12. Put on clean gloves that were placed on the portable machine before entering the room.

Rationale for steps 10, 11, and 12: Once you have touched the patient, your gloves are contaminated. To prevent the machine from being contaminated, change your gloves before touching it.

13. Make the exposure. If additional exposures are necessary, you may need to change gloves again. Place cassettes in contaminated plastic covers at the end of the patient's bed or on a bedside stand.

Rationale: The machine is not to be touched with contaminated gloves or it will be contaminated. The cassettes that have been placed near or against the patient are contaminated and cannot be replaced in the portable machine until the plastic covers are removed.

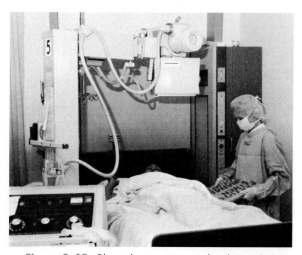

Figure 3–19. **Place the cassette under the patient.**

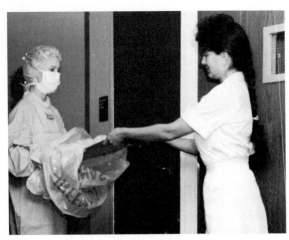

Figure 3–20. Slide the cassette from its covering, and allow the assistant to take it.

14. When radiographic exposures are completed and before you contaminate your gloves by removing the last cassette, push the machine out of the room, and notify your assistant to prepare to receive the cassettes.

15. Take the covered cassette or cassettes to the door of the unit where your assistant is waiting. Slide the plastic covering back from the cassette and allow the assistant to remove it. Discard the contaminated cassette cover in the waste receptacle in the patient's room (Fig. 3–20).

Rationale: Prevents contamination of cassettes that must be taken to another part of the hospital for processing.

16. Return to the patient. Make the patient comfortable. Place the bed in the low (closest to the floor) position, put the side rails up and the call button within the patient's reach.

Rationale: The patient's safety and comfort are the highest priority and must always be every health care worker's first concern.

17. Leave the patient's room, and return to the area prepared to receive your contaminated garments.

To remove contaminated garments:

1. Untie waist ties of gown (Fig. 3–21).

2. Remove your gloves according to the procedure for removing contaminated gloves, and place them in the waste receptacle (Fig. 3–22).

3. Untie top gown ties (Fig. 3–23).

4. Remove the first sleeve of the gown by placing your fingers under the cuff of the sleeve and pulling it over the hand (Fig. 3–24).

5. Remove the other sleeve with your protected hand inside the gown (Fig. 3–25).

6. Slip out of the gown, and hold it forward so that the inside of the gown is facing the outside (Fig. 3–26).

7. Place the gown in the waste container (Fig. 3–27).

8. Remove the cap and mask. Place them in the waste container, and leave the room (Fig. 3–28).

9. Wash your hands as previously described in this chapter.

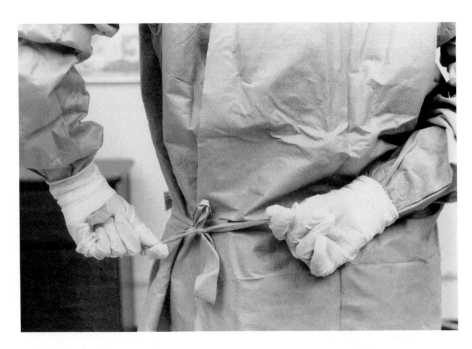

Figure 3–21. Untie lower waist ties of gown.

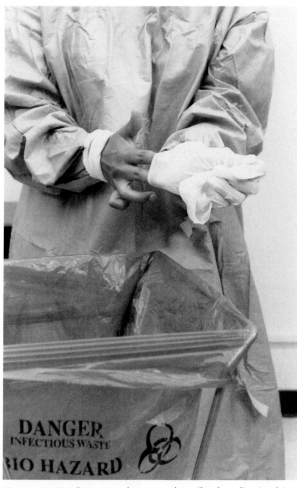

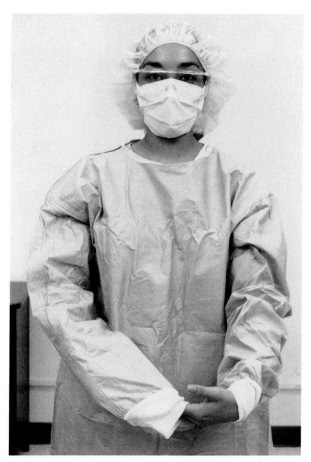

Figure 3–24. Remove the first sleeve.

Figure 3–22. Remove gloves as described earlier in this chapter.

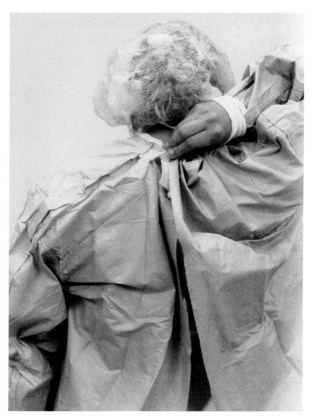

Figure 3–23. Untie top gown ties.

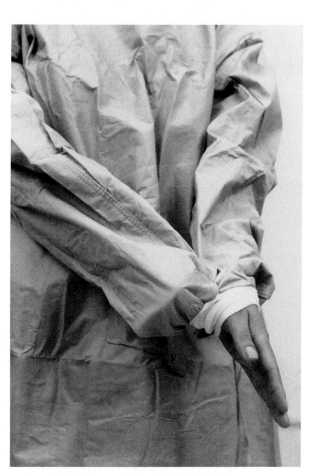

Figure 3–25. Remove the other sleeve.

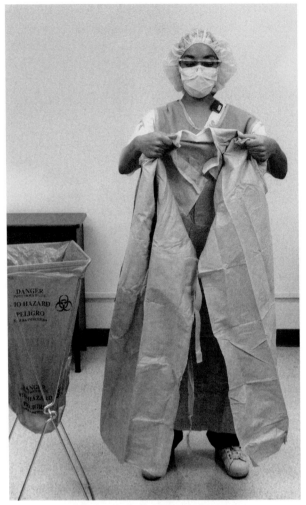

Figure 3–26. Fold the gown forward.

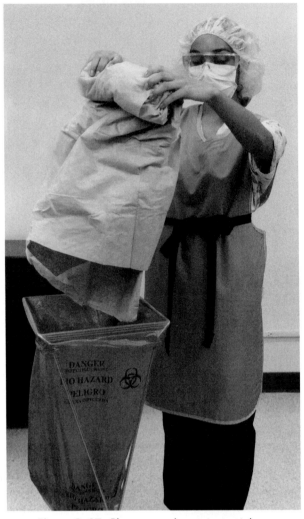

Figure 3–27. Place gown in waste container.

Transferring the Patient with a Communicable Disease

Occasionally, it is necessary for a patient with a communicable disease to come to the diagnostic imaging department for radiographs or treatment. The following precautions must be taken to prevent infecting anyone else and also to prevent contaminating a room or the equipment.

1. The patient must be transported by wheelchair or by gurney. If he or she has a disease that may be transmitted by droplet, airborne, or contact route, place a mask properly on the patient's face and wear a gown and mask to protect yourself. (Patients with tuberculosis must wear special masks as hospital policy directs.)

2. Place a sheet on the gurney or wheelchair, then cover it completely with a cotton blanket. Transfer the patient and wrap a cotton blanket around him or her (Fig. 3–29).

3. When the patient arrives at the destination, open the blanket without touching the inside.

4. Place a protective sheet on the radiographic table, transfer the patient to the table, and place a draw sheet over him or her. Make the necessary exposures. Arrange your work so that the patient does not have to spend more time than is necessary in the department.

5. Return the patient to the wheelchair or gurney. Wrap the cotton blanket around him or her and return the patient to the hospital room.

6. Adjust the bed to the position that is lowest to the floor, put the side rails of the bed up, and give the patient the call button.

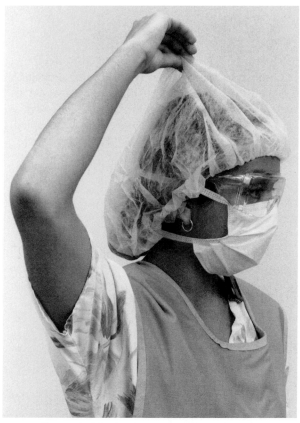

Figure 3–28. Remove your cap and mask.

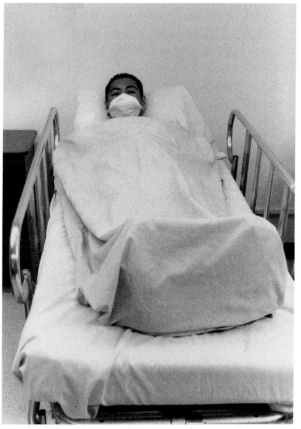

Figure 3–29. Place a particulate mask on a patient who has a disease that is spread by an airborne route.

Summary

Infection control is the obligation of all persons entering a health care facility. This includes hospital personnel, patients, and their visitors. Radiographers must learn the concepts and procedures for infection control, including Standard Precautions, before beginning to work in their chosen specialty area. It is your legal and ethical obligation as a radiographer to practice these procedures in all health care situations to prevent nosocomial infections and the spread of infectious diseases.

Nosocomial infections are caused by four basic types of microorganisms: bacteria, fungi, parasites, and viruses. Various forms of these microbes produce "hospital infections," which are becoming increasingly difficult to control in spite of the body's own elaborate defenses against disease. This may be due to the hospital environment, the patient's therapeutic regimen, or the lowered resistance of the patient to infectious agents.

The elements needed to transmit an infection are a reservoir, or an environment, in which pathogenic microbes can live and multiply; a portal of exit from the reservoir; a means of transmission; and a portal of entry into a new host. It is your duty as a radiographer to adhere strictly in your daily work to infection-control techniques to break the cycle of infection.

The threat of HIV and the disease that it produces, AIDS; the prevalence of HBV in health care institutions; and the increasing resistance of tuberculosis to standard treatments create an increased need for you as a radiographer to practice strict infection-control measures. This can be done by always adhering to Standard Precautions or blood and body substance isolation, by hand washing between each patient care situation, and by correct disposal of waste.

There are federal, state, and local agencies that control the safety of both patients and staff in health care institutions. You must be aware of the duties of each of these agencies and of your obligations to abide by their regulations.

In your personal life, you should maintain a health care regimen that includes adequate rest, a nutritious diet, and meticulous hygienic practices. This will help you to remain healthy and infection-free.

Chapter 3 Test

_____ 1. Jonas Goodstart has been a patient at Happy Valley Community Hospital for 5 days. During his stay in the hospital, he was taken to the diagnostic imaging department several times for diagnostic radiographic procedures. He was cared for each time he went to that department by a radiographer who had a severe upper respiratory infection. Two days after he returned home from the hospital, he also developed a severe upper respiratory infection. It would be appropriate to say that Mr. Goodstart had developed:
   a. An iatrogenic infection
   b. A nosocomial infection
   c. A community-acquired infection
   d. A blood-borne infection

_____ 2. Mary Mandura, an 82-year-old white female, has been hospitalized for several weeks as a result of multiple injuries suffered in an automobile accident. She has been treated with a series of broad-spectrum antibiotics to discourage infection. Ms. Mandura now has severe diarrhea, and the stool culture has produced _Clostridium difficile_. This would be called:
   a. A blood-borne infection
   b. A community-acquired infection
   c. A viral infection
   d. A superinfection

3. Match the following:
   1. The skin, the hair, the acidic condition of the stomach and intestines _____
   2. Antigen-antibody response _____
   3. Acquired immunity _____
   4. The inflammatory response _____
   5. Natural active acquired immunity _____
      a. Active production or receipt of antibodies
      b. The second line of defense against infection
      c. The first line of defense against infection
      d. Antibodies acquired by having a particular disease
      e. The third line of defense against infection

_____ 4. There is currently less reason to be concerned about contracting HIV because there is improved treatment and the disease is no longer fatal.
   a. True
   b. False

_____ 5. Hepatitis B and hepatitis C are blood-borne viral infections. When you are caring for persons known to have either of these diseases, use the following infection control techniques:
   a. Wear gloves if you may come in contact with blood or body substances.
   b. Wear goggles if there is a possibility of your being splashed with blood or body substances.
   c. Wear a particulate mask at all times.
   d. Wear a waterproof gown or apron if there is a possibility that your clothing may be splashed by blood or body substances.
   e. A and B are correct.

6. Explain the differences between Standard Precautions and transmission-based precautions.

_____ **7.** A person who has recently been infected with HIV may have no symptoms of disease but is able to transmit HIV to another person.
   a. True
   b. False

_____ **8.** HIV, or the disease that it produces, is transmitted by direct or indirect contact with infected blood or body substances.
   a. True
   b. False

9. Match the following agencies with their particular function:
   1. Food and Drug Administration _____
   2. Centers for Disease Control and Prevention _____
   3. World Health Organization _____
   4. Joint Commission on Accreditation of Healthcare Organizations (JCAHO) _____
      a. Conducts multicenter studies on diseases and publishes a weekly outline on the statistics of infectious diseases in the United States
      b. Receives data concerning infectious disease from all countries and compiles a report for every country
      c. Regulates the manufacture and sale of medications to protect health of U.S. citizens
      d. Sets requirements for hospital safety and infection control practices

_____ **10.** The radiographer should always dress for the workplace with infection control in mind. This means that
   a. Clothing must be washable; fingernails must be kept short; shoes must be comfortable and have closed toes; and no jewelry is worn except a wristwatch and a wedding band.
   b. The radiographer must look unattractive because anything that looks good spreads infection.
   c. A scrub suit must be worn at all times.
   d. The rules are to be followed when JCAHO is inspecting the institution in which you work.

_____ **11.** Microorganisms that need a host cell to reproduce and are virtually unresponsive to antimicrobial drugs are
   a. Bacteria
   b. Fungi
   c. Protozoa
   d. Viruses

_____ **12.** When a person is in the incubation period of the disease process, the radiographer has no control over its transmission.
   a. True
   b. False

_____ **13.** The radiographer must use strict infection-control measures that include blood and body substance precautions for
   a. Every patient who enters the diagnostic imaging department
   b. Patients who have known communicable diseases
   c. Only patients who have AIDS and hepatitis B
   d. Patients who seem ill

_____ **14.** Blood and body substance precautions include
   a. Use of clean, disposable gloves for sick persons

b. Use of clean, disposable gloves for contact of the hands with blood or body fluids, a mask and goggles if blood or body fluids may spray on your face, and a gown if the blood and body fluids may touch your clothing, for any patient care that may involve contact with blood or body fluids

c. Clean, disposable gloves as necessary

d. Gown, gloves, mask, and goggles for all patient care

_____ **15.** The most common means of spreading infection are
a. Soiled instruments
b. Infected patients
c. Human hands
d. Domestic animals

_____ **16.** The elements needed to produce an infection are a source, a host, and a means of transmission. An example of a source of infection might be
a. A radiography student who has a cold and comes to work
b. A visitor in the hospital who has a "fever blister" on her mouth
c. A patient who develops pneumonia
d. a, b, and c

_____ **17.** A safety precaution that must be taken when disposing of used hypodermic needles and syringes is
a. To place the needles in the waste basket as soon as possible
b. To recap the needle and dispose of it quickly
c. To place the syringe with the uncapped needle attached directly into the contaminated waste receptacle provided for them immediately after use
d. To detach the needle from the syringe and place only the needle in the contaminated waste receptacle

18. Match the following means of transmitting infection with the correct definition:
1. Touching objects that have been contaminated with disease-producing microbes
2. Ingesting contaminated water, food, drugs, or blood
3. Inhaling air contaminated with infectious microbes
4. Contact with secretions transferred by sneezing, coughing, or talking
5. Touching contaminated material with hands
a. Direct contact _____
b. Indirect contact _____
c. Droplet contact _____
d. Vehicle contact _____
e. Airborne contact _____

_____ **19.** When caring for a patient whom you know to be infected with HIV and who does not have AIDS, you use standard blood and body fluid precautions and
a. Share the information with the technologist in the next room who has no contact with the patient
b. Keep all information concerning the patient confidential
c. Keep the patient's chart in a place where it cannot be read by others
d. B and C are correct.

4

Basic Patient Care and Safety in Radiographic Imaging

Objectives

After studying this chapter, you will be able to:

1. Give clear verbal instructions to an ambulatory patient concerning the correct manner of dressing and undressing for a radiographic imaging procedure.

2. Correctly assess a patient's need for assistance to complete a radiographic procedure safely.

3. Demonstrate the correct method of moving and positioning a patient to prevent injury to yourself or the patient.

4. Demonstrate the correct method of assisting a disabled patient with dressing or undressing for a radiographic procedure.

5. List the safety measures that must be taken when transferring a patient from a hospital room to the radiographic imaging department.

6. Describe steps that you must take as the radiographer to protect the patient's integumentary system from injury.

7. Explain the criteria to be used when immobilization of a patient is necessary.

8. List the types of immobilizers available, and demonstrate the correct method of applying each one.

9. List the precautions to be taken if a patient is in traction or wearing a cast.

10. Demonstrate the correct manner of assisting a patient with a bedpan or urinal.

11. Explain your responsibilities as a radiographer concerning radiation safety.

12. List the departmental safety measures that you must take to prevent and control fires, patient falls, poisoning or injury from hazardous materials, and burns, as well as the measures to evacuate patients in case of a disaster.

Glossary

Ambulatory: Walking, or able to walk

Atrophy: Decrease in the size of the organ, tissue, or muscle

Catheter: A hollow, flexible tube that can be inserted into a vessel or cavity of the body to withdraw fluids

Chronic obstructive pulmonary disease (COPD): A progressive and irreversible condition that produces diminished inspiratory and expiratory lung capacity

Debility: Lack or loss of strength; weakness

Decubitus ulcer: A pressure sore or ulcer

Disinfectant: Any substance that inhibits the growth of bacteria

Dyspnea: Labored or difficult breathing

Fluoroscope: A device used for the immediate projection of a radiographic image on a fluorescent screen for visual examination

Hydrotherapy: The use of water immersion in the treatment of various mental or physical disorders

Intravenous infusion: Administering fluids or nutrients into the vein

Ischemia: Deficiency of blood in a part due to functional constriction or actual obstruction of a blood vessel

Range of motion: The range, measured in degrees of a circle, through which a joint can be extended and flexed

Sensory deprivation: A condition in which an individual receives less than normal sensory input

Tissue necrosis: Localized death of tissue due to injury or lack of oxygen

Ulceration: An area of tissue necrosis that penetrates below the epidermis; excavation of the surface of any body organ

---

Approaching your profession and your patients in a courteous and tactful manner can put your patients at ease and decrease their level of embarrassment so that the procedure can be performed in a smooth and timely manner. You, the radiographer, set the tone for the entire exchange when a patient arrives as an outpatient. And you are responsible for protecting yourself and your patients from injury in every way possible. Health care workers are often injured while moving and lifting patients, but almost all of these injuries are preventable if you use correct body mechanics and adhere to the rules of safety. Patients are also victims of injuries caused by being improperly moved or lifted. Most of these injuries can also be prevented.

Moving patients from the radiographic table to a gurney or wheelchair or from a hospital bed to a gurney or wheelchair requires some forethought regarding the safety of the patient as well as to the body mechanics you use. You need to take special care with the ancillary equipment that must be moved with the patient during a transfer. You must protect the patient's integumentary system from damage. This is of particular concern when the patient is unable to move by his or her own power. You must be aware of this potential for injury and use care to prevent skin damage.

Occasionally, you may have to immobilize a patient for his or her own safety during a radiographic procedure. Not only must you learn the institution-specific rules concerning immobilizers (restraints), you must be able to use various types of immobilizing devices safely.

The need for a bedpan or urinal may be a requirement that a patient may find embarrassing but unavoidable. As a professional radiographer, you will be able to put the patient at ease and proceed with tact and confidence that will facilitate the procedure to a swift conclusion. The different styles of bedpans require some knowledge as to correct placement under the patient. You need to understand how a bedpan feels underneath a patient and be understanding regarding the embarrassment that the patient experiences.

Adhering to the rules of radiation safety, preventing and controlling fires, using and disposing of hazardous chemicals correctly, and observing other rules of patient and departmental safety are important parts of your education as a radiographer.

Care of Patient's Belongings

A patient who comes to the radiographic imaging department as an outpatient is frequently required to remove all or some items of clothing and to put on a patient gown before an examination procedure or treatment can be performed. It is usually the radiographer who receives the patient and determines which items of clothing are to be removed. The patient's discomfort or embarrassment can be decreased if you approach this situation in a courteous and professional manner.

The patient should be taken to the specific dressing area and shown how to close the dressing room door or draw the curtain of the cubicle while undressing. Clearly explain that he or she is to put on the examining gown and point out where to go for the examination once prepared. (Remember that not everyone knows that some types of examining gowns open at the back rather than at the front; this information should be part of the explanation.) Doing this takes only a few moments, and it will make the patient feel more comfortable.

The patient should be given hangers for clothing. If it is permissible to leave clothing in the dressing room, explain this to the patient. If the patient cannot leave the clothing, show him or her what to do with it. Purses, jewelry, and other valuables should be treated with special care so that they will not be lost or stolen.

Many patients wear jewelry or carry a purse or other valuable items to the radiographic imaging department. The dressing rooms in most diagnostic imaging departments are not safe places to leave these items, and the patient may feel justifiably uneasy about leaving them there. Again, you must consider the patient's concern, and explain what must be done with personal items to keep them safe.

Metal items such as necklaces, rings, and watches are not to be worn for most diagnostic procedures and must be removed before the procedure can begin. An envelope or other container large enough to accommodate all such items should be offered to the patient. Identifying information should be written on a receipt, and you should tag all items and place them in the designated safety area. This procedure will prevent losses that may result in inconvenience and expense to both the patient and the department.

Do not place value on a patient's belongings. An item that may seem insignificant to you may be the patient's most treasured belonging. Every article of clothing or jewelry or other personal effect that a patient brings to the diagnostic imaging department should be treated with care.

Body Mechanics

Constant abuse of the spine from moving and lifting patients is the leading cause of injury to health care personnel in all health care institutions. You will be less fatigued and avoid injury to yourself and your patients if you follow the rules of correct body mechanics. These rules are based on the laws of gravity.

Gravity is the force that pulls objects toward the center of the earth. Any movement requires an expenditure of energy to overcome the force of gravity. When an object is balanced, it is firm and stable. If it is off balance, it will fall because of the pull of gravity. The center of gravity is the point at which the mass of any body is centered. When a person is standing, the center of gravity is at the center of the pelvis (Fig. 4–1).

Safe body mechanics require good posture. Good posture means that the body is in alignment, with all the parts in balance. This permits the musculoskeletal system (the bones and joints) to work at maximal efficiency with a minimal amount of strain on joints, tendons, ligaments, and muscles. Good posture also aids

other body systems to work efficiently. For instance, if the chest is held up and out (the musculoskeletal system), the lungs (the respiratory system) can work at maximal efficiency.

Rules for correct upright posture are as follows:

- Hold chest up and slightly forward with the waist extended. This allows the lungs to expand properly and fill to capacity.
- Hold head erect with the chin held in. This puts the spine in proper alignment, and there is no curve in the neck.
- Stand with the feet parallel and at right angles to the lower legs. The feet should be 4 to 8 inches apart. Keep body weight equally distributed on both feet.
- Keep the knees slightly bent; they act as a shock absorber for the body.
- Keep the buttocks in and the abdomen up and in. This prevents strain on the back and abdominal muscles.

When you move and lift objects, you must overcome the forces of weight and friction. You must determine the center of gravity and make a plan to surmount the weight of the object or person. You can do this by keeping the heaviest part close to the body. If this is not possible, one or more persons should assist you with moving or lifting the load.

The force of friction opposes movement. When you move or transfer a patient, reduce friction to the minimum to facilitate movement. You can do this by reducing the surface area to be moved or, in the case of a patient, by using some of the patient's own strength to assist with the move, if possible. If the patient is unable to assist, you can reduce friction by placing the patient's arms across the chest to reduce the surface area. The surface over which the patient must be moved must be dry and smooth. Pulling rather than pushing also reduces friction when moving a heavy object or person. A sliding board or pull sheet placed under an immobile patient also reduces friction. Directions for the use of these items are presented later in this chapter.

To avoid self-injury when moving heavy objects, remember to keep your body's line of balance closest to the center of the load.

Protective belts to support the back are available in some workplaces. These are somewhat controversial and should be worn only if prescribed by a physician or if it is the policy of the institution. The following are guidelines for picking up or lifting heavy objects:

- When picking up an object from the floor, bend the knees and lower your body. Do not bend from the waist (Fig. 4–2).

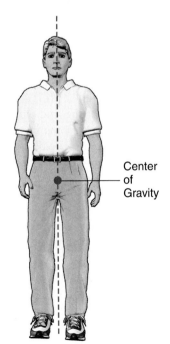

Figure 4–1. When a person is standing, the center of gravity is at the center of the pelvis.

Center of Gravity

- The biceps are the strongest arm muscles and are effective when pulling; therefore; pull heavy items or patients rather than push them.
- When assisting a patient to move, balance the weight over both feet. Stand close to the patient, flex your gluteal muscles, and bend your knees to support the load. Use your arm and leg muscles to assist in the move.
- Always protect your spine. Rather than twisting your body to move with a load, change your foot position instead. Always keep your body balanced over your feet, which should be spread to provide a firm base of support.
- Make certain that the floor area where you are working is clear of all objects.

CALL OUT!

To prevent lower back injury, always keep your center of gravity, your knees flexed, and your weight over both feet. Do not bend at the waist!

Moving and Transferring Patients

You may be called on to transfer or assist in transferring a patient from a hospital room to the diagnostic imaging department. At times, you may be the person appointed to instruct a porter in the correct method of transferring a patient.

CALL OUT!

Never move a patient without enough assistance to prevent injury to yourself and the patient!

Whatever the case, you need to take several precautions when moving a patient from the hospital room to the imaging department. They are as follows:

1. Establish the correct identity of the patient. You may accomplish this by going to the nurses' station on the unit housing the patient, identifying yourself, and giving the patient's name and the type of procedure for which he or she is being sought. In addition, when you approach the patient, identify yourself, state your purpose, and ask to see the patient's identification wristband.

   Rationale: The correct patient must receive the correct procedure.

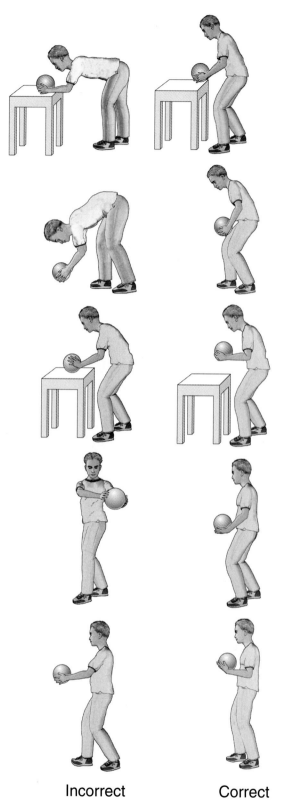

Incorrect   Correct

Figure 4–2. Keep your body balanced over your feet to provide a broad base of support.

2. Request pertinent information concerning the patient's ability to comply with the physical demands of the procedure while at the nurse's station.

   Rationale: Many radiographic imaging procedures require the patient to move about on a relatively narrow surface. You should be informed of the patient's condition and apprised of any mind-altering medications that the patient may have received during the previous 2 hours that may prevent complying with the demands of the procedure without special assistance.

3. Request information concerning the patient's ability to ambulate and any restrictions or precautions to be taken concerning the patient's mobility.

   Rationale: If a patient has restrictions in movement or weight bearing, you must know this so that you do not violate any of these restrictions and cause the patient injury. If you need help moving the patient to and from the bed to the gurney or wheelchair, request it at this time. A radiographer or a porter must never attempt to transfer a patient from a bed to a gurney to a bed without assistance. Furthermore, a patient must never be allowed to transfer to or from a wheelchair without assistance.

4. Move the patient to the imaging department according to the necessary restrictions after greeting and identifying him or her and providing an explanation of what is to occur.

   Rationale: The patient must always be a part of the planning process and given an opportunity to refuse a treatment or procedure. The correct patient must be taken for the correct procedure. The patient in the hospital wears an identification band, usually on the wrist. Procedures require that you, the radiographer, request that the patient state his or her name and then check the name against what is written on the identification band.

> ## CALL OUT!
> Never move a patient without assessing the patient's ability to assist!

When the procedure is completed, return the patient to the hospital room using the following procedure:

1. Stop at the appropriate nurses' station, return the chart, and inform the unit personnel that the patient is being returned to the room. If you need help, request it at this time.

   Rationale: If the unit personnel are not informed of the patient's return, they may not know that the patient has returned and may overlook his or her care.

2. Return the patient to the room, help the patient get into bed, and make him or her comfortable and safe. Place the patient's bed in the position that is closest to the floor, with the side rails raised and the call button within reach in case the patient needs assistance.

   Rationale: Never allow the patient to transfer from a wheelchair without assistance. The patient's safety is a concern. By placing the bed in the lowest position and securing the side rails, you assure yourself that the patient will not be accidentally injured by falling from a height.

> ## CALL OUT!
> Always lower the bed to the lowest position, and secure the rails in the upright position when you return the patient to bed.

Assessing the Patient's Mobility

Before you begin to move a patient, you must use your skills in critical thinking and problem solving to plan the most effective manner of accomplishing this task. The expected outcome of this plan will be to accomplish the move without causing additional pain or injury to the patient or to yourself. This is done by using interviewing skills and assessment skills.

You must look for the following as you assess the patient:

1. *Deviations from correct body alignment.* Deviations in normal physiologic body alignment may result from the following: poor posture, trauma, muscle damage, dysfunction of the nervous system, malnutrition, fatigue, or emotional disturbance. Support blocks or pillows, which are used to assist the patient during the procedure, must be available.

2. *Immobility or limitations in range of joint motion.* Any stiffness, instability, swelling, inflammation, pain, limitation of movement, or atrophy of muscle mass surrounding each joint must be noted and considered in the plan of care.

3. *The ability to walk.* Gait includes rhythm, speed, cadence, and any characteristic of walking that may result in a problem with balance, posture, or

independence of movement. You must plan for the amount of assistance needed to complete the move and the procedure safely.

4. *Respiratory, cardiovascular, metabolic, and musculoskeletal problems.* You must consider in your plan obvious respiratory or cardiovascular symptoms that impair circulation and signal potential problems in positioning. Metabolic problems such as diabetes mellitus or rheumatoid arthritis may be discovered during the interview process and planned for as necessary (symptoms and care of patients with medical problems are discussed in Chapter 7).

Other assessment considerations are as follows:

1. *The patient's general condition.* How well or how poorly is he or she functioning?

2. *Range of motion and weight-bearing ability.* Has the patient had a surgical procedure that restricts motion or limits weight bearing until it is healed?

3. *The patient's strength and endurance.* Will the patient become fatigued and be unable to complete the transfer with only stand-by assistance?

4. *The patient's ability to maintain balance.* Can the patient sit or stand for as long as the procedure requires?

5. *The patient's ability to understand what is expected during the transfer:* Is he responsive and alert?

6. *The patient's acceptance of the move:* Does the patient fear or resent the transfer? Will the transfer increase the pain? Does the patient feel that the move is unnecessary?

7. *The patient's medication history:* Has the patient received a sedative, hypnotic, or other psychoactive drug in the past 2 or 3 hours? Will any medication that he or she has taken affect the ability to move safely? (Medications are discussed in Chapter 12.)

You must decide how the patient can be transferred safely and comfortably, whether by gurney or by wheelchair. Hospitalized patients are seldom allowed to walk to and from the diagnostic imaging department for reasons of safety.

Before going to the patient, a consultation with the nurse in charge of the patient is recommended so that the patient's condition and limitations can be understood. If assistants are needed, they must be on hand. A patient must never be moved without adequate assistance; to do so may cause injury to the patient or to you. As the radiographer, you must always be at the patient's side as he or she moves. The following rules should be observed during a move:

1. Give only the assistance that the patient needs for comfort and safety.

2. Always transfer a patient across the shortest distance.

3. Lock all wheels on beds, gurneys, and wheelchairs before the move begins.

4. Generally, it is better to move a patient toward his or her stronger side while assisting on the patient's weaker side.

5. The patient should wear shoes for standing transfers, but not slippery slippers.

6. Inform the patient of the plan for moving and encourage him or her to help.

7. Give the patient short, simple commands and help the patient to accomplish the move.

Methods of Moving Patients

There are essentially three ways of transferring patients: by gurney, by wheelchair, and by ambulation.

By Gurney

When a patient is moved from a gurney to a radiographic table, or the reverse, great care must be taken to prevent injury. If the patient is unconscious or unable to cooperate in the move, the patient's spine, head, and extremities must be well supported. Convenient and safe ways to do this are by using a sliding board or a sheet to slide the patient from one surface to another.

SHEET TRANSFER

To place a sheet under a patient, use the following procedure: Obtain a heavy draw sheet or use a full bed sheet and fold it in half. If you need an assistant, have one person on each side of the bed or table. Turn the patient onto his or her side toward the distal side of the bed or table. Place the sheet on the table or bed with the fold against the patient's back (Fig. 4–3*A*). Roll the top half of the sheet as close to the patient's back as possible (see Fig. 4–3*B*). Inform the patient that he or she will be turned onto the side toward you and will be moving over the rolled sheet. Then turn the patient across the sheet roll and have your assistant straighten the sheet on the distal side (see Fig. 4–3*C*). You may then return the patient to a supine position, and the transfer may begin.

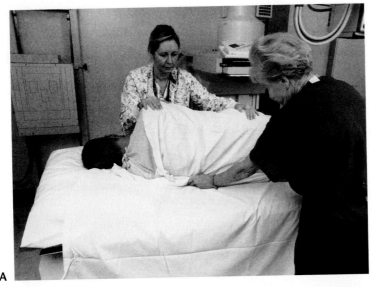

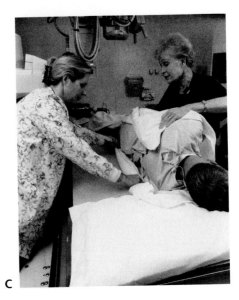

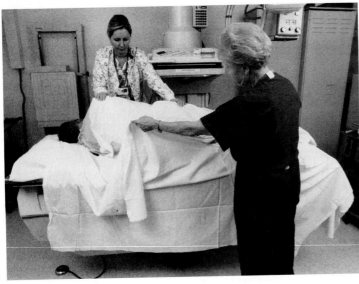

Figure 4–3. Pull sheet. **(A)** Place the sheet on the table with the fold against the patient's back. **(B)** Take the top half of the sheet and roll it against the patient. **(C)** After the patient is rolled to the opposite side, the rolled half of the sheet is straightened out.

If the patient is an adult, three or four people should participate in the maneuver. One person stands at the patient's head to guide and support it during the move, with another at the side of the surface to which the patient will be moved and a third person at the side of the surface on which the patient is lying. If there are four people, two may stand at each side. The sheet is rolled at the side of the patient so that you can easily grasp it in your hands close to the patient's body. In unison (usually on the count of three), the team transfers the patient to the other surface (Fig. 4–4).

If the radiographic table is stationary, extra padding should be placed over the metal parts of the table's edge to protect the patient from being bruised while being moved. Some tables have a floating top and should be moved forward, close to the edge of the gurney.

Tube housing positioned above the radiographic tables should be moved out of the way when patients are being moved in order to protect both you and the patient from bumping into them. To avoid bumping into a device such as a fluoroscopic unit, warn the patient not to sit up. You must also be careful not to injure yourself.

SLIDING BOARD TRANSFER

The sliding board (also called a smooth mover and a smoothie) is a glossy, plasticized board approximately 1.7 meters (5 feet 10 inches) in length and about 75 centimeters (2 feet 6 inches) wide. This item facilitates moving patients from one surface to another, usually from a gurney to an examining table. The sliding board usually requires fewer personnel to make the

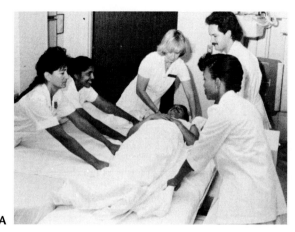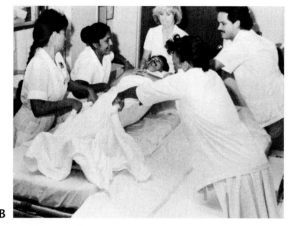

Figure 4–4. In unison, transfer the patient to the other surface.

move because it creates a firm bridge between the two surfaces over which the patient can be easily moved. The sliding board transfer procedure is as follows:

1. Obtain the sliding board, and spray it with antistatic spray, if necessary.

2. Enlist the assistance of one other person if the patient is of average size and weight; if the patient is large, three people may be necessary to move the patient safely.

3. Move the patient to the edge of the gurney. One person should hold the sheet that the patient is lying on over the top of the patient to keep the patient from possibly rolling off the gurney.

4. Move the gurney up against the radiographic table; lock the wheels of the gurney.

5. Assist the patient to turn onto his or her side, away from the table, and place the sliding board under the sheet upon which the patient was lying.

6. Create a bridge with the board between the edge of the radiographic table and the edge of the gurney (Fig. 4–5A).

7. Place the sheet over the board, and allow the patient to roll back onto the board.

8. With one person at the side of the radiographic table and the other at the side of the gurney, slide the patient onto the radiographic table (see Fig. 4–5B).

9. Assist the patient to roll toward the distal side of the radiographic table, keeping the patient secure by holding onto the sheet on which he or she was lying. The person standing on the side of the gurney should remove the sliding board from under the patient (see Fig. 4–5C).

10. Remove the gurney and perform the radiographic procedure.

11. When the procedure is completed, the patient can be transferred back to the gurney by repeating the steps above.

12. Once the patient is back on the gurney, place a pillow under the patient's head, if this is permitted, and put the side rails of the gurney up. Place a soft immobilizer over the patient. The patient may then be transferred.

13. When the move is complete, discard the soiled linen that was used on the radiographic table, and clean the sliding board and the table with a disinfectant spray.

14. Wash your hands and place clean linen on the table.

CALL OUT!

Always obtain enough assistance to move a patient, even with a smooth mover. This is for the safety of both the patient and the radiographer.

LOG ROLL

Occasionally, it is necessary to turn a patient without flexing his or her neck or back. This type of move is called a log roll. Five persons are necessary to negotiate this patient move safely, so you must call for four assistants. Two persons stand at each side of the table or bed on which the turn will take place. One person keeps the patient's head and neck immobile by placing the hands flat against the sides of the patient's face with palms held firmly at the angle of the jaw. Two assist with maintaining alignment of the torso and two with

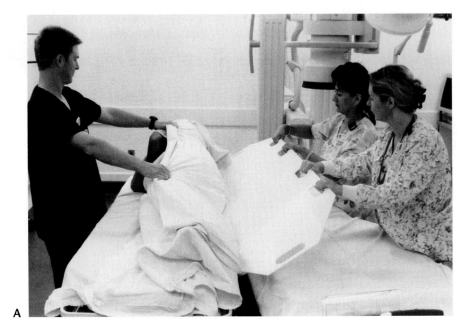

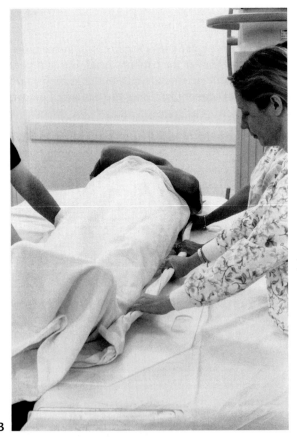

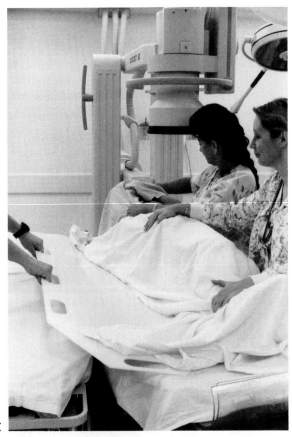

Figure 4–5. (A) Position the patient on his side and place the sliding board under the sheet on which the patient is lying. **(B)** Roll the sheet close to the patient, and slide the patient onto the table. **(C)** Remove the sliding board while safely securing the patient.

the legs. Use the sheet that is under the patient as a turnsheet. Prepare the patient for the move as follows:

1. Place the patient's arms across the chest and ask him or her to hold rigid if unable to assist.

2. Place a pillow or support bolster between the patient's knees to prevent pressure and to assist with maintenance of body alignment as the patient is turned.

3. Place another bolster in the place where the patient's head will rest when the turn is complete to support the head and neck in alignment.

When the patient is prepared and each member of the team understands his or her duty as the patient is turned, move the patient as follows:

1. Bring the sheet up over the patient's distal side. The sheet should be grasped by the two persons on that side close to the patient's body. The person in charge of the head and neck stands at the side of the table and positions the hands for firm support. The fourth member of the team assists with maintenance of the patient's torso alignment.

2. In unison, the team rolls the patient to the desired side as if the patient were a log, keeping the head, neck, and torso immobile during the move (Fig. 4–6).

3. When the turn is complete, the patient's head should be resting on the bolster positioned before the move began. The back must be firmly supported with bolsters or pillows. The upper leg may be flexed after the move is completed.

By Wheelchair

If a patient must be moved from a bed or radiographic table to a wheelchair, or the reverse, he or she must be helped. You should never allow a patient to get off a table or onto a wheelchair without some assistance. The patient is often not as strong as he or she thinks. The sudden movement may cause dizziness, and the patient may fall.

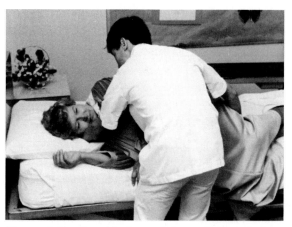

Figure 4–7. Stand in front of the patient and place on arm under her shoulders and the other across her knees. Assist her to a sitting position.

If the patient has been in a supine position and is to be helped to a sitting position, you should have the patient turn to the side with knees flexed. You then place yourself in front of the patient with one arm under the shoulders and the other across the knees.

1. If the patient can assist, instruct him or her to push up with the upper arm when told to do so (Fig. 4–7).

2. Then, on the count of three, move or help the patient to a sitting position at the edge of the table. Before helping the patient to stand, allow him or her to sit for a moment and regain a sense of balance. While the patient is "dangling," place nonskid slippers on the patient's feet.

3. If the patient needs minimal assistance to get off the table, you may stand at the patient's side and take the patient's arm to help.

4. If the radiographic table is high, never allow a patient to step down without providing a secure stepping stool. Always stay at the patient's side to assist. A telescoping table must be placed in the lowest position before a patient is assisted to move off of it.

5. The wheelchair must be close enough so that the patient can be seated in the chair with one pivot. Have the foot supports of the chair up and the wheels locked.

6. The footrests on the wheelchair should then be put down and the wheels unlocked. A safety belt should be put across an unsteady patient.

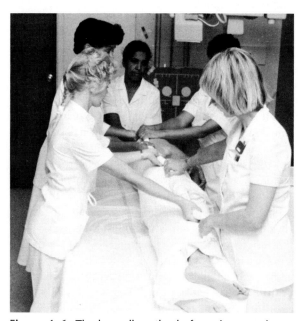

Figure 4–6. The log roll method of moving a patient.

CALL OUT!

When moving a patient from hospital bed to wheelchair, always place nonskid slippers on the patient's feet, provide assistance to prevent falls, and secure the seatbelt on the wheelchair.

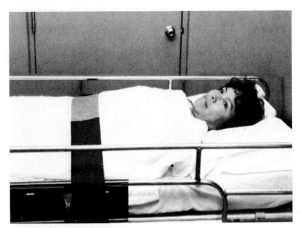

Figure 4–8. Keep the side rails of the gurney up and the safety strap attached.

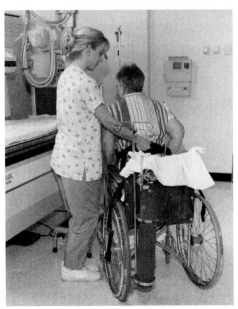

Figure 4–9. Place fingers through the back of the belt in an underhand grasp.

Once placed on the radiographic table, cover the patient with a protective sheet. Do not allow the patient to become chilled.

A patient who has received a narcotic, hypnotic, or other type of psychoactive medication; a confused, disoriented, unconscious, or head-injured person; or a child must never be left alone on a radiographic table or gurney. If the patient's behavior cannot be predicted or if the patient is in a wheelchair, observe him or her carefully. A soft immobilizer belt should be placed over any patient on a gurney or in a wheelchair. The side rails of the gurney must always be up (Fig. 4–8).

Using a Gait or Transfer Belt

In some institutions, a gait or transfer belt is required when moving or walking with a disabled patient. In other institutions, it is a matter of choice. You must learn the policy of the institution in which you are working.

A transfer or gait belt is a belt made of a sturdy material, either leather or a heavy fabric that is about 54 to 60 inches long. Its purpose is to assist in stabilizing the patient during ambulation. It is placed around the waist of the patient to be transferred when in a sitting position and fastened securely. Some of these belts have a hand grip for the health care worker to grasp at the back while assisting the patient.

1. Before applying the belt, explain its use to the patient and inform him or her that it will be worn for a very brief time.

2. Be certain that the belt is positioned at waist level and is not resting on bare skin. Be certain that it is not placed over an open wound, an operative site, a colostomy, or a patient's breast tissue. The belt should be secured so that there is only enough space for your fingers to slip through it in the rear.

3. After the belt is in place, place your fingers through the back of the belt in an underhand grasp (Fig. 4–9). Then support the patient during the move by holding onto the belt.

Use of Immobilizers

The ethical and legal restrictions concerning use of immobilizers (often called restraints) in patient care are discussed in Chapter 1. As the radiographer, you must remember that immobilizers must be ordered by the physician in charge of the patient's care and applied in compliance with institutional policy.

The Joint Commission on Accreditation of Healthcare Organization (JCAHO) states that immobilizers should be used only after less restrictive measures have been attempted and have proved ineffective in protecting the patient. Remember this and use your critical thinking skills to avoid the use of immobilizers if at all possible. Immobilizers are defined as any manual method or physical or mechanical device, material, or equipment attached or adjacent to the person's body that the person cannot remove easily that restricts freedom of movement or normal access to one's body (Omnibus Reconciliation Act, 1989).

The most effective method of avoiding the need to restrain an adult patient is the use of therapeutic communication to explore the patient's fears. If a patient seems fearful or is striking out or moving in an unsafe manner, you should assure the patient that the procedure will be carried out quickly and in a manner that keeps him or her as comfortable as possible. If this

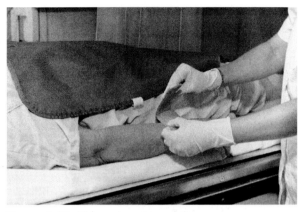

Figure 4–10. Velcro strap immobilizer.

does not reassure the patient, other less restrictive devices, such as soft Velcro straps, sandbags, and sponges, may be used to remind the patient to refrain from moving (Figs. 4–10 and 4–11). If immobilizers are to be used, you must be certain that they are being used to protect the patient's safety and that their use is the only alternative.

There are various types of immobilizing devices that may be used for adult patients. Immobilizers for use with children are discussed in Chapter 9. Reasons for application of immobilizers in the care of an adult patient include the following:

1. To control movement of an extremity when an intravenous infusion or diagnostic catheter is in place

2. To remind a patient who is sedated and having difficulty remembering to remain in a particular position

3. To prevent a patient who is unconscious, delirious, cognitively impaired, or confused from falling from a radiographic table or a gurney; from removing a tube or dressing that may be life sustaining; or from injuring himself by impact with diagnostic imaging equipment

When you are caring for a patient who has been immobilized, explain the reason for using immobilizers to the patient and to anyone who may accompany the patient. After immobilizers are applied, do not leave the patient unattended, and inform the patient that he or she is not alone and is not being punished. You should also explain that the immobilizers are only temporary and that as soon as the procedure is finished, the immobilizer will be removed.

A calm, reassuring manner often soothes an agitated or confused patient who has been immobilized. Patients in this state need repeated orientation as well as a quiet and quick explanation to complete the procedure and return the patient to the hospital room or wherever he or she is to be taken on completion of the radiographs.

Always apply immobilizers carefully and in the manner prescribed by the manufacturer of the device. The type of immobilizer to be used is dictated by need. All radiographers must document application of immobilizers as explained in Chapter 1. The following are rules for application of immobilizers:

1. The patient must be allowed as much mobility as is safely possible.

2. The areas of the body where immobilizers are applied must be padded to prevent injury to the skin beneath the device.

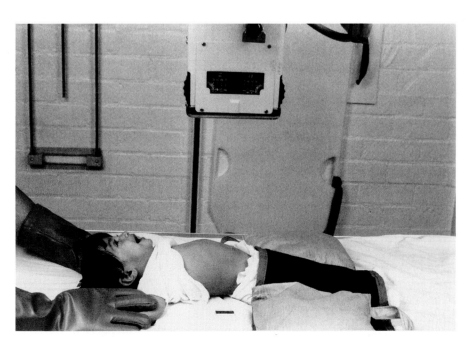

Figure 4–11. Sandbags can be used to hold lead shielding in place, which immobilizes the patient at the same time.

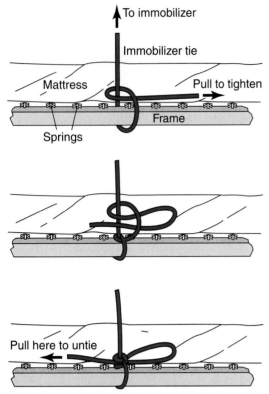

Figure 4–12. Following this sequence will result in tying a half-bow knot. The knot will remain secure until the free end is pulled. It is a safe knot that can be quickly released.

3. Normal anatomic position must be maintained.

4. Knots that will not become tighter with movement must be used (a half-knot is recommended) (Fig. 4–12).

5. The immobilizer must be easy to remove quickly, if this is necessary.

6. Neither circulation nor respiration must be impaired by the immobilizer.

7. If leg immobilizers are necessary, wrist immobilizers must also be applied to prevent the patient from either unfastening the device or, in an attempt to leave the radiographic table or gurney, accidentally hang him- or herself.

Although as the radiographer, you are not usually the health care worker who applies immobilizers or who monitors a patient in immobilizers for long periods of time, you must understand that immobilizers must be removed at least every 2 hours. After removal, the joints affected by the immobilizer must be put through range of motion. It may be necessary to remove one immobilizer at a time and reapply one before releasing another. Immobilizers must always be applied to the frame of the gurney, bed, or table, not to a moveable part of the equipment. Any use of immobilizers requires documentation of the type of immobilizer used, the time it was applied and removed, the reason for its application, and an assessment of the patient at each stage.

There are various types of immobilizers that may be used, including the following:

1. Limb holders or four-point restraints (Fig. 4–13*A*)

2. Ankle or wrist immobilizers (see Fig. 4–13*B*)

3. Immobilizing vest for keeping a patient in a wheelchair (see Fig. 4–13*C*)

4. Waist immobilizer, which keeps the patient safe on an examining table or in a bed, but allows the patient to change position (see Fig. 4–13*D*)

At times, a patient who is aggressive and delusional may need to have waist, wrist, and ankle immobilizers

Figure 4–13. (A) Limb holders restrain this patient's arms and legs. **(B)** Immobilizers for the ankle or wrist are soft and padded to prevent injury to the patient's skin. **(C)** An immobilizing vest prevents the patient from leaving the wheelchair and helps support him. The waist belt on this immobilizer adjusts to fit the size of the patient without restricting his breathing. **(D)** *Left:* This waist immobilizer is effective for keeping the patient in bed, while still allowing her to turn from side to side and to sit up in bed. *Right:* This safety belt allows freedom to move but not to fall from the bed.

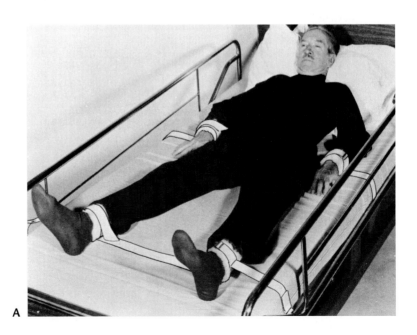

A

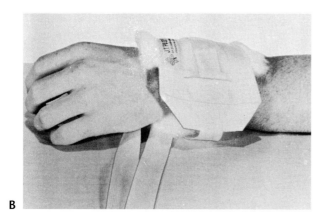

B

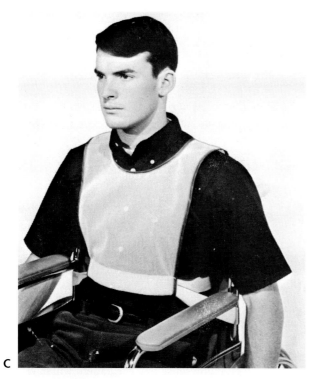

C

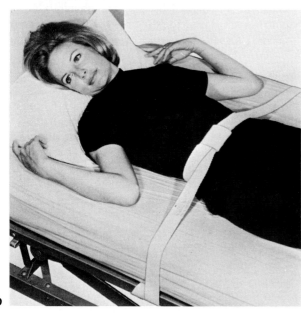

D

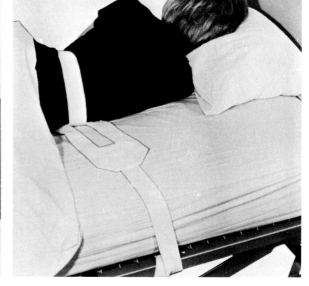

Figure 4–13. (continued)

that are stronger than those shown in Figure 4–13 *B, C,* and *D.* Immobilizers of this type also have locks. If this type of immobilizer is necessary, one or more security officers should be called to assist with application. A radiographer alone or with only the assistance of one other radiographer must never attempt to apply immobilizers to an extremely aggressive or combative patient. Persons who have been trained to deal with this type of patient problem must do this. When this type of immobilization is necessary, the rules of immobilizer application still apply.

Positioning the Patient for Diagnostic Imaging Examinations

When a patient must spend a long period of time in the diagnostic imaging department, it is your duty as the radiographer to assist the patient to maintain his or her body in normal alignment for comfort and to maintain normal physiologic functioning. There are several protective positions that the body may assume or be assisted to assume for comfort. There are also several positions that the patient may be requested to assume to facilitate diagnosis or treatment. You must familiarize yourself with all these positions and the problems that may be encountered with each in order to assist the patient as the need arises. The positions are as follows:

Supine or dorsal recumbent position. Patient is flat on the back. The feet and the neck will need to be protected when the patient is lying in this position. A pillow may be placed under the head to tilt it forward. The feet should be supported to prevent plantar flexion or footdrop (Fig. 4–14A).

Lateral recumbent position. Patient is on the right or the left side with both knees flexed. This position relieves pressure on most bony prominences. The patient may be supported with pillows or sandbags to maintain the position (see Fig. 4–14B).

Prone position. Patient lies face down. A small pillow should support the head to prevent flexion of the cervical spine. The patient may be moved down on the table so that the feet drop over the edge, or a pillow may be placed under the lower legs at the ankles to prevent footdrop (see Fig. 4–14C).

High Fowler's position. Patient semi-sits with head raised at an angle of 45 to 90 degrees off the table. This position is used for patient in respiratory distress (see Fig. 4–14D).

Semi-Fowler's position. Patient's head is raised at an angle of from 15 to 30 degrees off the table. The arms must be supported to prevent pull on the shoulders, and the feet must be supported to prevent plantar flexion or footdrop. Pillows or blocks under knees must be removed after a brief time (15 to 20 minutes) to prevent circulatory impairment (see Fig. 4–14E).

Sims' position. Patient lies on either left or right side with the forward arm flexed and the posterior arm extended behind the body. The body is inclined slightly forward with the top knee bent sharply and the bottom knee slightly bent. This position is frequently used for diagnostic imaging of the lower bowel as an aid in inserting the enema tip (Fig. 4–14F).

Trendelenburg position. The table or bed is inclined with the patient's head lower than the rest of the body. Patients are occasionally placed in this position during diagnostic imaging procedures and for promotion of venous return in patients with inadequate peripheral perfusion caused by disease.

Patients in respiratory distress or who have COPD must not be left in a prone, supine, or Sims' position for more than brief periods of time to avoid becoming increasingly dysgenic.

Assisting the Patient to Dress and Undress

The patient may arrive in the diagnostic imaging department alone if he or she comes from outside the hospital. As you are making an initial assessment of the patient's condition, you may observe that the patient will need help in removing clothing. This assistance may be necessary if the patient is in a cast or brace, is very young, or is in too weakened a condition to help him- or herself. The patient may have a contracture of an extremity or poor eyesight. Whatever the problem, if you sense that the patient will have difficulty undressing if left alone, you should offer assistance and stay near the dressing room to provide help when it is needed.

If a trauma patient is brought to the diagnostic imaging department from the emergency unit, removing the clothing in the conventional manner may cause further injury or pain. You may consider cutting away garments that interfere with acceptable radiographs; however, clothing must not be cut without the patient's consent except in extreme emergencies. If the patient is unable to give consent, a family member should do so in writing for your protection.

If clothing must be cut off, try to cut into a seam if at all possible. The clothes should not be automatically thrown in the trash. They should be offered to the patient and placed with the patient's other belongings.

1. If the patient is very young and is accompanied by a familiar adult, he or she will be more relaxed

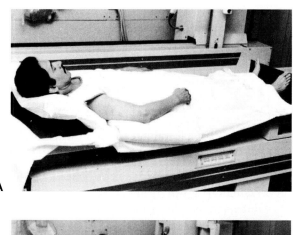
A

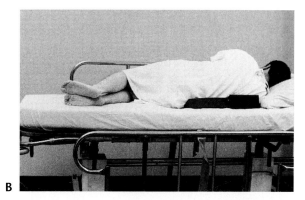
B

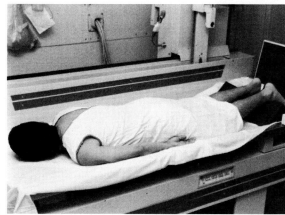
C

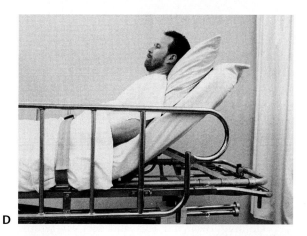
D

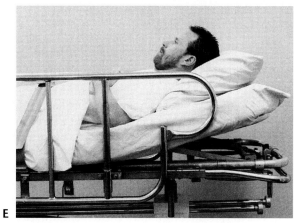
E

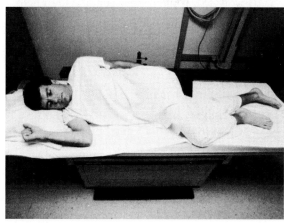
F

Figure 4–14. (**A**) Supine position. (**B**) Lateral recumbent position. (**C**) Prone position. (**D**) High Fowler's position. (**E**) Semi-Fowler's position. (**F**) Sims' position.

and cooperative if the adult helps him to dress and undress. Explain to the adult how the child should be dressed for the procedure, arrange a meeting place, and leave them alone.

2. If you must assist a patient who has a disability of the lower extremities, the clothing should be removed from the top part of the body first.

3. Place a long examining gown on the patient. Instruct him to loosen belt buckles, buttons, or hooks around the waist and slip his trousers over his hips. If he cannot do this for himself, reach under the gown and pull the trousers down over the hips.

4. Have the patient sit down. You may have to squat in front of the patient and gently pull the

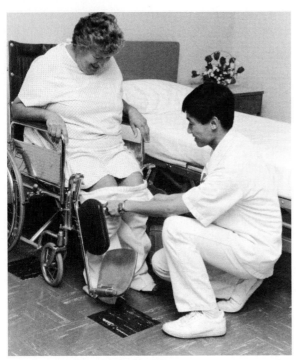

Figure 4–15. Squat in front of the patient, and remove the clothing over the feet and legs.

clothing over the legs and feet to remove it (Fig. 4–15). If the patient is not able to help, call for an assistant.

Some dresses may be removed in the same way. If this method is not practical, however, and the dress must be pulled over the woman's head, proceed as follows:

1. Place a draw sheet over the patient and then help her to remove her slip and brassiere.

2. Help her to put on an examining gown, then remove the draw sheet.

The following are steps to re-dress a patient with a paralyzed leg, a leg injury, a cast, or a brace:

1. Slide the clothing (pants or skirt) over the feet or legs as far as the hips while the patient is sitting and still wearing an examining gown.

2. Have the patient stand, and pull the clothing over the hips if he or she can tolerate it.

3. If the patient is not able to pull the clothing over the hips alone, have an assistant raise the patient off the chair so that you may slip the clothing over the hips and waist.

4. Remove the patient's arms from the sleeves of the gown. Have the patient hold the gown over his or her chest, and carefully pull the shirt over the head, or put it on one sleeve at a time.

5. When the outside items of clothing are on the patient, remove the gown from under the clothes.

The Disabled Patient

If the patient is on a gurney or the radiographic table and you must change the patient's clothing, you can most easily accomplish this with the patient in a supine position.

1. Cover the patient with a draw sheet and have an examining gown ready. Explain what is to be done and ask the patient to help if he or she is able. If the patient is paralyzed or unconscious, summon help before beginning the procedure.

2. Remove the clothing from the less affected side first. Then remove the clothing from the more affected side and place the clean gown on that side, making sure to keep the patient covered with the draw sheet.

3. Next place the clean gown on the unaffected side and tie the gown at the back, if practical (Fig. 4–16).

4. If the patient is wearing an article of clothing that must be pulled over the head, roll the garment up above the waist. Then remove the patient's arms from the clothing, first from the unaffected side and then from the affected side.

5. Next, gently lift the clothing over the patient's head. One person alone should not attempt to undress a disabled patient; to do so may cause further injury or discomfort.

6. To remove trousers, loosen buckles and buttons and have the patient raise his buttocks as you slip the trousers over his hips. If the patient is unable to help, have an assistant stand at the opposite side of the table. After the trousers have been loosened, have the assistant pull the patient toward him or her, then slide the trousers off one side of the hip. Next, draw the patient toward you and have the assistant slide the trousers off the other hip.

7. Slip the trousers below the knees and off (Fig. 4–17).

8. Fold the clothing and place it in a paper bag on which the patient's name has been printed. If the patient is accompanied by a relative or a friend, ask that person to keep the patient's clothing. If the patient is alone, you will be responsible for caring for the clothing.

When a patient's gown becomes wet or soiled in the radiology department, it is your duty to change it. If a patient is allowed to remain in a wet or soiled gown,

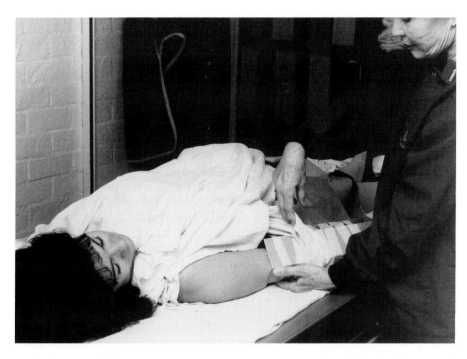

Figure 4–16. Place the clean gown on the unaffected side, then tie it behind the patient's neck.

the skin may become damaged, or he or she may become chilled.

When changing the gown of a patient who has an injury or is paralyzed on one side, remove the gown from the unaffected side first. Then, with the patient covered by the soiled gown, place the clean gown first on the affected side and then on the unaffected side. Pull the soiled gown from under the clean one.

Always make sure that the patient is covered during the process.

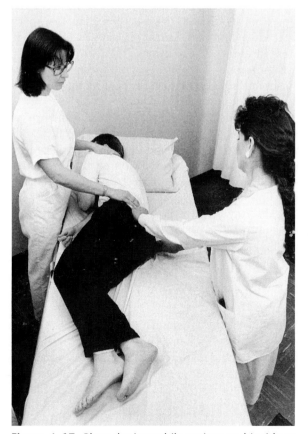

Figure 4–17. Place the immobile patient on his side to begin removing his trousers.

> ## CALL OUT!
>
> When changing a disabled patient's gown, allow enough material to work with by removing the unaffected side first or by placing the gown on the affected side first.

The Patient with an Intravenous Infusion

Frequently, patients are taken to the diagnostic imaging department with an IV infusion in place.

1. If the patient's gown must be changed, slip the clothing off the unaffected side first.

2. Carefully slide the sleeve of the unaffected side over the IV tubing and catheter, then over the container of fluid. For this step, the container must be removed from the stand.

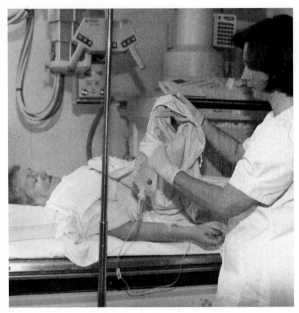

Figure 4–18. Place the clean gown over the IV container.

3. When replacing the soiled gown with a clean one, first place the sleeve on the affected side over the container of fluid, then over the tubing and onto the arm with the venous catheter in place (Fig. 4–18). Rehang the bottle of fluid and complete the change.

4. When moving the arm of a patient who has an IV catheter in place, support the arm firmly so that the catheter does not become dislodged. Remember to keep the bottle of fluid above the infusion site to prevent blood from flowing into the tubing.

If the intravenous infusion is being controlled by a pump and the patient's gown becomes wet or soiled and must be changed, do not attempt to disengage the IV tubing from the pump. In this case, you should:

1. Remove the gown from the unaffected arm, and place the soiled gown to one side of the table until the nurse in charge of monitoring the infusion can remove it.

2. Then replace the soiled gown with a clean gown over the unaffected side and the chest only.

Skin Care

As the radiographer, you are responsible for the care of your patient's skin or integumentary system while in the diagnostic imaging department. Skin breakdown can occur in a brief period of time (1 to 2 hours) and result in a decubitus ulcer that may take weeks or months to heal. Mechanical factors that may predis-

pose the skin to breakdown are immobility, pressure, and shearing force.

Immobilizing a patient in one position for an extended period of time creates pressure on the skin that bears the patient's weight. This, in turn, restricts capillary blood flow to that area and can result in tissue necrosis.

Moving a patient to or from a diagnostic imaging table too rapidly or without adequately protecting the patient's skin may damage the external skin or underlying tissues as they are pulled over each other creating a shearing force. This, too, may lead to tissue necrosis.

Another factor that contributes to skin breakdown is friction caused by movement back and forth on a rough or uneven surface such as a wrinkled bed sheet. Allowing a patient to lie on a damp sheet or remain in a wet gown may lead to skin damage. Similarly, urine and fecal material that remain on the skin act as an irritant and are damaging to the skin.

Early signs that indicate imminent skin breakdown are blanching and a feeling of coldness over pressure areas. This condition is called *ischemia*. Ischemia is followed by heat and redness in the area as the blood rushes to the traumatized spot in an attempt to provide nourishment to the skin. This process is called *reactive hyperemia*. If, at the time of reactive hyperemia, the pressure on the threatened area is not relieved, the tissues begin to necrose, and a small ulceration soon becomes visible. Ischemia and reactive hyperemia are difficult to observe in patients who are dark-skinned. In these cases, you must feel the skin to assess for threat of skin damage.

A shearing injury to the skin may cause it to appear bluish and bruised. If such an area is not cared for, necrosis and ulceration will occur.

Persons who are most prone to skin breakdown are the malnourished, the elderly, and the chronically ill. A patient who is elderly and in poor health may have dehydrated skin, an accumulation of fluid in the tissues (edema), increased or decreased skin temperature, or a loss of subcutaneous fat that acts to protect the skin. Any of these factors can contribute to skin breakdown, and you must be particularly cautious when moving or caring for this type of patient.

Preventing Decubitus Ulcers

Protection of the integumentary system must always be a consideration when caring for patients in the diagnostic imaging department. The tables on which the patients must be placed for care are hard, and often the surface is unprotected. The areas most susceptible to decubitus ulcers are the scapulae, the sacrum, the trochanters, the knees, and the heels of the feet.

You should assist the patient who is on a gurney or diagnostic imaging table for a long period of time to change position, or change it for the patient if he or she is unable to do so. Keep pressure off the hips, knees, and heels by placing a pillow or soft blanket under the patient or by turning him or her to a different position whenever possible. This is done in the usual hospital situation every 2 hours. If the patient is lying on a hard surface, such as the radiographic table, it should be done every 30 minutes. If a patient is perspiring profusely or is incontinent of urine or feces, make certain that he or she is kept clean and dry, and take precautions when moving the patient to prevent skin abrasions.

Special precautions should be taken to protect the patient's feet and lower legs during a position change or transfer. The feet should be protected by shoes, and care should be taken to prevent bruising while the move is made. Circulatory impairment in the lower extremities is common, and the slightest bump may be the beginning of an ulceration.

Cast Care and Traction

Radiographic exposures of fractures that have been casted are often needed to determine correct positioning of musculoskeletal tissues. Casts may be made of plaster (gypsum), fiberglass, plastic, or cast-tape materials. The material used depends on the type of injury, the length of time needed for immobilization, and the physician's preference.

As the radiographer, you will often care for the patient who has a newly applied cast. Some of the materials used, particularly plaster, contain water and can accidentally be compressed. Compression of a cast may produce pressure on the patient's skin under the cast, and this, in turn, may lead to the formation of a decubitus ulcer at the site of cast compression. A cast that becomes too tight may cause circulatory impairment or nerve compression. To prevent these complications, you must be able to assess the patient for circulatory or neurologic impairment and must learn to move a cast with care.

When moving a patient who is wearing a cast, slide your opened, flattened hands under the cast. Avoid grasping the cast with your fingers, since this may cause indentations if the cast material is still damp. A cast must be supported at the joints when it is moved. A casted extremity must be moved as a unit with flat hands supporting it at the joints (Fig. 4–19). When moving a patient who has an abduction bar placed between the legs of a spica cast, it is imperative that the abduction bar not be used as a moving or turning device.

To position a patient who is in a cast, you need to have bolsters or sandbags on hand so that the cast can be well supported. A recently casted limb usually should be kept elevated. If a cast is allowed to put

pressure on the skin in any area, it may impede circulation or damage underlying nerves.

A patient with a cast who is in the diagnostic imaging department for any length of time should be assessed for signs of impaired circulation or nerve compression every 15 minutes. A cast applied to an arm may cause a circulatory disturbance in the hand; a leg or body cast may affect circulation in the feet, toes, or lower leg. Signs of impaired circulation or nerve compression that you may easily detect are as follows:

Pain. Sudden pain or pain that increases with passive motion may indicate nerve damage.

Coldness. Fingers or toes distal to a cast should feel warm.

Numbness. A cast that is too tight may cause numbness, another sign of nerve damage.

Burning or tingling of fingers or toes. These symptoms may indicate circulatory impairment.

Swelling. Indicative of edema, swelling may result in circulatory impairment or nerve compression.

Skin color changes (to a pale or bluish color). Skin should remain pink and warm. In dark-skinned persons, temperature and comparison with the normal extremity are evaluated.

Inability to move fingers or toes. All fingers and toes should be able to be moved, fully extended, and flexed.

Decrease in or absence of pulses. These changes may indicate circulatory impairment.

If you observe any of the latter changes, you must immediately notify the physician in charge of the patient. The physician may order a change in the patient's position in an attempt to relieve pressure.

If the patient in a body cast or a spica cast reports difficult respirations or nausea or is vomiting, notify the physician because this may indicate abdominal distress that requires immediate treatment.

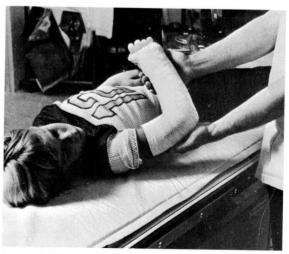

Figure 4–19. Support a cast at the joints when moving it.

If you are called on to take radiographic films of patients who are in traction, you will need to use a portable machine. When you are working with a patient in a traction device, you must never remove the traction apparatus or relieve the pull of the traction. To do so may cause a reduced fracture to become misaligned. If you are unable to complete the assignment because of a traction apparatus, you may have to enlist the help of the nurse in charge of the patient.

CALL OUT!

Never remove or move a traction bar from a patient while performing radiographic procedures.

Assisting the Patient with a Bedpan or Urinal

A patient may spend several hours in the diagnostic imaging department; often the patient is not able to postpone urination or defecation. He or she may be embarrassed about making the request and will wait until the last possible moment to do so. When a patient makes such a request, you should respond quickly yet treat it in a matter-of-fact manner.

1. If possible, help the patient to reach the lavatory near the examining room; this is the most desirable way to handle the situation. However, do not allow the patient to go to the toilet without assistance. Help the patient put on slippers or shoes, and wrap the draw sheet around him or her if no robe is available. Help the patient off the radiographic table or out of the wheelchair, and lead the patient to the lavatory. The patient may have been fasting or may have been given drugs that make him or her very unsteady; therefore, it is not safe to leave the patient unattended.

2. If the patient can help him- or herself in the lavatory, close the door and tell the patient that you will be just outside if you are needed. Each lavatory should be equipped with an emergency call button, and you should explain its use to the patient. If there is no emergency call button, check on the patient at frequent intervals to be certain that his or her condition is stable.

3. After the patient has finished using the lavatory, help him or her to wash hands if unable to do so.

4. Then accompany the patient back to the examination area.

5. Cover the patient and make him or her comfortable.

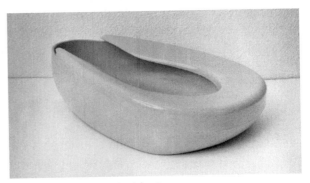

Figure 4–20. A standard bedpan.

6. Return to the lavatory and make certain that it is clean.

7. Wash your hands.

The Bedpan

The patient who is unable to get to the lavatory must be offered a bedpan or urinal. In the diagnostic imaging department, clean bedpans and urinals are usually stored in a specific place. Most departments stock disposable units. If not, you are charged with ascertaining that the bedpan or urinal to be used has been sterilized between uses.

There are two types of bedpans. The standard bedpan is made of metal or plastic and is approximately 4 inches high (Fig. 4–20). Most patients can use this type. However, a patient may have a fracture or another disability that makes it impossible to use a pan of this height. For these patients, the fracture pan is used. All diagnostic imaging departments should have these pans available (Fig. 4–21).

1. Before assisting the patient, wash your hands and then obtain tissue and a bedpan with a cover. If the pan is cold, run warm water over it; then dry it.

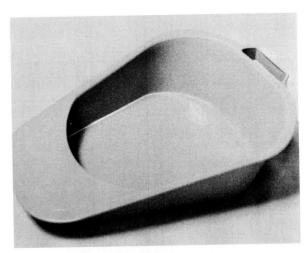

Figure 4–21. A fracture pan.

Close the examining room door, or screen the patient to ensure privacy. Always place a sheet over the patient while helping him onto the bedpan. Don clean, disposable gloves.

2. Next, approach the patient. Remove the bedpan cover, and place it at the end of the table. If the patient is able to move, place one hand under the lower back, and ask the patient to raise the hips.

3. Place the pan under the hips (Fig. 4–22). Be sure the patient is covered with a sheet. If unable to sit up, assist the patient to a sitting position. Do not leave a patient sitting on a bedpan—he or she is poorly balanced and may fall.

4. Remove your gloves and wash your hands. If you cannot stay with the patient or if the patient is not able to sit up, place two or three pillows behind the patient's shoulders and head so that he or she is comfortable. Leave the toilet tissue where the patient can reach it. Let him or her be alone, but remain nearby so that when finished you are on hand to be of assistance.

5. When the patient has finished using the bedpan, put on clean, disposable gloves and help the patient off the pan. Have the patient lie back, place one of your hands under the lumbar area, and have the patient raise the hips.

6. Remove the pan, cover it, and empty it in the designated area. Then rinse it clean with cold water and return it to the area where used equipment is placed.

7. Offer the patient a wet paper towel or washcloth to wash the hands and a dry paper towel to dry them.

8. Remove your gloves as described in Chapter 3, and wash your hands.

If a patient is unable to assist in getting onto and off a bedpan, do not attempt to help him or her alone. Enlist the aid of another team member. Have that person stand at the opposite side of the table. With the assistance of the second radiographer, turn the patient to a side-lying position. Place the pan against the patient's hips, then turn the patient back to a supine position while holding the pan in place. Be certain that the hips are in good alignment on the pan. Place pillows under the patient's shoulders and head and stay nearby. When the patient has finished using the pan, put on clean gloves and reverse the procedure to remove the pan.

If the patient is not able to clean the perineal area you will have to assist. Wear clean, disposable gloves to do this.

1. Take several thicknesses of tissue and fold them into a pad. Wipe the patient's perineum from front to back, then drop the tissue into the pan. If necessary, repeat the procedure until the perineum is clean and dry.

2. Cover the pan to take it to the bathroom and empty it. If the bedpan is disposable, and the patient will not be staying in the diagnostic imaging department long enough to use it a second time, you may place the bedpan in the trash. If the bedpan is nondisposable, place it in the soiled equipment area for re-sterilization.

3. Remove your gloves correctly and wash your hands.

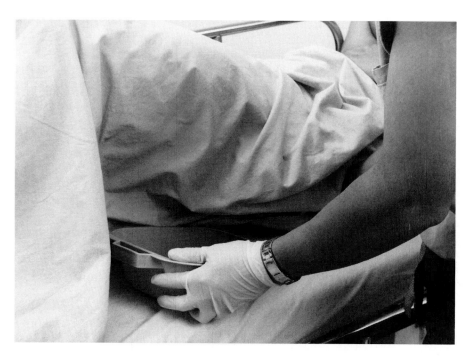

Figure 4–22. Place one hand under the patient's lower back, and ask the patient to raise the hips so you may place the pan.

If a patient has difficulty in moving or adjusting to the height of a regular bedpan, follow the same procedure using the fracture pan. The end with the lip is the back of the pan.

The Male Urinal

The male urinal is made of plastic or metal and is so shaped that it can be used by a patient who is supine, lying on the right or left side, or in Fowler's position (Fig. 4–23).). The urinal may be offered to the male patient who is unable to get off of the gurney or examining table to go to the lavatory.

1. If the patient is able to help himself, simply hand him an aseptic urinal and allow him to use it, providing privacy whenever possible.

2. When he has finished, put on clean, disposable gloves, remove the urinal, empty it, and rinse it with cold water. If the urinal is disposable and the patient will not be staying in the diagnostic imaging department long enough to use the urinal a second time, the urinal may be placed in the trash. If the urinal is nondisposable, place it with the soiled supplies to be re-sterilized.

3. Offer the patient a washcloth with which to cleanse his hands.

4. Remove your gloves and wash your own hands.

If a patient is unable to assist himself in using the urinal, you must position the urinal for him.

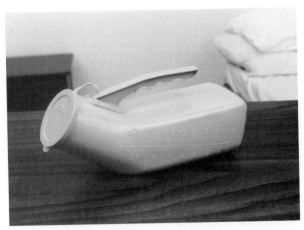

Figure 4–23. Male urinal.

1. Put on clean, disposable gloves; raise the cover sheet sufficiently to permit adequate visibility, but do not expose the patient unduly.

2. Spread the patient's legs and put the urinal between them.

3. Put the penis into the urinal far enough so that it does not slip out, and hold the urinal in place by the handle until the patient finishes voiding.

4. Remove the urinal, empty it, replace it, remove your gloves, and wash your hands.

Departmental Safety

Prevention of patient and personnel injury is the responsibility of all health care workers. It is your responsibility as a radiographer to practice safety in all aspects of your work. This includes fire and electrical safety, prevention of patient or staff falls, prevention of poisoning, and safe disposal of hazardous waste and toxic chemicals.

Institutional, local, state, and federal agencies regulate safety in health care institutions, and there are safety committees in all JCAHO-accredited health care agencies. Fire departments in all cities routinely evaluate the fire safety of health care and community institutions. Poison control centers advise health care institutions if poisoning is possible. The Nuclear Regulatory Commission enforces radiation safety and nuclear medicine standards, and the Environmental Protection Agency establishes guidelines for the disposal of radioactive waste.

Fire Safety

Your obligation as a radiographer is to learn the fire containment guidelines in any institution in which you work as a student or as an employee. You must know the following:

1. The telephone number of the institution for reporting a fire; the number must be posted in a clearly visible location next to the telephone.

2. The agency's fire drill and fire evacuation plan.

3. The location of the fire alarms.

4. The routes of evacuation in case of fire.

5. The locations of fire extinguishers and the correct type of extinguisher for each type of fire.

Carbon dioxide extinguisher: grease or electrical fire

Soda and acid water extinguisher: paper and wood fire

Dry chemical extinguisher: rubbish or wood fire

Antifreeze or water: rubbish, wood, grease, or anesthetic fire

6. A fire must be reported before an attempt is made to extinguish it, regardless of the size.

7. Hallways must be kept free of unnecessary equipment and furniture.

8. Fire hoses must be kept clear at all times.

9. Fire extinguishers must be inspected at regular intervals. Fire drills must be regularly scheduled for agency personnel.

10. Warning signs must be posted stating that, in case of fire, elevators are not to be used and stairways must be used instead.

If fire occurs, the correct procedure for patient safety must be followed:

1. Persons in imminent danger are to be moved out of the area first.

2. Windows and doors are to be closed.

3. If oxygen is in use, it must be turned off.

4. Patient and staff evacuation procedures must be followed.

General rules for the prevention of accidents involving electrical equipment should include the following:

1. Use only grounded electrical plugs (three-pronged) inserted into a grounded outlet.

2. Do not use electrical equipment when hands or feet are wet or when standing in water because water conducts electricity.

3. When removing an electrical plug from an outlet, grasp the plug at its base. Do not pull on the electrical cord.

4. Electrical cords must be unkinked and unfrayed. If they are not, don't use them.

5. Any electrical equipment must be in sound working order to be used for patient care. If it is not, the equipment must be returned to the manufacturer or to the area designated for repair service.

6. All electrical equipment must be tested before it is used for patient care.

7. Report any shocks experienced, and do not use equipment if a patient reports that it gives a tingling feeling or a shock.

8. Do not use a piece of electrical equipment that you do not understand.

9. To prevent falls, do not use extension cords that are not grounded and secured to the floor with electrical tape.

Prevention of Falls

Patient falls are one of the most common hospital accidents. You must always be on guard to prevent falls. No patient should be allowed to get out of a wheelchair or off a gurney or radiographic table without assistance from the radiographer or your designee.

The patients most prone to falls are the frail elderly, persons with neurologic deficits, persons who are weak and debilitated due to prolonged illness or lengthy preparation for procedures, persons with head trauma, persons with sensory deprivations, persons who have been medicated with sedating or psychoactive drugs, and confused patients. You must adhere to the following rules to prevent falls:

1. Learn the condition of your patient and determine whether he or she is safely able to enter, remain in, or leave the diagnostic imaging department without assistance.

2. Keep floors clear of objects that may obstruct pathways.

3. Keep equipment such a gurneys, portable radiographic machines, and wheelchairs in areas where they do not obstruct passageways.

4. Side rails must always be up when a patient is on a gurney.

5. A wheelchair must be locked if a patient is in it; a soft restraint may be needed if the patient is not reliable and may try to get up without assistance.

Poisoning and Disposition of Hazardous Waste Materials

The number of the nearest Poison Control Center must be posted near department telephones. As the radiographer, you must adhere to the following:

1. Any toxic chemical or agent that may poison patients or staff must be clearly labeled as such.

2. These substances must be stored in a safe area designated for them.

3. Emergency instructions to be followed in case of poisoning must be conspicuously posted in the diagnostic imaging department.

4. Chemicals must remain in their own containers marked as toxic substances.

5. Chemical and toxic substances must be disposed of according to federal mandates and institutional policy.

6. Restrictions for disposal of hazardous materials must be posted in a conspicuous area and followed by all in the department.

7. Contrast agents and other drugs must be kept in a safe storage area where access to them is not available to anyone not designated to use them.

8. All containers of hazardous substances must be clearly marked with the name of the substance, a hazard warning, and the name and address of the manufacturer.

9. Hazardous substances may be labeled with a color code that designates the hazard category, for instance, *health*, *flammability*, or *reactivity*.

You must read and fully understand all hazard warnings before using any product, and follow the guidelines as stated on the label. If there is no label or if the label is unclear, don't use the product.

If an accidental spill of a hazardous substance occurs, first aid guidelines are as follows:

Eye contact. Flush eyes with water for 15 minutes or until irritation subsides. Consult a physician immediately.

Skin contact. Remove any affected clothing; wash skin thoroughly with gentle soap and water.

Inhalation. Remove from exposure; if breathing has stopped, begin CPR; call emergency number and a physician.

Ingestion. Do not induce vomiting; call emergency number and Poison Control Center.

Diagnostic imaging personnel must understand the potential hazards of scalds or burns that may occur in their department. Although heating pads and hydrotherapy are not commonly dealt with by radiographers, you must be aware of their potential hazards and refer use of this type of equipment to nurses and those instructed to handle them safely.

Hot beverages must be kept away from children. Coffee and tea equipment used in staff lounges must be kept in safe working order and deactivated when empty or not in use. If a patient is offered a hot beverage, it should be at a temperature that will not scald him or her if it is accidentally spilled.

Radiation Safety

It is your responsibility as a radiographer to protect yourself, the patient, your co-workers, and any person in the vicinity from radiation exposure. While the benefit of rapid medical diagnosis by exposure of the patient to radiation outweighs the associated risks, you need to aim to consistently use the least amount of exposure necessary to achieve this diagnostic end.

Ionizing radiation in excessive amounts or in amounts higher than the accepted level in a brief time period can result in either illness to the recipient or a potential genetic disturbance to the descendants of the recipient. Other factors that can increase the risk of suffering the adverse effects of ionizing radiation are the patient's age at exposure, sensitivity of exposed cells, and the size and area of the body exposed. The very young, the very old, and pregnant women are the most vulnerable to adverse effects of radiation.

Your goal as a radiographer must be to limit the amount of ionizing radiation to acceptable limits in the patient, others in the vicinity, and yourself. To do this, you need to take the following precautions:

1. Maintain exposure to a level *as low as reasonably achievable* (ALARA).

2. Minimize the length of time the patient or others in the vicinity are placed in the path of the x-ray beam.

3. Maximize the distance between the source of the ionizing radiation and the person exposed to it.

4. Maximize the shielding from exposure of the patient and others in the vicinity of the radiation.

Time. Use the shortest exposure time possible. Remember that radiation dosage increases with fluoroscopic imaging.

Distance. The closer a person is to the radiation beam, the greater the exposure. The larger the field of radiation, the greater the risk of scattering the ionizing radiation and the greater the exposure risk. Increasing distance from the source greatly reduces the exposure risk of the radiographer and others in the vicinity.

Shielding. Shielding persons who are unable to reduce their exposure either by limiting time or increasing distance is the third alternative for protection from ionizing radiation. Shielding is done by setting up a protective barrier, usually lead or an equivalent, between the source of the ionizing radiation and the subject involved, whether the patient or others in the vicinity. There are primary and secondary barriers. Primary barriers are usually made of lead or similar material; they are designed to withstand being struck by the beam exiting the x-ray tube without allowing passage of ionizing radiation. Secondary barriers are designed to prevent passage of scatter and leakage, rather than direct, radiation.

The radiographer's obligation is to ascertain that all persons who are involved in or in the vicinity of a radiographic procedure are provided with appropriate protective apparel to shield them from ionizing radiation. This includes the patient, the physician, nurses, observers, and radiographers. Shielding can include a lead apron, lead gloves, a gonadal shield, a thyroid shield, and lead goggles (Fig. 4–24).

Use of gonadal shielding to protect male and female reproductive organs (ovaries and testes) is of vital importance. This is of particular importance when the patient is a child or an adult of childbearing age. There are several types of gonadal shields, including flat and molded contact shields (Fig. 4–25).

You must also use your technical expertise to minimize patient exposure to radiation. This includes beam limitation, technique selection, filtration, intensifying screens, and grids. Explanations of these techniques are beyond the scope of this text; their use is discussed in detail in other radiologic technology courses.

Your responsibility as a radiographer is to understand the technical aspects of the profession so that you can minimize the number of repeat radiographs necessary to achieve a diagnostic purpose. The need to frequently repeat exposures should influence you to put your critical thinking skills to work to assess and solve the problems you are encountering. You must assess your ability to clearly communicate with the patient as well as to keep pace with the necessary technical knowledge.

Estimates of patient exposure to ionizing radiation must be made available in the radiographic imaging department. These estimates denote the amount of radiation an average patient undergoing a given procedure would expect based on standard technique charts. The amount of exposure actually received is then compared with these estimates. All radiographic imaging equipment must also be inspected for radiation safety at regularly scheduled times.

Lead aprons and other protective apparel must be inspected periodically for quality control purposes. This apparel must be hung carefully over a wide bar or on special hangers when not in use. To fold or drop them may jeopardize their integrity.

Any health care worker, including the radiographer, who works in constant contact with ionizing radiation, must be monitored to assess the amount of exposure to it. This may be done by wearing a film badge sensitive to low radiation doses. The badge that you will wear is processed and analyzed at regular time periods. Two other devices that monitor radiation exposure are the thermoluminescent dosimeter and a pocket dosimeter. The thermoluminescent dosimeter is a plastic holder that contains crystals that absorb energy from radiation

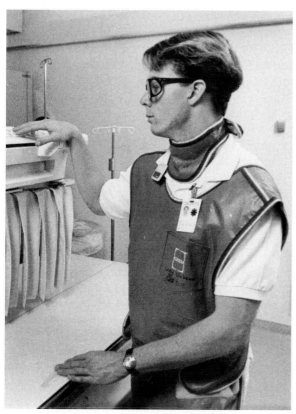

Figure 4–24. Lead apron, thyroid shield, lead goggles, and film badge, another type of shield, known as a shadow shield, is affixed to the tube housing. This type casts a shadow over the patient's body indicating where the shielding is taking place.

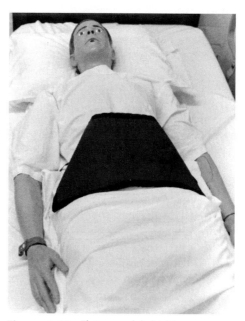

Figure 4–25. Flat gonadal shield.

exposure. The pocket dosimeter is shaped like a penlight and contains a metal electrode surrounded by air. The air, if exposed to ionizing radiation, is ionized and neutralized by the electrode.

Special precautions must be taken to prevent exposing pregnant patients and pregnant health care workers to ionizing radiation. This is particularly true during the early weeks of pregnancy, when particular fetal tissues are especially sensitive to radiation. There is a rule called "the 10-day guideline rule," which states that any woman in her childbearing years who is fertile should limit elective abdominal radiographs to the 10-day period following onset of menstruation. Since this is not a simple rule to follow, it may be used at the discretion of the physician in charge of the patient. Pregnant radiographers must limit their amount of exposure to radiation. The recommended dose limit (not to include medical exposure) for a fetus should not exceed 0.5 rem during the entire period of gestation, and the limit should not exceed 0.05 rem in any month.

To minimize your radiation exposure, you should not hold patients who cannot maintain a particular position during a radiographic procedure. If a patient cannot maintained a position, use bolsters or sandbags. If this is not feasible, a relative or a person who is not working regularly in radiography should be requested to assist.

Summary

When a patient from outside the hospital arrives in the diagnostic imaging department, it is often necessary for that patient to undress entirely or partially for the diagnostic examination or treatment. Always show the patient where and how to do so in a sensitive manner to spare the patient embarrassment.

It is also your responsibility as the radiographer to provide the patient with a safe place for personal belongings. Remember that an article of clothing or jewelry that may not seem valuable to you may be treasured by the patient. Everything that belongs to the patient must be treated as if it were of value.

You must always use correct body mechanics, beginning with good posture. When moving or lifting in the workplace, you should keep your weight close to the body and maintain a firm base of body support. This is accomplished by having your feet slightly spread out and knees flexed. You should twist or bend your body at the waist when lifting a heavy load. Weight should be pulled, not pushed. Use arm and leg muscles, not the spine, for lifting.

The three ways of moving patients are by gurney, by wheelchair, or by ambulation. When moving and lifting patients, you must assess the patient and resolve potential problems before beginning the transfer. The plan for moving the patient should be explained, and the patient's help should be enlisted before beginning. You must always notify the ward personnel when taking a patient to or from his or her room in the hospital. The use of enough assistant and equipment such as a smooth mover facilitates the move and protects you and the patient from possible injury.

When a patient is on the radiographic table or on a gurney in the diagnostic imaging department, his or her body must be in good alignment. If the patient is moved to a particular position for an examination, restore correct body alignment as soon as possible.

There are times when immobilizers must be used for the safety of the adult patient. When immobilizers are required, apply them according to the manufacturer's directions and the policy of the institution. Do not immobilize a patient without an order by a physician. When a patient is immobilized, you must attend to him or her at all times and release the immobilizers at least every 2 hours. You must follow the correct manner of documenting immobilizers.

Take care to prevent the patient's skin from being damaged while being cared for in the diagnostic imaging department. This can be done by preventing injury that may come from immobility, pressure, shearing force, or friction. Patients most susceptible to skin breakdown are the malnourished, the elderly, and the chronically ill. You must take special care to protect these patients from injuries to their integumentary system, because it may result in a decubitus ulcer that can take months to heal. You must also take extra precautions when caring for a patient who is wearing a plaster cast or who is in traction. Observe the patient's extremities for evidence of neurocirculatory impairment, which may result from the pressure of a cast on the skin. Some symptoms of neurocirculatory impairment that are easily detected are pain, coldness, numbness, burning or tingling of fingers or toes, swelling, color changes of the skin, and an inability to move fingers or toes. If you note these symptoms, change the patient's position and report the problem to the physician immediately. Do not release a traction apparatus while taking a radiographic image. If you cannot complete a procedure because of this, you must request assistance from the nurse in charge of the patient.

If a patient is unable to undress alone, you must offer assistance. You should give assistance in a matter-of-fact manner that does not violate the patient's privacy.

Patients must be kept clean and dry while in the diagnostic imaging department. It is the radiographer's duty to change the disabled patient's gown and covering if they become wet or soiled. Do this in a prescribed manner to ensure privacy, safety, and comfort.

Some examinations in the diagnostic imaging department are long and tedious. They often stimulate peristalsis and a need to defecate or urinate. Meeting these needs cannot be postponed. You must be prepared to assist with the bedpan or urinal if necessary, and you should do it in a way that ensures the patient as much privacy as possible.

You must take infection-control measures as you assist with bedpans and urinals. These items must be used for one patient only and then disposed of in the proper waste receptacle or, if not disposable, taken to an area for re-sterilization. You must put on clean, disposable gloves when assisting with the patient's elimination needs, and you must wash your hands after removing the gloves. The patient must not be left unattended while on a bedpan, gurney, or diagnostic imaging table. Patients must never be allowed to get on or off an examining table or out of a wheelchair without assistance. They must also be carefully attended on trips to the lavatory and in a dressing area after an examination or treatment.

You must be constantly on guard to protect patients and other staff members from accidents. Falls are the most common accident in hospitals. If you are knowledgeable about your patients' condition and attend to them carefully when they are in your care, most falls can be prevented.

As the radiographer, you must understand the precautions to take routinely to prevent fire and the correct procedures to follow if a fire occurs. Prevention of accidents due to faulty electrical equipment, poisoning, and correct use and disposal of hazardous materials is also your professional obligation.

You must protect yourself, the patient, and your co-workers from unnecessary exposure to ionizing radiation because excessive amounts, or amounts higher than the accepted level, may adversely affect the person or his descendants. The very young, the very old, and pregnant women are particularly susceptible to adverse effects of ionizing radiation. Precautions to prevent excessive exposure involve knowledge, technical expertise, and constant vigilance as you work.

Chapter 4 Test

_____ 1. When admitting a patient to the diagnostic imaging department, you should
   a. Take the patient to the dressing area and explain in some detail how he or she should dress (or undress) for the procedure
   b. Give the patient directions concerning how to care for purses or valuables brought to the department
   c. Assist any patient who appears to need assistance with preparation for an examination
   d. a and b
   e. a, b, and c

_____ 2. The most effective means of reducing friction when moving a patient is by
   a. Placing the patient's arms across the chest and using a pull sheet
   b. Pushing rather than pulling the patient
   c. Rolling the patient to a prone position
   d. Asking the patient to cooperate with you

_____ 3. When transporting a patient back to this hospital room, some safety measures to be used are
   a. Place the side rails up, the bed in "low" position, and the call bell at hand
   b. Inform the nurse in charge of the patient that the patient has been returned to the room
   c. Give the patient something to eat or drink
   d. a and b
   e. a, b, and c

4. List seven potential problems that you as the radiographer must consider when assessing a patient's ability to move.

_____ **5.** The following procedure(s) must be observed when assisting a patient with a bedpan:
   a. Respect the patient's privacy
   b. Seek assistance for an immobile patient
   c. Wear clean gloves to remove the bedpan
   d. a and c
   e. a, b, and c

6. Match the following patient positions with the correct definition:
   1. Patient on side with forward arm flexed and top knee flexed _____   a. Fowler's position
   2. Semi-sitting position with head raised 45 to 60 degrees _____   b. Supine position
   3. Patient lying flat on back _____   c. Semi-Fowler's position
   4. Patient on back with head lower than extremities _____ d. Trendelenburg position
   5. Patient on back with head raised 15 to 30 degrees _____ e. Sims' position

_____ **7.** Contributing factor(s) to skin breakdown are
   a. Turning every 1 to 2 hours
   b. Friction and pressure
   c. Frequent diagnostic imaging procedures
   d. An unstable environment

8. Two convenient and safe methods of moving a patient from a radiographic table to a gurney are _____ and _____.

9. Describe three legitimate reasons for application of immobilizers to an adult patient.

10. List seven rules to be followed if immobilizers are to be used during patient care in the diagnostic imaging department.

_____ **11.** If a patient who has a cast in place complains of pain that is sudden in onset and increases in intensity when the affected limb is moved, you should
   a. Complete the procedure and discharge the patient
   b. Elevate the affected limb
   c. Notify a physician immediately
   d. Find a nurse to administer pain medication

_____ **12.** When caring for a patient who has a new cast applied to an extremity, you must remember to
   a. Hold the cast firmly at a position between the joints when moving it
   b. Observe for signs of impaired circulation
   c. Support the cast with bolsters and sandbags
   d. a, b, and c
   e. b and c

_____ **13.** When caring for a patient who is disabled and is difficult to move, you must remember that it is essential to
   a. Keep the patient as quiet as possible
   b. Work quickly
   c. Obtain as much help as necessary to avoid injury to the patient and to you
   d. Move the patient by gurney

14. List four signs of circulatory impairment if a patient is wearing a plaster cast.

_____ **15.** The leading cause of work-related injuries in the field of health care is
   a. Bumping into misplaced equipment

b. Overexposure to radiation

c. Poor hand-washing techniques

d. Abuse of the spine when moving and lifting patients

16. List five general rules for correct upright posture.

_____ **17.** It is within your scope of practice as a radiographer to release a traction apparatus if you see fit to do so.

a. True

b. False

18. When moving a heavy object, you should _____ the weight, not _____ it.

19. List eight fire-prevention and containment guidelines that you must learn and use routinely.

20. List the rules to be followed concerning toxic chemicals in the diagnostic imaging department

21. Explain the first-aid precautions to be used in the event of eye or skin contact, inhalation, or ingestion of a toxic chemical.

22. List four precautions that you must use to protect yourself and others from overexposure to ionizing radiation.

_____ **23.** When moving a patient into an unnatural position for a radiographic examination, the patient should maintain that position

a. Until he or she asks to be moved

b. Until the film is developed and approved by the radiologist

c. Only for the time it takes to make the exposure

d. a and b

e. b and c

24. List the four areas of the body that are most susceptible to skin breakdown.

_____ **25.** Patients most prone to falls are

a. The frail elderly

b. The person who is confused

c. Persons who have been given a psychoactive drug

d. Persons with sensory deficits

e. a, b, c, and d

_____ **26.** A student radiographer must take repeat radiographs on patients several times owing to their poor quality. The student must question his or her

a. Technical knowledge

b. Lack of concern for the patient

c. Communication skills

d. a and b

e. a and c

27. Explain precautions to be taken by the radiographer who is 8 weeks pregnant.

_____ **28.** A 4-year-old girl is in the diagnostic imaging department for skull radiographs after falling out of a grocery cart. She is accompanied by her mother. The child is screaming and flailing about. You are assigned to her care and are concerned that you will be unable to obtain satisfactory radiographs. Her radiographs are important to her diagnosis because skull fracture is suspected; however, she is in danger of falling from the table in her agitated state. Your best approach to his problem would be to

a. Put on a lead apron and lead gloves and hold her yourself while another radiographer takes the radiograph

b. Ask another radiographer to hold the child

c. Send the child home until she is more tranquil

d. Ask the child's mother to hold her

e. Sedate her and then proceed

_____ **29.** Which is the best way to move a patient from a gurney to a radiographic table?

a. Log roll

b. Sheet transfer

c. Smooth mover and three assistants

d. Four assistants

30. Where is the radiographer's center of gravity?

_____ **31.** What is not a safety precaution that you must take when returning a patient to bed?

a. Lower the bed to its lowest point

b. Make sure the bedside table is over the side of the bed

c. Make sure that the side rails are in their upright and locked position

d. Place the call button within reach of the patient

32. Briefly describe how to move a patient who needs only minimal assistance from bed to wheelchair.

33. When assisting a patient on a bedpan, should the handle of the fracture pan be located toward the patient's back or between the patient's legs?

34. What are the three methods of reducing exposure to ionizing radiation?

35. Name three types of shields used in patient protection.

5

Surgical Asepsis and the Radiographer

Objectives

After studying this chapter, you will be able to:

1. Define surgical asepsis and differentiate between medical asepsis and surgical asepsis.
2. Explain the radiographer's responsibility for maintaining surgical aseptic technique when it is a required part of patient care.
3. Differentiate between disinfection and sterilization.
4. Explain the methods you must use as a radiographer to determine the sterility of an item or pack to be opened and used for an invasive procedure.
5. List the rules for surgical asepsis.
6. Demonstrate the correct method of opening a sterile

pack and of placing a sterile object on a sterile field.
7. Demonstrate the correct method of putting on a sterile gown and sterile gloves.
8. Demonstrate the skin preparation for a sterile procedure.
9. Explain your responsibilities for the safety of the surgical team, the patient, and yourself in the operating room.
10. Demonstrate the correct method of removing and reapplying a sterile dressing.

Glossary

Antimicrobial: Any substance or procedure that kills microorganisms or suppresses their multiplication

Depilatory agent: An agent that causes the falling out of hair

Fenestrated: Having one or more openings

Invasive: Involving puncture or incision of the skin or insertion of an instrument or injection of foreign material into the body

Ratchet: The section of the forceps that allows an instrument to remain closed and firmly locked until released

Surgical asepsis differs from medical asepsis. Medical asepsis is defined as any practice that helps reduce the number and spread of microorganisms. *Surgical asepsis* is defined as the complete removal of microorganisms and their spores from the surface of an object. The practice of surgical asepsis begins with cleaning the object in question using the principles of medical asepsis. A sterilizing process using the technique recommended for that item follows. Various applications of heat or chemical action accomplish total removal of microorganisms and spores.

Any medical procedure that involves penetration of body tissues (an invasive procedure) requires the use of surgical aseptic technique. This includes major and minor surgical procedures, administration of parenteral medications, invasive radiographic imaging procedures, catheterization of the urinary bladder, tracheostomy care, and dressing changes.

As a radiographer, you will be frequently required to go to the operating room (also called the OR or surgical suite) to perform diagnostic radiography during surgical procedures. Because surgical asepsis is also routinely practiced in the special procedures areas of the radiographic imaging department, you must be familiar with the required procedures.

Before any invasive procedure can be performed, the patient's skin must be prepared (skin prep). The purpose of a skin prep is to remove oils, dirt, and as many microorganisms as possible before the procedure. This prevents contamination of the operative site, thereby reducing chances of infection. Hair is considered to be a contaminant and is frequently removed from the skin surrounding the operative site. Because you may be responsible for the skin prep in your own department, you must learn to perform this procedure effectively.

Occasionally, a physician may request you to remove a patient's dressing or reapply a simple sterile dressing. If not performed correctly, this procedure is another potential source of contamination for the patient or for you.

You must be able to recognize breaches in aseptic technique and also be able to remedy the problem quickly. If not, contamination will go unrecognized, and infection may result. It is the duty of all health care workers who participate in procedures requiring the use of surgical asepsis to be able to maintain strict surgical aseptic technique at all times because the patient's well-being is at stake.

The Environment and Surgical Asepsis

To review, the methods of transmission are by direct and indirect contact, by droplet, by vehicle, and by airborne route. (The means of transmission of microorganisms are discussed in detail in Chapter 3.) Every possible effort is made in the surgical suite and in special procedures areas to protect the patient from infection. Creating an environment that establishes barriers that limit the source of contamination does this. All persons who enter the surgical suite are expected to follow the rules established to maintain these barriers.

Surgical departments have dress and behavior protocols that are strictly enforced. The radiographer who is assigned to work in this area is expected to follow these protocols. You should wear comfortable, supportive shoes. You should not wear clogs, sandals, and cloth shoes because they may not be safe. You must have meticulous personal hygiene, and you must take a shower shortly before reporting for work in the OR.

Jewelry, long fingernails, artificial fingernails, and polish are prohibited because they harbor microorganisms. Any health care worker who has an acute infection or open skin lesion must not work in the surgical suite or special procedures area because of an increased potential for infecting the patient.

There are three zones designated in the surgical suite to help decrease the incidents of infection. The first zone is considered to be an unrestricted zone, where persons may enter in street clothing. The second is a semirestricted zone, where only persons who are dressed in scrub clothing with hair covered and shoes covered may enter. The third zone is a restricted zone, and only persons wearing scrub suits, hair coverings, shoe covers, and masks are allowed. If a surgical or invasive procedure is in progress, the doors of this area are kept closed, and only persons directly involved in the procedure may be present. Those who are directly involved in the operation are dressed in sterile gowns and gloves.

All persons who expect to proceed from the unrestricted zone of the operating suite into the semirestricted zone must go into a dressing area, don a scrub suit, and tuck the blouse of the suit into the pants or wear a scrub blouse that is close to the body. The hair and beard or mustache, if present, must be covered with a surgical cap. All hair must be confined, since hair harbors many microorganisms that may be shed with movement (Fig. 5–1). Shoe covers are placed over shoes to reduce contamination in many institutions. You must then scrub your hands and arms as described for medical asepsis before proceeding into the restricted zone of the surgical suite, the special procedures room, the neonatal intensive care unit, or the neonatal nursery. It is believed that the bare skin may shed microorganisms. Because of this, in some surgical suites, persons in the OR who are not in sterile gown and gloves must wear a scrub jacket to help prevent any shedding from bare arms.

Before entering the OR when a surgical procedure is in progress, all personnel must don a surgical

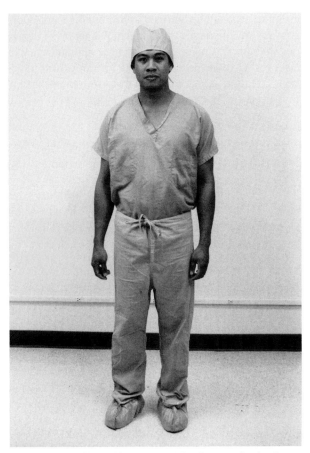

Figure 5–1. The scrub suit must fit close to the body. Cover all hair with a scrub cap.

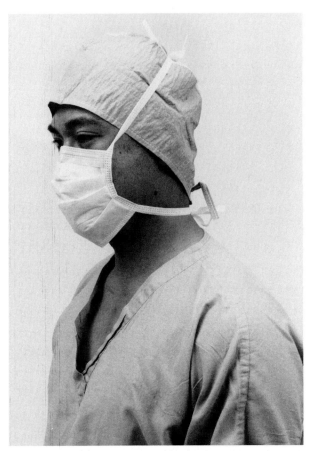

Figure 5–2. The mask must cover nose and mouth, and ties should not cross.

mask. The person participating in the surgical procedure must first perform a surgical scrub (described later in this chapter). The surgical mask protects the patient from droplet contamination by a health care worker; however, it also protects the health care worker from airborne pathogenic microbes that may be released during a surgical procedure. A single, high-filtration mask is recommended. It must cover the nose and mouth and must not gap. The ties should not cross because it may create venting (Fig. 5–2)). A mask is worn for only one procedure and then discarded. Never place a mask around your neck for re-use. When removing, handle masks only by the ties and discard them in a receptacle for this purpose, since they are considered highly contaminated (Fig. 5–3).

Sterile linens and other equipment and supplies used for sterile procedures must be packaged in a particular manner to be considered safe for use. They must also be stored in a manner that protects them from contamination.

Any break in sterile technique increases the patient's susceptibility to infection. Those involved in carrying out a sterile procedure must constantly be aware of which areas and articles are sterile. If a ster-

ile article is touched by a nonsterile one, it must be replaced by an article that is sterile. A contaminated area must be made sterile again. You need to learn and follow correct sterilization techniques. You must also learn correct methods of opening sterile packs and donning sterile gown and gloves.

The use of contaminated instruments or gloves, a wet or damp sterile field, and microorganisms blown onto a surgical site are the most common causes of contamination. Ventilating ducts must have special filters to prevent dust particles from entering the room.

Airflow in the OR should be unidirectional, and the air pressure in the room should be greater than in the outside corridors. Humidity in the OR should also be controlled to prevent static electricity. Doors to the OR must always be kept closed during a surgical procedure and traffic in and out of the room strictly controlled.

When you need to use radiographic equipment in the OR, you must clean it with a disinfectant solution before bringing it into the area. Many hospitals have radiographic equipment that is never removed from the surgical suite, and it is routinely cleaned by the housecleaning department before every use.

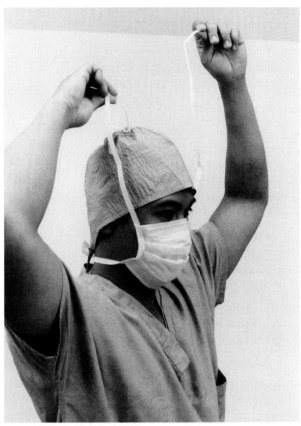

Figure 5–3. When removing, handle the mask only by the ties.

Conversation in the OR or special procedures rooms is kept to a minimum. You must always be aware that the surgeon is in charge while performing a surgical or invasive procedure. The environment is often tense because the patient's life is at risk and needless conversation is not welcome.

The radiographer or student radiographer whose work involves sterile procedures must develop a sense of responsibility and maintain the highest standards possible when practicing surgical asepsis. The patient's welfare depends on this.

The Surgical Team

The surgical team consists of a variety of staff members who serve the patient during surgery. They are as follows:

Surgeon: the physician who plans and performs the surgical procedure and makes the surgical decisions

Surgical assistant: usually another surgeon, who may be a resident physician; there may be several assistants if the patient's surgical needs require this

Anesthesiologist: a physician with special education in anesthesiology, who makes the decisions concerning type of anesthesia required

Nurse anesthetist: a registered nurse who has had special education in anesthesiology who administers anesthesia and monitors the anesthetized patient under the supervision of the anesthesiologist

Radiologic technologist: present to perform imaging procedures

Diagnostic imaging is increasingly used in surgical procedures. Some of the operative procedures that require the use of imaging either before surgical intervention or during the surgical procedure are operative cholangiograms, ureteral retrogrades, and ureteral stent placement; reconstructive orthopedics; tube and pacemaker placement; determination of the extent of trauma; and determination of the presence of foreign objects such as needles, bullets, and sponges.

Many of these procedures are planned, and the radiographer is in the OR during the entire surgery. On some occasions, the need for a radiographer is not planned, and you may be called to come to the OR at a moment's notice. Although you are not usually required to don sterile garments, you must wear a scrub suit, cap, and mask while in the surgical suite and scrub as for medical asepsis.

Many other members of the surgical team work behind the scenes to prepare surgical packs; procure, clean, and repair instruments; and limit contamination of the surgical suite.

Methods of Sterilization

Removal of microorganisms and their spores must be complete, or the article is not sterile. Methods used to attain sterilization depend on the nature of the item to be sterilized. All effective methods of sterilization have advantages and disadvantages. The packaging and sterilizing of items used for medical purposes has become a highly specialized field and is described only briefly in this text, since it is usually not in the scope of the radiographer's practice. Methods currently in use for sterilization are listed in Table 5-1.

Whatever method of sterilization is used, there are indicators placed in the center and outside of each pack to be sterilized. When the indicator changes color, it is proof that the contents of the pack have been exposed to the sterilization method sufficiently to change the color of the indicator. There are variations among indicators, and you must familiarize yourself with the types that are used in your place of employment.

Disinfection

All items that penetrate the skin or mucous membranes must be sterile. Articles or surfaces that cannot be sterilized in the OR or in the special procedures

---

TABLE 5-1
Methods of Sterilization

TYPE OF STERILIZER	USE
Steam sterilizers	Steam under pressure is effective and convenient for many items. They are called autoclaves and are manufactured to sterilize by the following methods: gravity-displacement; pulsing gravity; prevacuum; abbreviated prevacuum cycle; and high-speed, also called flash sterilization.
Chemical sterilization	Also referred to as *cold sterilization* and used for items that can not withstand heat to be rendered sterile. Aqueous glutaraldehyde and peracetic acid are the chemicals often used.
Gas ethylene oxide sterilization	Used for items that cannot withstand moisture and high temperatures. All items sterilized in this manner must be cleaned and dried since water united with ethylene oxide forms ethylene glycol, which cannot be eliminated by aeration and is toxic. All gas-sterilized items must be properly aerated before use.
Gas plasma sterilization	Plasma is a highly ionized gas usually made with vaporized hydrogen peroxide or peracetic acid. It provides a nontoxic, dry, low-temperature, time efficient means of sterilization for many items.

---

area must be disinfected. Tables, floors, walls, and equipment used in areas where the patient is to have an invasive procedure are included in this category. Skin around the area to be penetrated is also disinfected. When skin is disinfected, the solutions used are called *antiseptics*. The term *disinfection* means that as many microorganisms as possible are eliminated from the surfaces by physical or chemical means. Spores are often not destroyed by disinfection. *Germicides* are solutions that destroy microorganisms. Some germicides are antiseptics and disinfectants.

Chemical disinfectants are numerous and vary in their effectiveness for destroying microorganisms. The nature of the contamination and the area or object to be disinfected are also taken into consideration when a disinfectant is selected for use. The manufacturer's directions must be followed carefully when using any chemical.

Disinfectants are categorized as high level, intermediate level, or low level, according to their effectiveness. Some commonly used disinfectants are listed in Table 5-2). To destroy spores, the disinfectant must

---

TABLE 5-2
Commonly Used Disinfectants

HIGH LEVEL	
2% Activated glutaraldehyde	Effective against *Mycobacterium tuberculosis*, fungi, most bacteria, and spores at required length of time; used to disinfect surgical instruments that cannot withstand heat
INTERMEDIATE LEVEL	
Isopropyl alcohol 70% or 90%	Effective against vegetative bacteria, fungi, and viruses including HIV and HBV; used as a disinfectant and an antiseptic
Iodine and iodophor	Effective against vegetative bacteria, *Mycobacterium tuberculosis*, most viruses, and fungi; not sporicidal; used most often as an antiseptic
LOW LEVEL	
Hydrogen peroxide	Effective against some bacteria, fungi, and viruses; not used widely as a disinfectant
Phenolic compounds	Most are effective against the tubercle bacilli, bacteria, and fungi; used mostly for cleaning walls, furniture, and so on
Chlorine compounds	Effective against gram-negative bacteria, viruses, and *Pseudomonas*; used most often as a disinfectant for countertops and other surfaces to be disinfected

be one of high level, and the object to be disinfected must remain in the solution for a longer period of time. The tubercle bacillus and other vegetative bacteria are highly resistant to disinfectants. A high-level disinfectant must be used for a longer time interval to destroy these bacteria.

Physical methods of disinfecting are boiling in water and ultraviolet irradiation. Boiling may be used as a means of disinfection if no other method is available; however, many spores are able to resist the heat of boiling (212°F or 100°C) for many hours. To increase the effectiveness of boiling, sodium carbonate may be added to the water in quantity to make a 2% solution. It should not be added if the material being boiled is made of rubber, because sodium carbonate destroys the rubber. If an object is to be disinfected by boiling and sodium carbonate is added to the water, it should be boiled for 15 minutes. If sodium carbonate has not been added, boiling time should be 30 minutes.

Ultraviolet rays kill microorganisms when they come into direct contact with them. This is not a practical means of disinfecting for hospital use, because there is no assurance that the ultraviolet has actually come into contact with microbes, which are in a constantly mobile state because of air currents.

Packing and Storing Sterile Supplies

Several acceptable materials can be used for packaging items that are to be sterilized: cloth, nonwoven fabrics, paper, and plastic. Whichever material is chosen, the following restrictions must be considered:

1. The sterilizing agent must be able to penetrate the material.

2. The sterilizing agent must be able to escape at the end of the sterilizing procedure.

3. Items packaged must be covered completely by the wrapper and securely fastened with tape or a heat seal that does not lend itself to re-use.

4. Pins, staples, or other sharp, penetrating objects must not be used to fasten packages, because they allow a port for contaminants to enter the pack when removed.

5. Contents must be identifiable, and evidence of exposure to the sterilizing agent must be present. Indicator tape with stripes that change color when exposed to the sterilizing agent is the most frequently used.

6. Packaging must be impermeable to dust, microbe, and moisture and must be able to maintain the sterility of the contents until opened.

7. The wrapper must be strong enough to remain damage-free.

8. Items must be wrapped to allow opening and removing them without contamination.

9. The wrapping material must be free of toxic ingredients and dyes and must be economical.

A special area is designated in hospitals for the preparation of sterile supplies by a method that is followed at all times. Cloth wrappers are made of muslin of a specified weight. If this material is used for wrapping, it must be used in quadruple thickness, usually accomplished by using two double-thickness wrappers together. Nonwoven fabrics are available in three thicknesses: light, medium, and heavy. Lightweight nonwoven fabrics must be used in four thicknesses and medium-weight in double thickness. Heavyweight nonwoven material is usually used for surgical drapes in single thickness.

All sterile items are stored in the same place, separate from nonsterile items. A sterile package must have an expiration date printed on it. You must check the sterilization date carefully to be certain that the shelf life (the time that the package may be considered sterile while being stored) has not been exceeded. If there is no date on the package, consider it nonsterile.

All storage areas for sterile materials must be clean, dust-free, vermin-free, and draft-free. Generally speaking, items that have been sterilized in the hospital and wrapped in cloth or paper wrappers are considered sterile for 30 days if they are in a closed cupboard. If they are on an open shelf, they are considered sterile for 21 days. Extremes of temperature and humidity must be avoided, and traffic in the storage area should be light. Items sealed in plastic bags immediately after sterilization are considered sterile for 6 to 12 months, provided the seal is not broken.

Commercially packaged sterilized items are considered sterile until the seal is broken or the package has been damaged or until the expiration date on the package has passed.

Rules for Surgical Asepsis

The basic rules for surgical aseptic technique apply whenever and wherever the sterile procedure is done. You must commit these rules to memory and use them in your own department and in the OR:

1. Know which areas and objects are sterile and which are not.

2. If the sterility of an object is questionable, it is *not* to be considered sterile.

3. Sterile objects and persons must be kept separate from those that are nonsterile.

4. When any item that must be sterile becomes contaminated, the contamination must be remedied immediately.

5. When tabletops are to be used as areas for creating a sterile field, they must be clean, and a sterile drape must be placed over them.

6. Personnel must be clothed in a sterile gown and gloves if they are to be considered sterile.

7. Any sterile instrument or sterile area that is touched by a nonsterile object or person is considered contaminated by microorganisms.

8. A contaminated area on a sterile field must be covered by a folded sterile towel or a drape of double thickness.

9. If a sterile person's gown or gloves become contaminated, they must be changed.

10. A sterile field must be created just before use.

11. Once a sterile field has been prepared, it must not be left unattended, because it may become contaminated accidentally and be presumed to be sterile.

12. A nonsterile person does not reach across a sterile field.

13. A sterile person does not lean over a nonsterile area.

14. A sterile field ends at the level of the tabletop or at the waist of the sterile person's gown.

15. Anything that drops below the tabletop or a sterile person's waistline is no longer sterile. The only parts of a sterile gown considered sterile are the areas from the waist to the shoulders in front and the sleeves from 2 inches above the elbow to the cuffs.

16. The cuffs of the sterile gown are considered nonsterile because they collect moisture. Always cover the cuffs of the sterile gown with sterile gloves.

17. The edges of a sterile wrapper are not considered sterile and must not touch a sterile object.

18. Any part of a sterile drape that falls below the tabletop is considered nonsterile and is not brought up to table level.

19. Sterile drapes are placed by a sterile person, who drapes the area closest to him or her first to protect the sterile gown.

20. A sterile person must remain within the sterile area. He or she does not lean on tables or against the wall.

21. If one sterile person must pass another, they must pass each other back-to-back.

22. The sterile person faces the sterile field and keeps sterile glove hand above the waist and in front of the chest. The sterile person avoids touching any area of his or her own body.

23. Any sterile material or pack that becomes dampened or wet is considered nonsterile.

24. Any objects that are wet with sporicidal solution and are placed on the sterile field must be placed on a folded sterile towel for the moisture to be absorbed.

25. A wet area on a sterile field must be covered with several thicknesses of sterile toweling or an impervious drape.

26. All areas that are used for sterile procedures, including floors, should be well cleaned with disinfectant solution after each procedure. Mops should be disposable and used only one time.

27. Air-conditioning units must be kept clean, and filters should be changed frequently to prevent bacteria from blowing on sterile fields.

28. Ventilation ducts must have special filters to prevent particles from entering the OR or special procedures room.

29. When pouring a sterile solution, place the lid face upward and do not touch the inside of the lid or the lip of the flask. Pour off a small amount of solution before the remainder is poured into the sterile container.

30. When a sterile solution is to be poured into a container on a sterile field, the container is placed at the edge of the sterile field by the sterile person (Fig. 5–4).

CALL OUT!

If the sterility of an item is questionable, it is not to be considered sterile.

Opening Sterile Packs

You must be prepared to open sterile packs and either place their contents on the sterile field or hand them to the sterile person without contaminating them. There is a standard method for this procedure, which you will be able to do without difficulty after it is practiced.

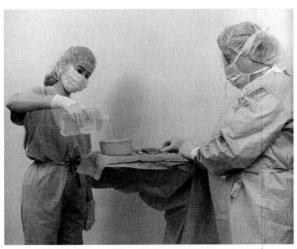

Figure 5–4. Place container at edge of sterile field, and pour from a distance that prevents contamination.

Cloth-Wrapped Packs

You should already have washed your hands. When a request for a sterile item is received, obtain the correct pack and return it to the procedures room. A cloth-wrapped pack is sealed with indicator tape. The lines in the tape are dark gray if the pack has been correctly sterilized.

Place the pack on a clean tabletop with the sealed end toward you (Fig. 5–5). Opening a sterile pack involves the following steps:

1. Remove the tape from a cloth wrapped pack and discard it. If it is a commercial pack, remove the outer protective wrapper and place it with the sealed end toward you (see Fig. 5–5A).

2. Open corner 1 back and away from the pack (see Fig. 5–5B).

3. Next, open corners 2 and 3 (see Fig. 5–5C and D).

4. Then, open corner 4, and drop it toward your body (see Fig. 5–5E).

5. Do not touch the sterile contents of the pack. This can now become a sterile field, and more sterile items may be placed in the center of the drape, or the sterile contents of the pack can now be placed on another sterile field.

6. To move the contents to another sterile field, grasp the underside of the wrapper and let the edges fall over your hand.

7. Hold the contents forward for the sterile person to grasp (see Fig. 5–5F). If it is preferable that you place the contents on the sterile field, grasp the corners of the wrapper with the other hand so that they do not brush the field.

8. While maintaining a safe margin of distance from the sterile field, grasp the ends of the open wrapper, and gently flip the object onto the sterile field being careful not to contaminate the field (see Fig. 5–5G).

Commercial Packs

Commercial packs are usually wrapped in paper or plastic wrappers. They are frequently sealed in plastic to ensure prolonged sterility. Directions for opening the containers in such a way that there is no contamination are printed on the pack and should be read before opening. The most common type of pack is sealed at the edges. The seal can be separated at the top and peeled back until the sterile article is exposed. The pack can either be opened completely and the contents made available for the sterile person to pick up, or the contents can be dropped onto the sterile field. Never cut packs open or pierce with a knife or sharp object. Do not tear packs open, and do not allow the contents to slide over the edges of the pack. They should be flipped or lifted out.

Sterile Forceps

A sterile forceps, usually a large, serrated ring forceps with ratchet closures, may be used to transfer an object from one sterile area to another. In this case, obtain a forceps packaged in a sterile wrapper. Open the wrapper as directed above, and proceed as follows:

1. Grasp the forceps by the handle with clean hands. Open the ratchet and grasp the object to be transferred with the serrated ring at the end of the forceps. Be careful not to contaminate the sterile end of the forceps.

2. Close the ratchet around the object to be transferred.

3. Transfer the object to the new location on the sterile field.

4. Open the ratchet and drop the sterile object onto the sterile field (Fig. 5–6).

5. Place the forceps into the soiled article container.

Do not use the forceps more than one time for each object to be transferred. If needed a second time, obtain another forceps.

The Surgical Scrub

Although as the radiographer you are not often the "sterile person" in the OR or special procedures room,

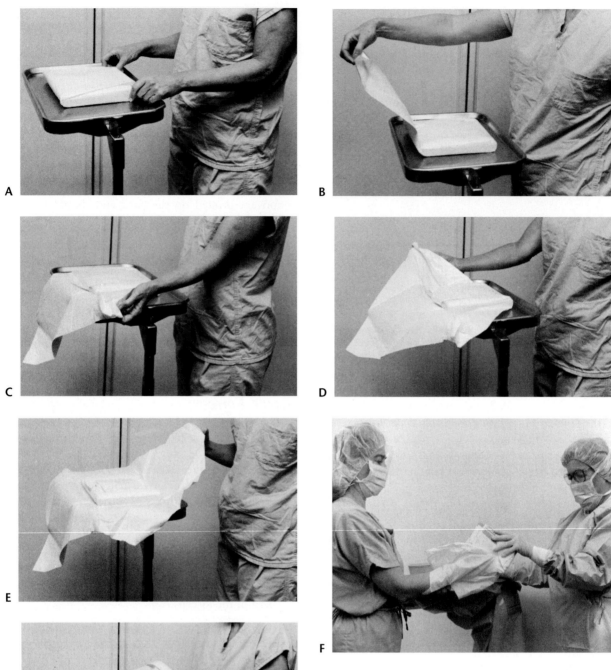

Figure 5–5. (**A**) Begin opening sterile pack with sealed end toward you. (**B**) Break seal and move first corner of wrapper back and away from you. (**C** and **D**) Open the next two corners of the pack to the left and right, respectively. (**E**) Open the fourth corner by dropping it toward you. (**F**) Contents of sterile pack are held out for the sterile person to grab. (**G**) Contents of sterile pack are flipped onto the sterile field.

you must be able to perform the surgical scrub if the situation calls for it. To begin, change regular exterior clothing for a scrub suit, and place shoe covers over your shoes. The shoe covers are made of heavy paper and have built-in conductive strip that prevents the production of static electricity. Then put on a surgical cap or hood to cover all hair. Hoods are used if the person has a beard. Remove all jewelry. If you are wearing pierced ear studs, make sure they are covered by the cap.

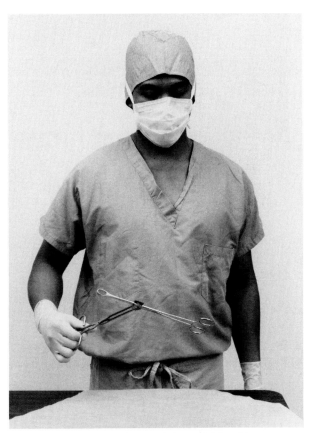

Figure 5–6. Open ratchet and drop sterile object on sterile field.

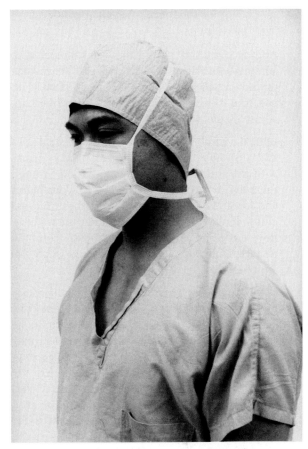

Figure 5–7. Mask must cover nose and mouth.

Fingernails must be short and in good condition. Open areas or lesions on or around the nails or hands harbor additional microorganisms that may infect the patient. Do not wear artificial nails or nail additives, since they may harbor additional microbes and fungi.

If the procedure to be performed in the OR or special procedures room involves fluoroscopy or if the team is unable to protect themselves while radiographic exposures are being taken, all must wear protective lead garments over the scrub suits and under the sterile gowns. These protective garments, which should include a lead apron, a thyroid shield, and special glasses, should be put on before the surgical scrub is begun.

Remove a face mask from the container. Handle this mask by the ties only. Place the mask on your face so that it covers your nose and mouth (Fig. 5–7). Tie it at the back of the head and neck, and check for comfort and security. Never touch the mask after it is in place, because it quickly becomes contaminated. Change masks between each procedure, and never wear it around the neck to be pulled up again over the face.

At this point, the procedure varies with the OR assignment. If you are to take radiographic exposures, you should scrub for 3 minutes with an antiseptic soap, dry your hands with paper towels, and proceed to your position in the OR. If you are to put on a sterile gown and gloves, you must do a surgical scrub. Scrub tops are not allowed to become wet during the scrub.

The procedure for the surgical scrub varies from hospital to hospital, but either the timed method or the brush stroke method is used. Some institutions require an initial 10-minute scrub and subsequent 5-minute or reduced brush stroke scrubs for each case after the initial scrub during a 24-hour period. The suggested number of brush strokes is 30 strokes to the nails of each hand and 20 strokes to each area of the hands and forearms. The fingers should be scrubbed as if they have four sides. The antimicrobial agents most commonly used for the surgical scrub at this time are an iodine complex and detergent (iodophor) and, in case of allergy, parachlorometaxylenol (chloroxylenol, PCMX).

The purpose of the surgical scrub is to remove as many microorganisms as possible from the skin of the hands and lower arms by mechanical and chemical means and running water before a sterile procedure. Before beginning the procedure, make sure your arms are bare to at least 4 inches above your elbows. You must put on a lead apron before beginning the scrub.

The procedure for the timed or stroke method surgical scrub is as follows:

1. Approach the sink. Adjust the water temperature and pressure. Most surgical scrub areas have knee or foot regulators for water faucets. If they do not, the faucet handles should be turned on, adjusted, and not touched again.

2. Obtain a scrub brush. Brushes must be single use and disposable. Combination sponge brushes with the antimicrobial agent permeated through them are most commonly used. Wet your hands and forearms to approximately 2 inches from the elbow. Hold your hands up and allow the water to flow downward toward your elbows from the cleanest area to the least clean area, and apply the antimicrobial agent (Fig. 5–8*A*).

3. Scrub your hands and arms using a firm rotary motion. Fingers, hands, and arms should be considered to have four sides, all of which must be thoroughly cleaned. Follow an anatomical pattern, beginning with the thumb and proceeding to each finger. Next, do the dorsal surface of the hand, the palm, and up the wrist, ending 2 inches above the elbow. Wash all four sides of the arm. Scrubbing for the OR always begins with the hands because they are in direct contact with the sterile field (see Fig. 5–8*B*).

4. A nail cleaner is included with the scrub brush. After the first hand and arm scrub, clean under each fingernail with this nail cleaner and dispose of it (see Fig. 5–8*C*). Rinse hands and arms, and rescrub in the same pattern until all brush strokes are complete or until the time is up (see Fig. 5–8*D*).

5. When you have completed the scrub, drop the brush into the sink or a receptacle prepared to receive the used brushes. Do not touch the sink or the receptacle. Remember to hold your hands up above the waist and higher than the elbows during and after the surgical scrub.

6. Proceed to the area where a sterile towel, sterile gown, and sterile gloves have been prepared for you.

7. Pick up the sterile towel, which is folded on top of the sterile gown, by one corner, and let it unfold in front of you at waist level. Do not let the towel touch your scrub suit (see Fig. 5–8*E*).

8. Dry one hand and one arm with each end of the towel. Do not go back over areas already dried.

9. When your hands and arms are thoroughly dry, drop the towel to the floor or into a receptacle for this purpose, being careful to keep hands held up above the waist (see Fig. 5–8*F*).

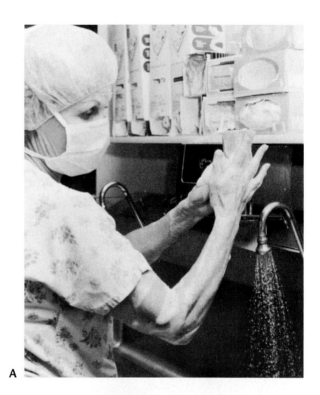

A

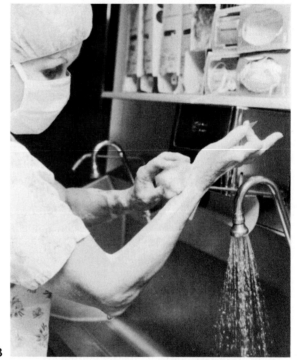

B

Figure 5–8. Radiographer must don lead apron prior to surgical scrub. (**A**) Hold hands upward during surgical scrub and allow water to flow towards the elbows. (**B**) Begin surgical scrub by washing all sides of the hands. (**C**) Clean under each fingernail with nail cleaner in package. (**D**) Rinse hands and arms beginning with the hands. (**E**) Pick up sterile towel and allow it to unfold. Do not let towel touch scrub suit. (**F**) Do not go over area already dried. Drop towel when drying complete.

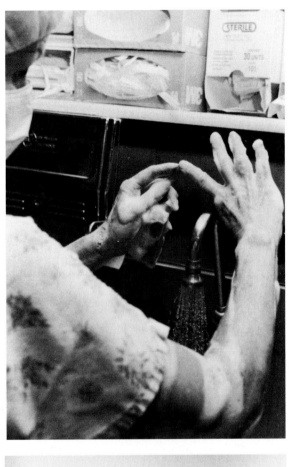

C

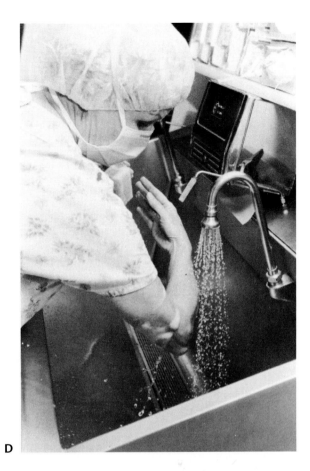

D

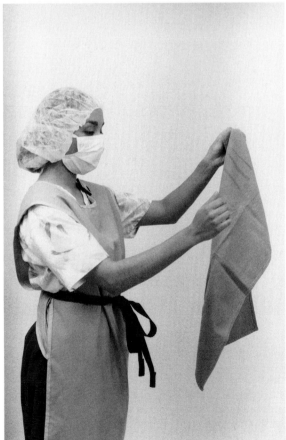

E

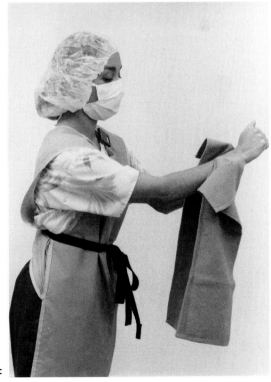

F

Figure 5–8. (continued)

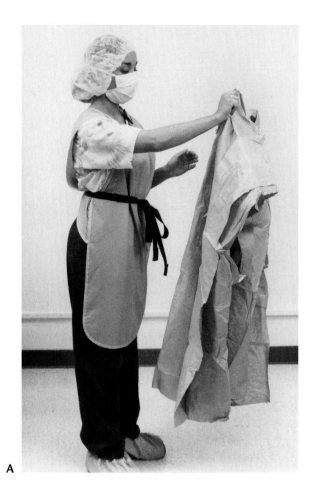

A

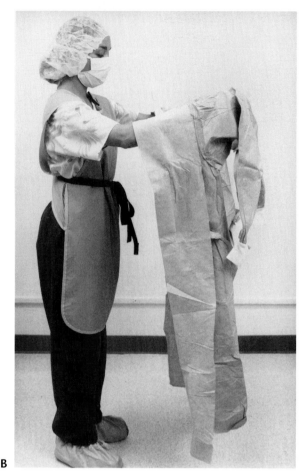

B

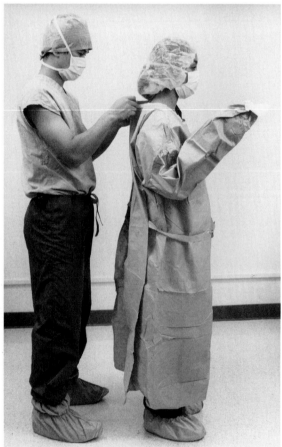

C

Figure 5–9. (**A**) Pick up the sterile gown by holding it at the shoulder seams and then allow it to unfold in front of you. (**B**) Place both arms into the armholes and wait for assistance. (**C**) Cuffs of gown sleeves are left covering the hands if closed-gloving technique is to be used.

Sterile Gowning and Gloving

If you must open your own sterile gown and glove packs, do this before the surgical scrub. Usually, an assistant is on hand to do this for the person who is scrubbing.

Gowning

The sterile gown is made either of a synthetic nonwoven material or of cloth. To put it on, follow these simple steps:

1. Grasp the gown and remove it from the table.

2. Step away from the table. The gown will be folded inside out.

3. Hold the gown away from your body, and allow it to unfold lengthwise without touching the floor (Fig. 5–9*A*).

4. Open the gown and hold it by the shoulder seams. Place both arms into the armholes of the gown and wait for assistance (see Fig. 5–9*B*).

5. Your assistant or the circulating nurse will place your hands into the inside of the gown at the shoulders and pull the gown over your shoulders and arms until your hands are exposed if open-gloving technique is to be used. If closed-gloving technique is to be used, the cuffs of the gown sleeves will be left to cover your hands (see Fig. 5–9*C*).

Gloving

There are two methods of gloving for sterile procedures: open and closed. For the radiographer's purposes, the open method is more practical. Setting up for a sterile procedure, as well as performing certain minor sterile procedures, requires the use of sterile gloves, but not a sterile gown. In this case, you should wash your hands according to the rules of medical sepsis described in Chapter 3 and proceed with gloving by the open method.

Open the glove wrapper, and expose the gloves. Sterile gloves are always packaged folded down at the cuff and powdered so that they may be put on more easily.

1. Glove the dominant hand first. Assuming that the right is your dominant hand, pick up the right glove with the left hand at the folded cuff and slide the right hand into the glove, leaving the cuff of the glove folded down.

2. When the glove is over your hand, leave it and pick up the left glove with your gloved right hand under the fold (Fig. 5–10*A*). Pull the glove over

your hand and over the cuff of the gown in one motion (see Fig. 5–10*B*).

3. Then place the fingers of your gloved left hand under the cuff of the right glove, and pull it over the cuff of the gown. After the cuffs of the gloves cover the cuffs of the sterile gown, you can adjust the gloves (see Fig. 5–10*C* and *D*).

Closed Gloving

Closed gloving must be practiced several times before it is perfected. As the radiographer, you must not be discouraged if you contaminate your gloves the first few times that you put them on. The important thing is to notice when the gloves become contaminated and to ask for another pair.

The closed method is restricted for use when a sterile gown has already been put on and the hands remain enclosed within the cuffs of the gown. The sterile glove pack is opened before the procedure begins.

1. With your left hand (or nondominant hand) covered by the gown sleeve cuff, pick up the right glove and place it palm-side down on the palm of your right hand, which is also covered by the cuff of the second sleeve. The fingers of the glove should be pointing toward the elbow (Fig. 5–11*A* and *B*).

2. Grasp the cuff of the glove through the gown with your right hand. Your covered left hand pulls the glove over your right hand, gently inserting your fingers into the finger spaces of the glove. Be certain that the cuff of the glove covers the cuff of the gown (see Fig. 5–11*C* and *D*).

3. With the gloved right (or dominant) hand, pick up the next glove, and place it on the palm of the left hand with the fingers pointing to the elbow.

4. Grasp the cuff of the glove through the sleeve cuffs with your gloved right hand and pull the second glove into place (see Fig. 5–11*E*).

Taking Radiographic Films in the Operating Room

As the radiographer, you are responsible for protecting yourself and all persons in the OR from radiation. You are also expected to be knowledgeable concerning the areas that are sterile and protecting them and the patient from contamination in the process of your work.

Usually, three types of radiographic imaging equipment are used in the OR: fixed ceiling or table

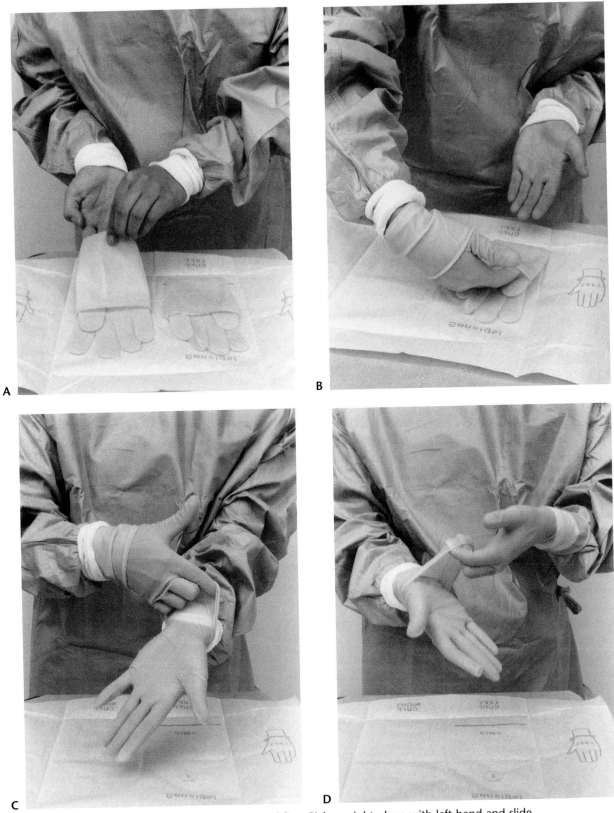

Figure 5–10. (**A**) Glove dominant hand first. Pick up right glove with left hand and slide right hand into glove. Leave cuff of glove folded down. (**B**) Next, pick up left glove with gloved right hand under fold of left glove. (**C**) Pull first the left cuff of glove over cuff of gown cuff. (**D**) Then place fingers of gloved left hand under cuff of right glove and pull it over gown cuff.

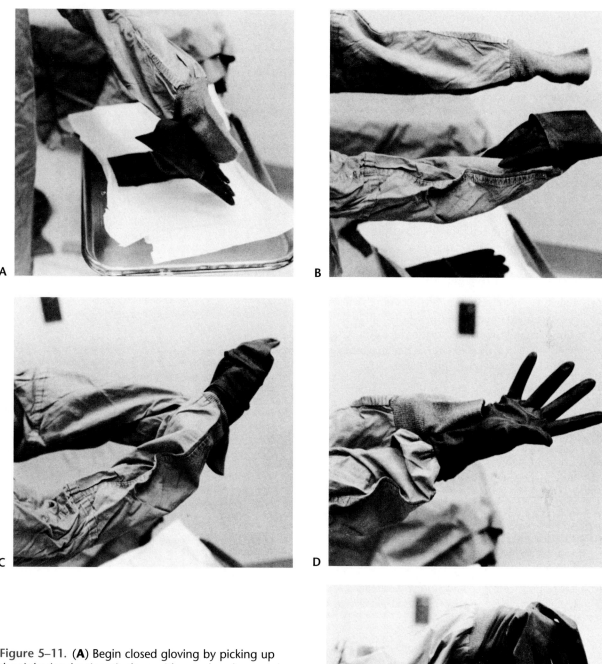

Figure 5–11. (**A**) Begin closed gloving by picking up the right (or dominant) glove with your hand covered by the cuff of the gown. (**B**) The fingers of the glove must be pointing toward your elbow. (**C**) Grasp the cuff of the glove through the sleeve of the gown on the opposite arm and pull on the glove. (**D**) Pull the glove on and make certain that the cuff of the glove covers the cuff of the gown. (**E**) Grasp the cuff of the second glove with the glove hand and pull it on.

mounted, portables, and image intensifiers or C-arms for fluoroscopy. You are responsible for making certain that any radiographic equipment used during a surgical procedure is clean and dust-free before use in the OR. Following are some guidelines for working in the surgical suite and OR:

1. Overhead units must be cleaned with a disinfectant solution and the portable radiographic machine and the image receptors to be used must be cleaned with a disinfectant solution before you change into a scrub suit and scrubs.

2. Maintain sterile technique for all items and persons involved in the invasive surgical procedure.

3. If possible, place image receptors and take scout films before draping the patient for the procedure.

4. If the image receptors must be placed after the procedure is begun, you may pass the image receptor to the scrub nurse. The scrub nurse receives the image receptor in a sterile plastic bag and places it at your direction (Fig. 5–12*A*).

5. If you place the image receptor yourself, the surgical team must make room for you. You may place the image receptor by raising the sterile drapes touching only the inside of the drape; or, the circulating nurse may lift the drapes and assist in placing the cassette into the image receptor holder (see Fig. 5–12*B*).

6. During a filming series, all personnel who are not scrubbed must leave the OR if at all possible. The scrubbed members of the team must wear protective radiation apparel. They may also step behind protective lead-lined screens (Fig. 5–13).

7. When hands are directly exposed to radiation, as they may be during fluoroscopy, leaded sterile gloves as well as all other protective equipment must be worn.

8. Pregnant female personnel should not be present in the OR when radiographic imaging is in progress.

9. Wear radiation detection badges on the outside of the lead apron and under the sterile gown during radiographic imaging procedures, and check at prescribed intervals.

10. During imaging, *remove all unnecessary instruments from the operative field and place a sterile drape over the open incision.*

Skin Preparation for Sterile Procedures

As the radiographer, you may be called on to prepare the patient's skin for an invasive procedure in the special procedures area. This is often referred to as a "skin prep" in the field of medicine. The purpose of the skin prep is to remove as many microorganisms as possible by mechanical and chemical means to reduce the potential for infection. The antimicrobial agent used for this purpose may vary; however, it must prevent tissue irritation and the rebound growth of microbes. There are two aspects to skin preparation for a sterile procedure: mechanical and chemical, as described in the text that follows.

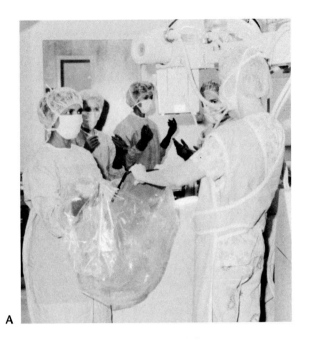

A

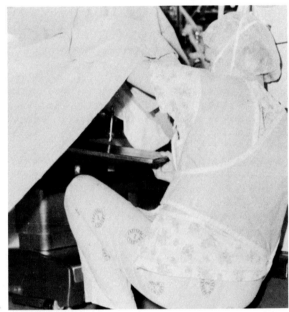

B

Figure 5–12. (A) Place the image receptor in the protective bag, being careful not to contaminate the outside of the scrub nurse's gloves. **(B)** Place the image receptor by lifting the underside of the sterile drapes.

Mechanical Methods of Skin Preparation

The mechanical aspects of skin preparation may include the removal of hair and always includes a friction scrub with antiseptic soap and water. At present, it is felt that hair is best left at the invasive site in most cases, since its removal often causes injury to the dermal layers of the skin. It must be done only with an order from the physician in charge of the patient and

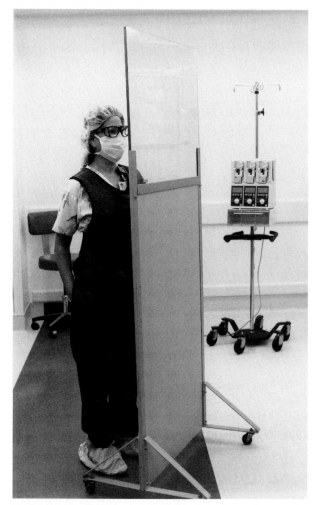

Figure 5–13. A lead screen shields members of surgical team.

as close to the time of the procedure as possible to prevent growth of microorganisms resulting from traumatized skin.

If hair removal at the potential surgical site is ordered, the two most recommended methods that may be used are a depilatory agent or clipping. A depilatory ointment may be applied to the area and then removed with the hair. An electric battery-operated clipper with a disposable or removable head that can be disinfected between uses is ideal, if available, because it prevents cutting or abrading the skin.

If neither of these methods is available, a sharp safety edge razor may be used to wet shave the area. The procedure is explained to the patient, who is then placed in a comfortable position. Before any skin preparation with antiseptics, you must ask the patient if he or she is allergic to iodine or any other antiseptic solutions. If the answer is positive, you must inform the physician, who will choose a substitute. Following is the procedure for hair removal:

1. Obtain clean gloves, a prep set that includes a small basin, a sponge permeated with antiseptic soap, one or two safety edge razors, a sponge for rinsing, and a small towel.

2. Put on clean gloves.

3. Shave the skin using short, firm strokes. Hold the skin taut and shave in the direction of hair growth. Remove only as much hair as necessary, being careful not to nick or cut the skin since bacteria proliferate in these areas.

4. After you have removed all unwanted hair, rinse the area with sterile water and pat it dry with the towel.

After hair removal or if hair removal is not required, a sterile skin prep is begun. The procedure for the sterile skin prep involves scrubbing the skin with a disinfectant soap and rinsing with sterile water. This is a sterile procedure, and all items used must be kept sterile. The person performing the scrub wears sterile gloves. Often, prepackaged prep trays are available for special procedures that contain two small basins (one for sterile water and one for antiseptic), a set of large sponges, sterile towels, sterile gloves, and the antiseptic detergent solution. A flask of sterile water must also be on hand to be poured into the basin before you don sterile gloves. The antiseptic detergent solutions most commonly used for skin preparation are iodophor, chlorhexidine gluconate, and, in special circumstances, parachlorometaxylenol with a physician's order. Chlorhexidine gluconate should not be used near the eyes, nose, or mouth. The sterile skin prep procedure is as follows:

1. Explain the procedure to the patient, and be certain he or she is not allergic to the antiseptic to be used.

2. Assemble the equipment needed, and open the sterile pack.

3. Pour sterile water into one of the basins. If the antiseptic agent is not in the sterile set, pour it into the other sterile basin.

4. Put on the sterile gloves using the open gloving technique.

5. Drape the area to be prepped with sterile towels to designate the upper and lower limits of the area to be prepped. The physician will explain how large an area must be prepped. Usually, it is an area approximately 6 to 10 inches in diameter around the invasive area.

6. Wet a sponge with sterile water and then with the soap solution, and begin scrubbing in the center of the area to be prepared, working slowly outward in a circular motion. Use a firm stroke, since friction is as important in the removal of microorganisms as

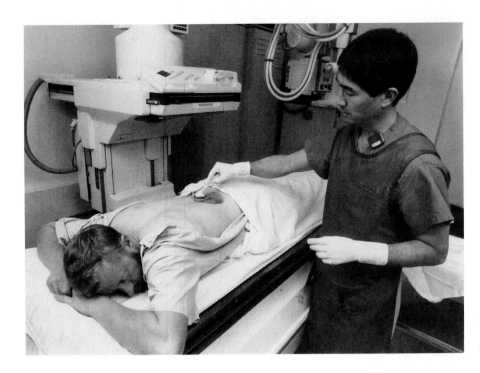

Figure 5–14. Begin at center of field to be prepped and move out. Repeat procedure with second sponge.

is the antiseptic soap. Do not go back over the skin that has already been scrubbed with this sponge. When you reach the edges of the area being scrubbed, remove the sponge from the sterile field, discard it, and obtain another sponge. Repeat the procedure using the other sponge (Fig. 5–14). If the umbilicus is to be prepared, clean it with cotton applicators soaked in the antiseptic detergent.

7. The scrubbing procedure should last approximately 5 minutes. Then rinse the skin well with sterile water, or wipe away the lather without rinsing. The routine varies depending on the procedure to be performed, the antiseptic used, and the policy of the institution. Blot the skin dry with sterile towels or sponges.

8. Carefully inspect the patient's skin during the skin prep. If the skin shows any sign of irritation or rash, stop the procedure and thoroughly rinse off the antiseptic with sterile water. Notify the physician of the patient's sensitivity so that another antiseptic may be chosen that is not harmful.

9. Do not allow solution to drain off the area being prepped and pool under the patient during the procedure, because this may burn the skin.

Chemical Method of Skin Preparation

After the mechanical aspects of skin prep are complete, the skin around the area to be penetrated is often paint-ed with an antiseptic solution. This destroys some of the remaining microbes and acts as a deterrent to further microbial growth for a brief period of time. Agents commonly used include chlorhexidine and hexachlorophene. The choice of solution depends on the institutional policy and the patient's tolerance of the product. Never use alcohol on mucous membranes or on an open wound because it coagulates protein and may cause harm.

If the patient's skin is to be painted with antiseptic after the scrub, do this in a circular motion beginning at the center of the area to be prepped and working outward (Fig. 5–15). Many special procedure sets have long-handled sponges and a receptacle for this purpose. If there are no special skin-prep sponges, you may use gauze sponges, folded and grasped in a sterile ring forceps and dipped into a small sterile container of antiseptic.

CALL OUT!

Maintain sterile technique during skin prep for invasive procedures!

Draping for a Sterile Procedure

After the skin has been mechanically and chemically prepared and allowed to dry, sterile drapes may be applied. Place drapes around the area of skin that has been prepared. The type of sterile drape to be used differs with each procedure. In the diagnostic imag-

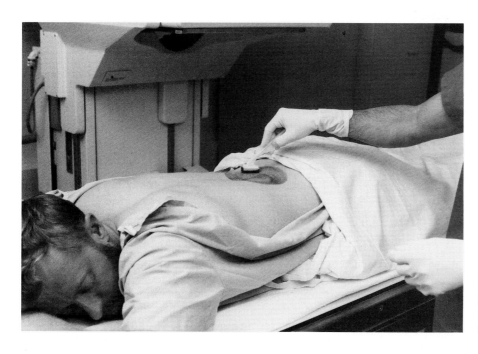

Figure 5–15. Paint with antiseptic solution in circular motion beginning at center of area to be prepped.

ing department, the drapes are usually a single-thickness, impermeable, disposable material. A fenestrated drape is often used, and, if so, the drape should be applied in such a way that the opening leaves only the operative site exposed. Handle sterile drapes as little as possible. Do not flip or fan sterile drapes.

If sterile towels are used, place them so that they are well within the limits of the area prepared, and fold and place them so that they overlap and the folds face the operative site.

Usually, the physician places the sterile drapes after donning sterile gloves for the procedure. As the radiographer, you must have the sterile pack that contains the drapes open and ready. Many prepackaged procedure sets contain sterile drapes. If you are the one to place the sterile drapes, you must first open a set of sterile gloves for yourself. Then, open the pack containing the drapes. Put on the sterile gloves, and place the drapes. Place first the part of the drape that is closest to you so that the sterility of your gloves is maintained, or hold the drape to protect your gloves (Fig. 5–16). Once the drape is in place, it may not be moved, because the underside of the drape would then be contaminated by touching the patient's skin. If a drape is contaminated during

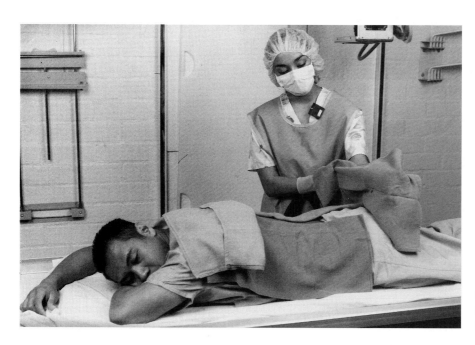

Figure 5–16. Place sterile towels folded so that they overlap. Folds face operative area.

the draping procedure, remove it at once and replace it with another sterile drape.

A plastic adhesive drape may be chosen for use. This type of drape adheres to the patient's skin and does not slip as the procedure progresses. The scrub nurse and the surgeon or the surgeon's assistant place this drape after the usual skin prep. After it is in place, the incision is made through the drape. Removal of this type of drape requires care to prevent injury to the patient's skin as it is pulled away.

Changing Dressings

You must not remove or reapply dressings without an order from the physician caring for the patient. When the physician does request that a dressing be removed for a procedure in the diagnostic imaging department, you must be able to remove it without contaminating the wound or yourself in the process.

All dressings must be treated as if they are contaminated, because drainage from wounds may harbor pathogenic microorganisms. Before removing or replacing a dressing, obtain the following materials:

Clean gloves

A bag for infectious waste and a bag closure

When these items are prepared, follow this procedure:

1. Wash your hands as for a medical aseptic procedure.

2. Place the patient in a comfortable position and explain the procedure.

3. Provide privacy for the patient by closing the door and keeping all of the body covered except the area where the dressing is in place.

4. Before putting on the clean gloves, loosen the tape holding the patient's dressing in place. (It is difficult to manage tape while wearing gloves.) Remove the tape with care; if it adheres to the skin and the patient complains of pain, use a commercial tape remover. Pull the tape off toward the wound while supporting the skin with the non-dominant hand.

5. Put on the clean gloves, and remove the dressing carefully (Fig. 5–17A). Be cautious when removing the dressing because it may adhere to the wound or because there may be a drain in place. If the dressing adheres to the wound, stop the procedure and inform the physician. Do not forcefully remove a dressing. To do so may damage the tissues around the wound or dislodge a tissue drain.

6. Assess the soiled dressing for drainage or blood. Inform the physician if you see a large amount of either on the dressing.

7. Place the soiled dressing into the bag prepared for it (see Fig. 5–17B). Remove the gloves correctly.

8. Place your hands under the cuff in the bag and unfold it upward; close the bag with a closure and place it into a receptacle for contaminated waste (see Fig. 5–17C).

9. Wash your hands.

When a dressing is reapplied, sterile technique must be used. The procedure is as follows:

1. Assemble the necessary equipment and wash your hands. Equipment needed will be:
   A sterile towel or small sterile drape
   Sterile gauze dressings of the appropriate size
   Tape
   A refuse bag and closure
   Sterile gloves
   If the area around the wound is soiled or the wound is draining, additional sterile gauze sponges, a sterile forceps, and sterile normal saline solution may be needed to cleanse the skin around the wound. A small, sterile receptacle must be obtained in which to pour the normal saline solution. Do not cleanse the wound itself.

2. Approach the patient and explain what is to be done.

3. If the soiled dressing has not been removed, remove it in the manner described above.

4. Open the sterile towel or drape to double thickness, and use it as a sterile field on which to place the sterile dressings.

5. Open the dressings and drop them onto the sterile field without contaminating them (Fig. 5–18A).

6. Prepare the tape by having it cut or torn into the lengths needed to keep the fresh dressing in place. Place these lengths of tape in a convenient place away from the sterile field.

7. Cleanse the skin around the wound with sterile normal saline, if necessary, in the following manner:

   Pour normal saline into the sterile receptacle prepared for it.
   Moisten the gauze sponges with sterile normal saline, and gently cleanse the skin, beginning in the area closest to the wound and moving outward.
   Drop the soiled sponges into the refuse bag, being careful not to contaminate your gloves. A sterile forceps may be used to hold the pads.
   Do not wash the wound itself, and do not apply medication or antiseptics.

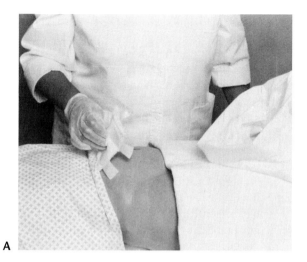

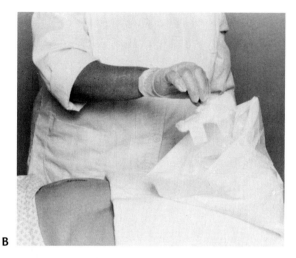

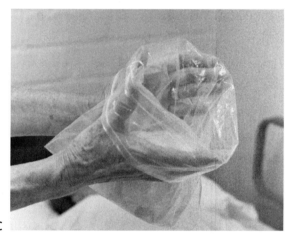

Figure 5–17. (**A**) Remove the old dressing carefully. Wear clean gloves to do this. (**B**) Place soiled dressing in an impermeable bag that has been prepared for it. (**C**) Place your hands under the fold, and bring the bag to a close without touching the folded edge.

Use as many pads as necessary to cleanse the skin.

8. Allow the skin to dry. Then apply the new sterile dressings (see Fig. 5–18*B*). If there is drainage, apply additional dressings to absorb the drainage.

9. Remove your gloves and drop them into the refuse bag. Apply tape to hold the dressing in place. Place tape so that gentle pressure is applied in both directions away from the injury and tape covers both ends of the dressing. Do not allow the tape to pull against the patient's skin.

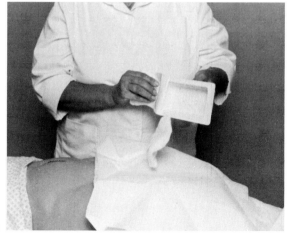

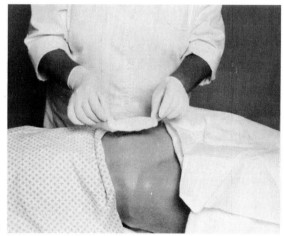

Figure 5–18. (**A**) Drop sterile dressings on sterile field without contaminating them. (**B**) Allow antiseptic to dry; then apply the new dressing.

10. Cover the patient and make him or her comfortable.

11. Dispose of the waste material correctly and wash your hands.

Summary

As the radiographer, you must participate in examinations that require the use of sterile technique, both in the surgical suite and in your own department. Any health care worker who participates in sterile procedures must practice meticulous surgical asepsis to prevent contamination that may result in patient infection. The most common means of spreading microorganisms in the OR during special procedures are by using contaminated instruments and gloves, by allowing a sterile field to become damp, and by failing to control air currents across sterile fields. All these situations are avoidable.

There are several methods of rendering an article sterile, that is, completely removing microorganisms and their spores. These methods are steam under pressure, chemical sterilization, gas ethylene oxide, and gas plasma sterilization.

Sterilization indicators are used inside and outside packs before they are exposed to the sterilization process. They are an indication that the article has been exposed to a particular sterilization process. You must be able to read and understand the indicators used in the institution in which you work.

Mechanical and chemical methods are used to disinfect objects and surfaces that cannot be sterilized. To ensure their effectiveness, the manufacturer's directions must be followed exactly.

Mechanical disinfecting methods are boiling and ultraviolet irradiation. Boiling is used as a means of disinfection only if no other method is available, because many microorganisms and their spores can withstand the boiling temperature for many hours. Ultraviolet rays kill microorganisms when they come into direct contact with them; however, it is an inefficient method of disinfection and is seldom used in hospitals.

You must learn the rules of surgical asepsis, because all invasive medical procedures require its use. You must learn to differentiate sterile objects from nonsterile objects and to open sterile packs correctly to prevent contamination. When there is a question about the sterility of an item, it is always considered to be nonsterile.

The surgical team comprises the surgeon, the surgical assistant, the anesthesiologist, the nurse anesthetist, the circulating nurse, the scrub nurse or surgical technologist, and the staff who prepares and maintains the surgical suite.

A surgical scrub is performed in the OR before a sterile gown and gloves are donned for a surgical procedure. The radiographer is not usually the sterile person in the OR because he or she will be there to take radiographic images for operation of the fluoroscope. You are expected to assist with special procedures in your own department, which requires the use of surgical aseptic technique and, in some instances, a surgical scrub.

Preparation of the skin for surgical penetration involves removing as many microorganisms as possible from the operative site. This reduces the possibility of infection from the procedure. Mechanical and chemical methods are used to prepare the skin, followed by application of sterile drapes around the operative area.

As the radiographer, you may be required to remove or reapply a dressing. You should perform these procedures using aseptic technique. Any dressing that is removed must be assumed to harbor pathogenic microorganisms. Soiled dressings must not be touched with bare hands; gloves must be used. The soiled dressings must be wrapped in a waterproof bag and disposed of properly to prevent contamination.

When dressings are removed or reapplied, the patient must be protected from infection. You must also protect yourself and others in your department. Use of aseptic technique and proper methods of waste disposal will accomplish these goals.

Chapter 5 Test

_____ 1. Which of the following is the best definition of surgical asepsis?
   a. Removing as many microorganisms as possible by mechanical and chemical methods
   b. Removing as many microorganisms and spores as possible by autoclaving
   c. Complete removal of microorganisms and spores
   d. Scrubbing, gowning, and gloving to prevent contamination

_____ **2.** Which of the following procedures does not require the use of surgical aseptic technique
  a. An intramuscular injection
  b. An intravenous injection
  c. An intrathecal procedure
  d. An arteriogram
  e. A gastrointestinal series

_____ **3.** All items that penetrate the skin or mucous membranes must be
  a. Disinfected
  b. Sterile

_____ **4.** You are the new radiographer in charge of maintaining a special procedures suite at the local community hospital. Since most procedures in this suite demand sterile technique, you must consider
  a. The type of disinfectant solutions that the housekeepers will use to clean the area before and after each procedure
  b. How often the air filters are changed
  c. How sterile packs and instruments are packaged and stored
  d. a and b
  e. a, b, and c

_____ **5.** Any dressing removed in the diagnostic imaging department should be considered
  a. Sterile
  b. Surgically aseptic
  c. Contaminated
  d. Medically aseptic

_____ **6.** Sterile drapes are placed by the sterile person. They drape
  a. The area farthest away from them first
  b. The area nearest the invasive site first
  c. The area closest to them first

_____ **7.** The skin is disinfected before beginning all invasive procedures to
  a. Protect the sterile drapes from contamination
  b. Decrease the possibility of introducing microorganisms into the open wound
  c. Protect the health worker from infection
  d. Ensure the success of the procedure

_____ **8.** Removal of hair is done in preparation for an invasive procedure
  a. As close to the time of the invasive procedure as possible
  b. The night before the procedure
  c. Any time at all

_____ **9.** Common means of transmitting microorganisms in the OR or special procedures room include
  a. Use of contaminated gloves or instruments
  b. Allowing a sterile field to become wet or damp
  c. Allowing microorganisms to be blown onto a surgical suite
  d. None of the above
  e. a, b, and c

_____ **10.** To maintain a sterile field, the person who has created it must never leave it unattended.
  a. True
  b. False

_____ **11.** If an object on a sterile field drops below the "sterile person's" waistline, it may still be considered to be sterile.
   a. True
   b. False

_____ **12.** The edges of a sterile wrapper may be considered sterile.
   a. True
   b. False

_____ **13.** Match the following:
   1. Surgeon _____

   2. Scrub nurse _____

   3. Radiographer _____

   4. Nurse anesthetist _____

   5. Circulating nurse _____

   a. Monitors the patient during anesthesia
   b. Ensures radiation safety in the OR
   c. Performs the surgical procedure
   d. Monitors the patient in the OR
   e. Arranges the sterile field

_____ **14.** When preparing the skin for a sterile procedure, you should scrub
   a. From the outside inward
   b. In a back and forth motion
   c. In a circular motion from inside to outside

_____ **15.** Before you use a sterile pack, you must check its
   a. Shelf life
   b. Expiration date
   c. List of contents
   d. Method of sterilization

_____ **16.** Boiling is an acceptable means of sterilization.
   a. True
   b. False

6

Vital Signs and Oxygen Administration

Objectives

After studying this chapter, you will be able to:

1. Define vital signs and explain when you are responsible for their assessment.
2. List the rates of temperature, pulse, respiration, and blood pressure that are considered to be within normal limits for a child and for an adult, male and female.
3. Identify sites and methods available for measuring body temperature and correctly read a clinical thermometer.
4. Accurately monitor pulse rate.
5. Accurately monitor respirations.
6. Accurately monitor blood pressure.
7. Identify the most common types of oxygen administration equipment, and explain their potential hazards.
8. Describe the equipment that must be available and functional in all radiographic imaging departments to monitor blood pressure and to administer oxygen.
9. List the precautions that must be taken when oxygen is being administered.

Glossary

Chronic obstructive pulmonary disease (COPD): Disease of the lungs in which inspiratory and expiratory lung capacity is diminished

Diencephalon: The posterior part of the forebrain

Dyspnea: Difficulty breathing resulting from insufficient airflow to the lungs

Hypothalamus: The portion of the diencephalon lying beneath the thalamus at the base of the cerebrum and forming the floor and part of the lateral wall of the third ventricle

LPM: Liters per minute

Radiolucent: Permitting the passage of radiant energy such as x-ray, yet offering some resistance to it

Tympanic: Bell-like; resonance pertaining to tympanum

Volatile: Easily vaporized or evaporated; unstable or explosive in nature

Measuring Vital Signs

Taking a patient's vital signs (also called cardinal signs) is an important part of a physical assessment and includes measurement of body temperature, pulse, respiration, and blood pressure. As the radiographer, you must know how to measure each vital sign to be prepared in case you encounter an emergency situation in which these skills are needed. It is also important to learn what the patient's vital signs are under normal circumstances because everyone has some variation from what is considered normal for their particular age group. After you know the patient's usual, or baseline, vital signs, you can judge whether your patient's vital signs are deviating from that baseline. Changes in vital signs can be an indication of a problem or a potential problem. A patient's baseline vital signs cannot be established with one reading of pulse, respiration, or blood pressure because of the many variables that can make one reading unreliable. You must also measure the patient's vital signs if he or she comes to the diagnostic imaging department for an extensive procedure or examination without a chart and no registered nurse is available.

Oxygen is an essential physiologic need for survival. It comes from the environment to the lungs, then is transported to the bloodstream and body tissues. The human brain cannot function for longer than 4 to 5 minutes without an adequate oxygen supply.

It is occasionally necessary to administer oxygen in the diagnostic imaging department, and you may be expected to assist in its administration. Also, a patient receiving oxygen therapy in the hospital room may be unable to leave the room to go to the diagnostic imaging department for necessary procedures. In this instance, you will be required to make portable radiographic exposures at the bedside. Because oxygen is a potentially toxic and volatile substance, you need to understand the precautions that are to be taken when assisting with oxygen administration or when using radiographic equipment while oxygen is in use.

It is your responsibility as the radiographer to make certain that there is a functioning sphygmomanometer, a stethoscope, and the equipment necessary to administer oxygen in each diagnostic imaging room at the beginning of each shift. Emergencies requiring these items arise, and there is no time to look for this equipment.

A physician's order is not required for vital signs to be measured. Unless a registered nurse is present to do so, you should take vital signs when a patient is admitted to the diagnostic imaging department for any invasive diagnostic procedure or treatment, before and after the patient receives medication, any time the patient's general condition suddenly changes, or if the patient reports nonspecific symptoms of physical distress such as simply not feeling well or feeling "different."

Body Temperature

Body temperature is the physiologic balance between heat produced in body tissues and heat lost to the environment. It must remain stable if the body's cellular and enzymatic activities are to function efficiently. Changes in the body's physiology occur when the body temperature fluctuates even 2 to 3 degrees. Body temperature is controlled by a small structure in the basal region of the diencephalon of the brain called the *hypothalamus*, sometimes referred to as the body's thermostat.

Body heat is produced by chemical processes that result from metabolic activity. When the body's metabolism increases, more heat is produced. When it decreases, less heat is produced. Both normal and abnormal conditions in the body can produce changes in body temperature. The environment, time of day, age, weight, hormone levels, emotions, physical exercise, digestion of food, disease, and injury are some factors that influence body temperature. The body's cellular functions and cardiopulmonary demands change in proportion to temperature variations outside of normal limits.

A patient whose body temperature is elevated above normal limits is said to have a fever, or *pyrexia*. Fever indicates a disturbance in the heat-regulating centers of the body, usually as a result of a disease process. As body temperature increases, the body's demand for oxygen increases.

The normal body temperature remains almost constant; however, a variation of 0.5 to 1 degree above or below the average is within normal limits. The normal body temperature of infants and children up to 13 years of age varies somewhat from these readings. Average body temperature in well children from ages 3 months to 3 years is from 99°F (37.2°C) to 99.7°F (37.7°C). From 5 years to 13 years, the normal temperature is from 97.8°F (36.7°C) to 98.6°F (37°C).

Symptoms of a fever are increased pulse and respiratory rate, general discomfort or aching, flushed dry skin that feels hot to the touch, chills (occasionally), and loss of appetite. Fevers that are allowed to remain very high for a prolonged period of time can cause irreparable damage to the central nervous system.

A person with a body temperature below normal limits is said to have hypothermia, which may be indicative of a pathological process. Hypothermia may also be induced medically to reduce a patient's need for oxygen. It is rare for a person to survive with a

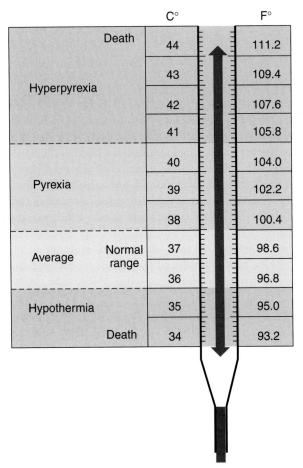

	C°		F°
Death	44		111.2
	43		109.4
Hyperpyrexia	42		107.6
	41		105.8
	40		104.0
Pyrexia	39		102.2
	38		100.4
Average — Normal range	37		98.6
	36		96.8
Hypothermia	35		95.0
Death	34		93.2

Figure 6–1. The range of human temperature as measured orally. (Taylor C, Lillis C, LeMone P: *Fundamentals of Nursing: The Art and Science of Nursing Care.* Philadelphia: JB Lippincott, 1989.)

body temperature between 105.8°F (41°C) and 111.2°F (44°C) or below 93.2°F (34°C) (Fig. 6–1).

Measuring Body Temperature

There are four areas of the body in which temperature is usually measured: the oral site, the tympanic site, the rectal site, and the axillary site.

Oral temperature is taken by mouth under the tongue; the average oral temperature reading is 98.6°F (37°C). The axillary temperature is taken in the axilla or armpit. The average axillary temperature is 97.6°F to 98°F (36.4°C to 36.7°C). Rectal temperature is taken at the anal opening to the rectum. The average rectal temperature is 99.6°F (37.5°C).

The site selected for measuring body temperature must be chosen with care depending on the patient's age, state of mind, and ability to cooperate in the procedure. Because the reading will vary depending on where it is measured, be sure to specify the site used when reporting the reading. Temperature

readings are reported in most health care facilities as follows:

A rectal temperature of 99.6°F is written 99.6 R

An oral temperature of 98.6°F is written 98.6 O

An axillary temperature of 97.6°F is written 97.6 Ax.

A tympanic temperature of 97.6°F is written 97.6 T.

Whatever method of measuring body temperature is chosen, as the radiographer, you must assemble the necessary equipment, wash your hands, put on clean gloves if contact with blood or body fluids is possible, and position the patient appropriately.

The Tympanic Membrane Thermometer

The tympanic membrane thermometer (also called an *aural thermometer*) is a small, hand-held device that measures the temperature of the blood vessels in the tympanic membrane of the ear (Fig. 6–2*A*).This provides a reading close to the core body temperature if correctly placed. The procedure for its use is as follows:

1. Place a clean sheath on the probe that is to be inserted into the external auditory canal (see Fig. 6–2*B*). The patient may be sitting upright or in a supine position.

2. Place the probe into the external auditory canal, and hold it firmly in place until the temperature registers automatically on the meter held in the nondominant hand.

3. Remove the probe and read the indicator.

4. Remove the probe cover and dispose of it correctly. Remove your gloves and wash your hands.

5. Record the reading. Immediately report any abnormal temperature to the radiologist in charge of the procedure.

The Electronic Thermometer for Oral Temperature

The procedure for the electronic thermometer is the same as for the tympanic membrane thermometer except that the probe is placed under the patient's tongue and held in place until the instrument signals that it has registered a temperature (Fig. 6–3).

Oral Temperature, Glass Thermometer

The mouth is an accessible site for measuring body temperature if a tympanic membrane thermometer is

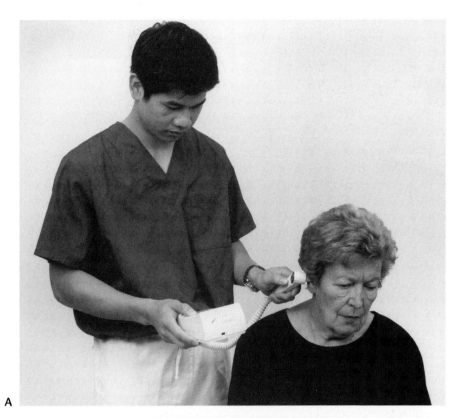

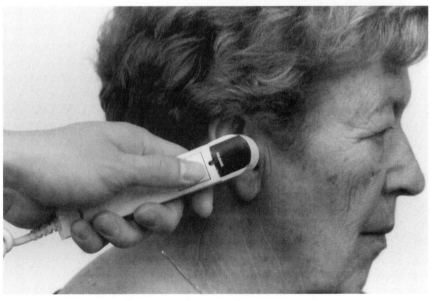

Figure 6–2. (**A**) Measuring temperature with a tympanic thermometer. (**B**) A clean sheath is placed on the probe, and the probe is placed inside the external auditory canal.

not available. This site should not be used if the patient is apt to be injured during the procedure by biting down on the thermometer or if the patient is unable to hold the instrument under the tongue with lips closed for the specified period of time. Patients who fall into this category include those who are delusional, disoriented, or delirious; those who have facial injuries or have had oral surgery; those with a history of convulsions; those unable to breathe with the mouth closed; and young children.

When measuring oral temperature with a glass clinical thermometer, the procedure is as follows:

1. Wash your hands. Put on clean gloves.

2. Select a sterilized thermometer with an elongated tip.

3. Shake the thermometer down to a mercury reading of 96°F (35°C).

4. Approach the patient, explain the procedure, and place the thermometer tip under the patient's tongue.

5. Have the patient close the lips over the tip of the thermometer, and leave it in place for 3 to 5 minutes.

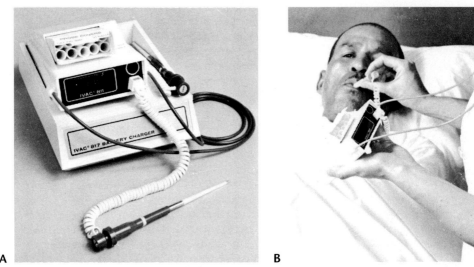

A   B

Figure 6–3. (**A**) An electronic thermometer. There are interchangeable oral and rectal probes. The cylindrical objects near the top of this model are disposable probe covers. (**B**) The radiographer reads the thermometer on the clock-like face when the thermometer signals that peak temperature has been reached.

6. Remove the thermometer, wipe it with a tissue, read it, and place it with the soiled equipment.

7. Remove your gloves and wash your hands.

The oral glass type of thermometer must be held at eye level by the blunt end and turned until the mercury column can be seen and read. The point on the marked scale where the mercury stops indicates the temperature to be recorded. Each long line on the thermometer represents one full degree of body temperature and is numbered accordingly. The short lines each represent two tenths (0.2) of one degree of body temperature; these lines are not numbered (Fig. 6–4).

After reading the thermometer, record it on the patient's chart, and report an abnormal temperature to the radiologist.

Taking an Axillary Temperature

Use of the axillary site is the safest method of measuring body temperature because it is noninvasive. It is particularly useful when measuring an infant's temperature. Unfortunately, the time and precision of placement needed to obtain an accurate reading make this method somewhat unreliable. When it is necessary to measure temperature using the axillary site, an electronic, disposable, or a glass thermometer with a blunt tip may be used. The procedure is as follows:

1. Obtain the instrument to be used; if it is a glass thermometer, shake it down.

2. Wash your hands. Put on clean gloves.

3. Dry the patient's armpit with a paper towel or a dry washcloth.

4. Place the thermometer into the center of the armpit.

5. Place the patient's arm down tightly over the thermometer with the arm crossed over his chest. Gently hold the arm of a child or a restless adult in place until the thermometer has registered. A

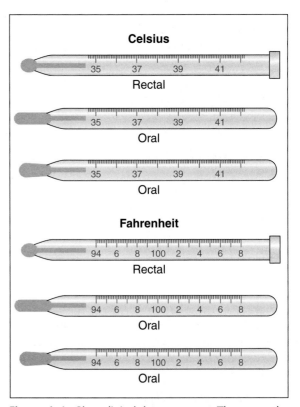

Figure 6–4. Glass clinical thermometers. The upper three thermometers are calibrated to measure degrees Celsius. The lower three thermometers measure in the Fahrenheit scale. Those with blunt bulbs are rectal thermometers.

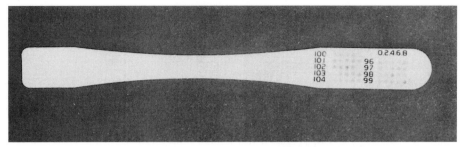

Figure 6–5. Disposable thermometer.

glass clinical thermometer must be held in place for 5 minutes, whereas electronic and disposable thermometers are held for 1 minute.

6. Remove the thermometer and the probe cover, or wipe the glass thermometer.

7. Read the thermometer; report and record the reading.

8. Dispose of the thermometer as appropriate.

Taking a Rectal Temperature

The rectal site is considered to provide the most reliable measurement of body temperature because factors that can alter the results are minimized. It is also in close proximity to the pelvic viscera or "core" temperature of the body. Body temperature should not be measured rectally if the patient is restless or has rectal pathology such as tumors or hemorrhoids.

To take a rectal temperature, use a thermometer with a blunt tip. Never use an oral thermometer, whether glass or electronic, to take a rectal temperature. Probe covers are often colored red for rectal temperature. The procedure is as follows:

1. Wash your hands.

2. Obtain a thermometer with a blunt tip. If a probe cover is used, apply it.

3. Put on clean gloves.

4. Ensure the patient's privacy. Place the patient in Sims' position and cover with a drape sheet.

5. Expose the patient only as much as is necessary for clearly viewing the rectal area.

6. Lubricate the thermometer tip with lubricating jelly. If the tip is covered with a probe cover, apply lubricant over the cover.

7. Separate the patient's buttocks with the heel of your hand so that the rectum is clearly visible.

8. Gently insert the tip of the thermometer into the rectum above 1 to 1½ inches, and hold it in place for 2 to 3 minutes. Do not leave a patient with a rectal thermometer in place. You must hold the thermometer.

9. When the time has passed, remove the thermometer and return the patient to a comfortable position.

10. Remove the probe cover or wipe the thermometer with a tissue. Read it and dispose of it as appropriate.

11. Remove your gloves in the specified manner and wash your hands.

Other Instruments Used to Measure Body Temperature

Temperature-sensitive patches are available that can be placed on the abdomen or forehead of infants or children to measure temperature. If they indicate an abnormal temperature, you should use another method to ascertain the actual reading.

If a patient's behavior is unreliable or if re-sterilization of equipment is not convenient, an unbreakable, disposable, single-use thermometer can be used (Fig. 6–5). Wear gloves as in previous descriptions. The thermometer is removed from its wrapper, and the indicator end is placed under the patient's tongue for 1 minute. The beads change color, indicating the patient's temperature. After recording the temperature, discard the thermometer. The accuracy of these instruments is uncertain.

Pulse

As the heart beats, blood is pumped in a pulsating fashion into the arteries. This results in a throb, or pulsation, of the artery. At areas of the body in which arteries are superficial, the pulse can be felt by holding the artery beneath the skin against a solid surface such as bone. The pulse can be detected most easily in the following areas of the body:

- *Apical pulse:* over the apex of the heart (heard with a stethoscope) (Fig. 6–6A)

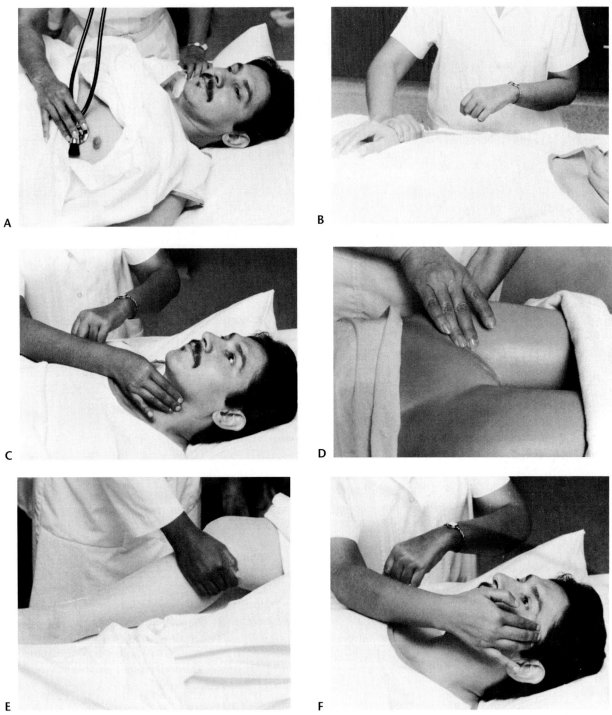

Figure 6–6. (**A**) Apical pulse. (**B**) Radial pulse. (**C**) Carotid pulse. (**D**) Femoral pulse. (**E**) Popliteal pulse. (**F**) Temporal pulse. (**G**) Dorsalis pulse. (**H**) Posterior tibial pulse. (**I**) Brachial pulse.

- *Radial pulse:* over the radial artery at the wrist at the base of the thumb (see Fig. 6–6B)
- *Carotid pulse:* over the carotid artery at the front of the neck (see Fig. 6–6C)
- *Femoral pulse:* over the femoral artery in the groin (see Fig. 6–6D)
- *Popliteal pulse:* at the posterior surface of the knee (see Fig. 6–6E)

- *Temporal pulse:* over the temporal artery in front of the ear (see Fig. 6–6F)
- *Dorsalis pedis pulse (pedal):* at the top of the feet in line with the groove between the extensor tendons of the great and second toe (may be congenitally absent) (see Fig. 6–6G)
- *Posterior tibial pulse:* on the inner side of the ankles (see Fig. 6–6H)

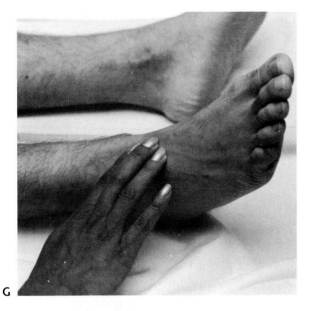

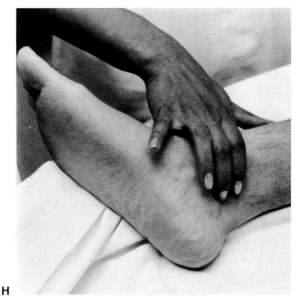

G

H

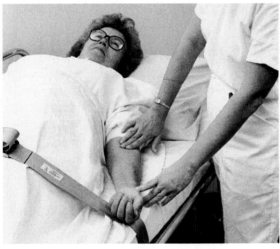

I

Figure 6–6. (Continued)

- *Brachial pulse:* in the groove between the biceps and triceps muscles above the elbow at the antecubital fossa (see Fig. 6–6*I*)

Usually, the pulse rate is rapid if the blood pressure is low and slower if the blood pressure is high. The patient who is losing blood has an unusually rapid pulse rate and a very low blood pressure. The normal average pulse rate in an adult man or woman in a resting state is between 60 and 90 beats/min. The normal average pulse rate for an infant is 120 beats/min. A child from 4 to 10 years of age has a normal average pulse rate of 90 to 100 beats/min.

Assessment of the Pulse

The pulse rate is a rapid and relatively efficient means of assessing cardiovascular function. *Tachycardia* is an abnormally rapid heart rate (over 100 beats/min), and *bradycardia* is an abnormally slow heart rate (below 60 beats/min). If a registered nurse is not present to take the pulse rate be prepared to make this assessment before beginning any invasive diagnostic imaging procedure in order to establish a baseline reading and to reassess it frequently until the procedure is complete and the patient leaves the department. The radial pulse is usually the most accessible and can be taken most conveniently on an adult patient. It should be counted for 1 full minute. If there is any irregularity of the radial pulse rate, take the apical pulse. The apical pulse is also monitored if the patient's radial pulse is inaccessible.

For infants and children, the apical pulse is the most accurate for cardiovascular assessment. The femoral, popliteal, and pedal pulses are assessed bilaterally if peripheral blood flow is to be assessed.

When assessing pulse rate, report the strength and regularity of the beat as well as the number of beats per minute. The normal rhythm of the pulse beat is regular, with equal time intervals between beats. The pressure of the fingers should not obliterate the pulse. When this does happen, report the pulse as weak or thready. If the beat is irregular, unusually rapid, unusually slow, or unusually weak, immediately report this to the physician in charge of the patient. You must also report changes in pulse rate during a procedure.

To assess the pulse, you need a watch with a second hand and a pad and pencil to record the findings. For monitoring the apical pulse, you need a stethoscope, along with alcohol sponges for wiping the earpieces and the bladder of the instrument. To assess the radial, femoral, carotid, popliteal, pedal, and temporal pulses, observe the following guidelines:

1. Wash your hands, approach the patient, and lightly place your index finger and middle finger flat over the artery chosen for assessment. Do not press too hard, or your fingers will compress the artery and you will not feel the beat.

2. When you feel the throbbing of the artery, count the throbs for 1 minute. Do not use the thumb when counting the pulse rate, because it too has a pulse that may be mistaken for the patient's pulse.

CALL OUT!

Be careful not to press too hard with the fingers or you won't be able to feel the pulse.

CALL OUT!

Do not use your thumb to count the pulse because it has its own pulse.

The pedal, popliteal, and femoral pulses are often monitored during special diagnostic imaging procedures to ascertain that the patient's circulatory status in the lower extremities is satisfactory. When this is done, the pulses are not always counted. Instead, they are palpated and assessed as present and strong, weak, regular, or irregular. The areas where the pedal and popliteal pulses are palpated are sometimes indicated with a marker or a pen so that they may be easily found to be checked as necessary. You must become proficient in finding and assessing these pulses.

Apical Pulse

To assess the apical pulse, you need a stethoscope and alcohol wipes. The procedure is as follows:

1. Clean the earpieces and the bladder of the stethoscope with alcohol wipes. Wash your hands.

2. Approach the patient and place him or her in a semi-Fowler's or supine position.

3. Drape the patient so that the lower chest area is exposed.

4. Place the bladder of the stethoscope at the fifth intercostal space 5 cm from the left sternal margin (the nipple of the breast can be used as a landmark for 5 cm).

5. If the beat cannot be heard, move the stethoscope slightly in every direction until it can be heard.

6. Count the beats for 1 minute, and assess the heartbeats for regular rate and rhythm.

7. Remove the stethoscope; wipe the earpieces and bladder with alcohol. Cover the patient and make him or her comfortable.

8. Wash your hands. Report any irregularities to the physician and record the pulse rate.

When recording pulse rate, use the abbreviation P for pulse. Record AP for apical pulse. For example, P 80 equals a pulse rate of 80 beats/min. AP 88 equals an apical pulse rate of 88 beats/min. Record any abnormalities and immediately report these to the patient's physician, for example, *P 94, thready (or weak) and irregular*.

Respiration

The function of the respiratory system is to exchange oxygen and carbon dioxide between the external environment and the blood circulating in the body. Oxygen is taken into the lungs during inspiration. It passes through the bronchi, into the bronchioles, and then into the alveoli, which are the gas-exchange units of the lungs. Oxygen is transported to the body tissues by the arterial blood. Deoxygenated blood is returned to the right side of the heart through the venous system. It is then pumped into the right and left pulmonary arteries and reoxygenated by passing through the capillary network on the alveolar surfaces. The blood is then returned to the left side of the heart through the pulmonary veins for recirculation. During this process, carbon dioxide is also deposited in the alveoli and exhaled from the lungs during expiration.

The average rate of respiration (one inspiration and one expiration) for an adult man or woman is 15 to 20 breaths/min; for an infant, 30 to 60 breaths/min. Respirations of fewer than 10 breaths/min for an adult may result in cyanosis, apprehension, restlessness, and a change in level of consciousness, because the supply of oxygen is inadequate to meet the needs of the body.

Normal respirations are quiet, effortless, and uniform. Medication, illness, exercise, or age may increase or decrease respirations, depending on the body's metabolic need for oxygen. When a patient is using more than the normal effort to breathe, he or she is described as dyspneic or as having dyspnea.

Assessment of Respiration

As with other vital signs, it is important to establish a baseline respiratory rate because changes in respiration are often an early sign of a threatened physiologic state. Remember, however, that the rate of respiration increases with physical exercise or emotion. Respiration is also quicker in newborns and infants. When assessing respiration, observe the rate, depth, quality, and pattern. The assessment procedure is as follows:

1. *Keep patient in present position.* The patient remains in a sitting or supine position for assessment of the pulse. He or she should be in a quiet state and not be aware that you are observing the respirations. If the patient is aware that you are assessing the respirations, he or she may consciously or unconsciously alter the pattern.

2. *Observe the chest wall for symmetry of movement.* There should be an even rise and fall of the chest with no involvement of muscles other than the diaphragm. In the adult patient, abdominal, intercostal, or neck muscle involvement in breathing is a sign of respiratory distress and should be noted. Other signs of respiratory distress in an adult patient include the need to assume a sitting position or the need to lean forward and place the arms over the back of a chair or on the knees in order to breathe easily.

3. *Observe skin color.* Cyanosis, or bluish discoloration, is easily observed around the mouth, in the gums, in nailbeds, or in the earlobes. Cyanosis may be a sign of respiratory distress.

4. *Count the number of times the patient's chest rises and falls for one full minute.* The most convenient time to count respirations is immediately after the pulse count as you appear to be continuing to count the pulse rate but are observing respiratory movement instead. An easy way to count respirations is to cross the patient's arm across the chest and count the rise and fall of the arm. When recording respiration, use the abbreviation R. R 20 equals 20 rises and falls of the chest wall. Any abnormalities or deviations from the baseline should be reported to the physician in charge of the patient immediately and recorded, for instance, *R 28, shallow and labored.*

> ### CALL OUT!
> The patient should be unaware that you are counting the respirations.

Blood Pressure

In general terms, pressure is defined as the product of flow times resistance. Blood pressure is the amount of blood flow ejected from the left ventricle of the heart during systole and the amount of resistance the blood meets due to systemic vascular resistance. Maintenance of blood pressure depends on peripheral resistance, pumping action of the heart, blood volume, blood viscosity, and the elasticity of the vessel walls.

If the volume of blood decreases because of hemorrhage or dehydration, the blood pressure falls because of a diminished amount of fluid in the arteries. Fluid or blood replacement reverses the problem.

The viscosity of the blood is determined by the number of red blood cells in the blood plasma. With an increased number, the blood thickens or becomes more viscous and subsequently increases the blood pressure.

The arteries are normally elastic in nature; however, age or a build-up of atherosclerotic plaque reduces the flexibility of the arteries and increases blood pressure.

The peripheral blood vessels distribute blood ejected into the circulatory system to the various body organs. When the peripheral blood vessels are in a normal physiologic state, they are partially contracted. If this normal physiologic state is changed because of changes in environmental factors such as heat or cold, medication, disease, or other obstructive conditions, peripheral blood vessel resistance may increase. This increase causes an increase in blood pressure. Or, the peripheral blood vessel resistance may decline, thus causing a decrease in blood pressure.

Blood pressure normally varies with age, gender physical development, body position, time of day, and health status. As a person ages, the blood pressure usually increases as the body systems that control blood pressure deteriorate.

Physiologic factors that may increase blood pressure are increased cardiac output, increased peripheral vascular resistance, increased blood volume, increased blood viscosity, and decreased arterial elasticity. Physiologic factors that decrease blood pressure are decreased cardiac output, decreased peripheral vascular resistance, decreased blood volume, decreased blood viscosity, and increased arterial elasticity.

Blood pressure is usually lower in the morning after a night of sleep than later in the day after activity. Blood pressure increases after a large intake of food. Emotions and strenuous activity usually cause systolic blood pressure to increase.

Men usually have higher blood pressure than women. Infants generally have higher blood pressure than adults, and adolescents have the lowest overall blood pressure. Because the range of blood pressure varies in these age groups, measurements for infants and children should be taken in series.

The instrument used to measure blood pressure is called a *sphygmomanometer.* Two numbers, read in millimeters of mercury (mm Hg), are recorded when reporting blood pressure: systolic pressure and diastolic pressure. The systolic reading is the highest point reached during contraction of the left ventricle of the heart as it pumps blood into the aorta. The diastolic pressure is the lowest point to which the pressure drops during relaxation of the ventricles and indicates the minimal pressure exerted against the arterial walls continuously.

The normal systolic pressure in men and women ranges from 110 to 140 mm Hg, and the normal diastolic pressure ranges from 60 to 80 mm Hg. Children's blood pressure ranges from 90 to 120 mm Hg for systolic pressure and from 50 to 70 mm Hg for diastolic pressure. Adolescent patients' blood pressure ranges from 85 to 130 mm Hg systolic and 45 to 85 mm Hg diastolic.

Pulse pressure is the difference between the systolic and diastolic blood pressure and is an indicator of the stroke volume of the heart (the amount of blood ejected by the left ventricle during contraction). Pulse pressure decreases when a patient is in a state of hypovolemic shock.

You must have a patient's baseline blood pressure reading so that you may evaluate the patient's blood pressure effectively if necessary. A patient is considered to be hypertensive if the systolic blood pressure is consistently greater than 140 mm Hg and if the diastolic blood pressure is consistently greater than 90 mm Hg. A patient is considered hypotensive whose systolic blood pressure is less than 90 mm Hg.

Equipment Needed to Measure Blood Pressure

There are two types of sphygmomanometers, a mercury manometer and an aneroid manometer (Fig. 6–7). Each has a cloth cuff, which comes in a variety of sizes. Within the cuff is an inflatable bladder, which should be nearly long enough to encircle the arm. Each also has a pressure manometer, a thumbscrew valve to maintain or release the pressure, a pressure

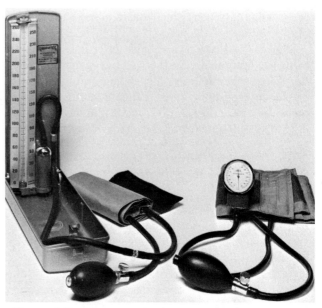

Figure 6–7. Two types of sphygmomanometers. (**Left**) A mercury manometer. (**Right**) An aneroid manometer with self-securing cuffs. There are several varieties of aneroid manometers.

bulb to inflate the bladder, and rubber tubings that lead to the gauge and to the pressure bulb. The bulb and the tubing must be free of leaks.

The mercury manometer is the more accurate of the two, but it is less convenient to use. The aneroid manometer needle should point to zero before the bladder of the cuff is inflated, and its calibration should be checked for accuracy and recalibrated by means of a perfectly accurate mercury manometer at least once each year.

The blood pressure cuff should be selected according to patient size. A cuff that is too large or too small for the patient's arm will give an incorrect reading.

A good-quality stethoscope has a bladder and a bell, strong plastic or rubber tubing 12 to 18 inches (30 to 40 cm) in length that leads to firm but flexible binaurals (the metal tubings leading to the earpieces), and earpieces that fit snugly and securely into the ears. You can use either the bladder or the bell of the stethoscope for assessing blood pressure. The bell transmits low sounds and should be held lightly against the skin; the bladder transmits high-pitched sounds and is held firmly against the skin (Fig. 6–8).

An automated vital sign monitor is used during special diagnostic imaging procedures when it is necessary to know the patient's circulatory status at all times. The pulse and blood pressure and mean arterial pressure are measured with this instrument. (Many types of Doppler and electronic blood pressure monitoring devices are used in clinical practice. Their methods of operation vary and are not discussed in this chapter.)

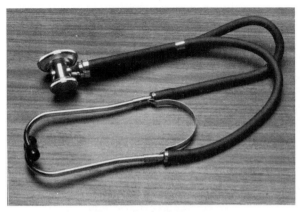

Figure 6–8. Stethoscope.

Measuring Blood Pressure

Have the patient sitting in a chair with his or her arm supported or reclining in a supine position. Although a pressure can be taken while the patient is standing, it is not recommended. You will most frequently encounter the need to take a blood pressure while the patient is lying down.

The room should be as quiet as possible to facilitate hearing the pulsations. Make sure that no clothing is between the blood pressure cuff and the skin. The bladder and bell of the stethoscope and the earpieces should be cleansed with alcohol sponges before and after each use to prevent passing infection indirectly from one person to another.

The procedure for taking blood pressure is as follows:

1. Roll up the patient's sleeve, if necessary. *The brachial artery must be free of clothing.*

2. Place the deflated sphygmomanometer cuff evenly around the patient's upper arm above the elbow; secure it so that it will not work loose. Make sure that the cuff is facing the correct direction and that the arrow indicating the artery is placed appropriately.

3. Place the bladder or bell of the stethoscope over the brachial artery. This artery is located at the center of the anterior elbow and may be identified by feeling its pulsations. Place the instrument flat against the brachial artery (Fig. 6–9). *Do not allow the stethoscope or the tubing to touch the patient's clothing because it will create sounds that may confuse your reading.*

4. Place the gauge of the sphygmomanometer on a flat surface or attach it to the top edge of the cuff so that you can easily read it.

5. Place the earpieces of the stethoscope in your ears. They must fit snugly.

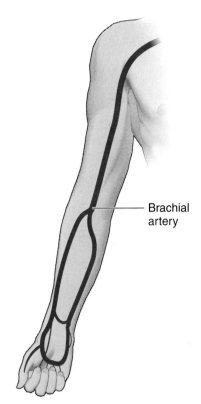

Brachial artery

Figure 6–9. The bell or bladder of the stethoscope is placed over the brachial artery.

6. Tighten the thumbscrew of the pressure bulb, and pump the bulb until the indicator or mercury reaches 180 mm Hg or until you are no longer able to hear a pulse beat (Fig. 6–10).

7. Open the valve by slowly loosening the thumbscrew. Allow the indicator to fall slowly as you listen for the first audible pulse beat. Listen carefully for the pulse beat to begin, and take the reading on the gauge where it is first heard. *This first reading is the systolic blood pressure.*

8. Continue to listen to the pulsations until they become soft or the sound changes from loud to very soft or is inaudible. Note where the sound changes or is no longer heard. *This is the diastolic reading.*

When you listen for the diastolic pressure, you may frequently detect a change in intensity of the sound before the sound is completely muffled. Note the point at which you can hear this softer sound, and then note the point at which you no longer hear a pulsation. This reading is a more accurate indication of intra-arterial diastolic pressure. Record both readings, but record the softer sound first. There are times when you may hear extraneous sounds such as tapping, knocking, or swishing. These are known as Korotkoff sounds, and you must record these as well.

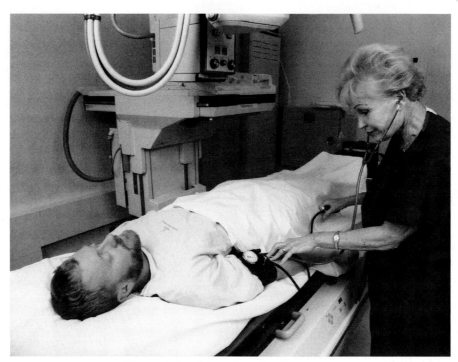

Figure 6–10. Measuring blood pressure.

Record blood pressure in the following manner: if the systolic reading is 120 and the diastolic reading is 80, it is written *BP 120/80* and is read "one twenty over eighty." If the diastolic reading is soft at 80 and then completely muffled at 60, it should be written 120/80/60 (the 60 reading being the Korotkoff sound).

Blood pressure measurement for infants and small children is a more complex procedure and requires a smaller sphygmomanometer cuff and less pressure exerted upon inflation. A physician or nurse educated in this skill should perform this. Usually, a nurse is on hand to monitor when invasive diagnostic imaging procedures are to be done for patients in this age group.

Oxygen Therapy

An adequate oxygen supply is essential to life. Because oxygen cannot be stored in the body, the supply from the external environment must be constant. When a human being's oxygen supply is suddenly interrupted or interfered with in any manner, it is an emergency that must be dealt with immediately to prevent a life-threatening situation. This type of emergency may occur in the diagnostic imaging department; therefore, you may be the first person to observe such a problem. It is your responsibility to ensure that the equipment needed to administer oxygen is available at all times and in functioning condition in your work area. It is also your responsibility to assist with oxygen administration in emergency situations. You must also become acquainted with the methods of oxygen administration that you may encounter in other areas of patient care.

The lungs supply oxygen and remove carbon dioxide from the body. Oxygen and carbon dioxide are carried to and from the various body systems in the blood. Only small amounts of oxygen are carried in solution in the blood. The major supply of oxygen is carried in chemical combination with hemoglobin. The oxygen capacity of the blood is expressed in percentage of the volume. The amount of oxygen in either air or blood is called the oxygen tension (partial pressure) and is written PO_2. Carbon dioxide is described similarly as PCO_2.

Carbon dioxide diffuses into the plasma of systemic capillary blood, but the major part enters the red blood cells. Carbon dioxide also is carried in combination with hemoglobin, which assists with its removal from the body. When there is an excessive build-up of carbon dioxide in the bloodstream, the pH (acidity or alkalinity) of the blood changes, often with dire physiologic effects. Prevention of excessive acidity of the blood is achieved through the presence of a bicarbonate (HCO_3) buffer in the bloodstream.

The effectiveness of pulmonary function (the lungs' ability to exchange oxygen and carbon dioxide efficiently) is most accurately measured by laboratory testing of arterial blood for the concentrations of oxygen, carbon dioxide, bicarbonate, acidity, and the saturation of hemoglobin with oxygen (SaO_2).

Laboratory values (called *arterial blood gases*) considered within normal limits are as follows:

pH: 7.35 to 7.45

$PaCO_2$: 32 to 45 mm Hg

PaO_2: 80 to 100 mm Hg

HCO_3: 20 to 26 mEq/L

SaO_2: 97%

When pulmonary function is disturbed, the level of oxygen in the arterial blood becomes inadequate to meet the patient's physiologic needs. This condition is referred to as *hypoxemia*. Carbon dioxide may be retained in the arterial blood, which results in a condition called *hypercapnea*. When the PaO_2 is below 60 mm Hg or the hemoglobin saturation is less than 90%, it can be assumed that adequate oxygenation of the blood is not taking place. You will usually rely on observation of physical symptoms of this problem (discussed in Chapter 7), because hypoxemia occasionally occurs with little warning and not enough time for laboratory analysis of arterial blood gases.

Pulse Oximetry

A pulse oximeter is frequently used to monitor the oxygen saturation of hemoglobin (SaO_2). This is a fast, noninvasive method of monitoring the patient for sudden changes in oxygen saturation, such as when a patient has just been removed from a ventilator. A sensor is attached to a fingertip or an earlobe (Fig. 6–11). A photodetector attached to the sensor is able to distinguish between oxygenated and deoxygenated hemoglobin of the blood pulsing through the tissue at the location of the sensor. Normal SaO_2 values are 95% to 100%. Values of less than 85% indicate that the tissues are not receiving adequate oxygen. The pulse oximeter is used in all areas of acute health care as well as in the special procedures areas of radiographic imaging.

Hazard of Oxygen Administration

Oxygen is considered to be a medication and, like all other forms of medical therapy, must be prescribed by a physician. Excessive amounts of oxygen may produce toxic effects on the lungs and central nervous system or may depress ventilation.

Varying degrees of oxygen toxicity may result from inhalation of high concentrations of oxygen for more than a brief period of time. Mild oxygen toxicity may produce reversible tracheobronchitis. Severe oxygen toxicity may cause irreversible parenchymal lung injury. Because of the potential for adverse effects from excessive amounts of oxygen, oxygen should be administered as prescribed and in the lowest possible amount to achieve adequate oxygenation.

Special care is necessary when oxygen is administered to patients who have chronic obstructive pulmonary disease (COPD). You must remember that excessive oxygen in the blood of the patient who has COPD may depress the respiratory drive, and the patient may stop breathing. This occurs because patients with a chronic lung disease have chemoreceptors that no longer respond to the stimulus of CO_2 to breathe, as occurs in a healthy person. They must rely on hypoxemia as a respiratory stimulus. If they receive an excessive amount of oxygen, hypoxia is no longer present and respiration ceases.

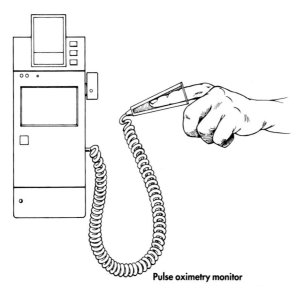

Pulse oximetry monitor

Figure 6–11. Pulse oximetry is an effective tool for measuring subtle changes in oxygen saturation (SaO_2). The finger, earlobe, or bridge of the nose can be used. A sensor detects changes in oxygen saturation levels in the blood pulsing through the tissue where the probe is attached. (Fuller J, Schaller-Ayers J: *Health Assessment: A Nursing Approach,* 2nd ed. Philadelphia: JB Lippincott, 1994.)

> ### CALL OUT!
> High flow rates of oxygen are toxic to patients who have COPD because their respiration is controlled by the higher levels of carbon dioxide in the blood.

Infection and bacteria thrive in oxygenated environments. Therefore, the equipment used to deliver oxygen is a potential source of infection to the patient. Be certain that the tubing, cannulas, and masks for oxygen delivery are used for one patient only and then discarded. Oxygen supports combustion; therefore, take care to prevent sparks or flames from being where oxygen is being administered. Smoking is prohibited in rooms where oxygen is in use, and anything that may produce sparks or flames must be used with extreme caution. Take precautions when your equipment is to be used in the presence of pure oxygen to be certain that it will not produce sparks.

CALL OUT!

Oxygen is combustible, so take great care to prevent sparks from being near electrical equipment.

Oxygen Delivery Systems

Oxygen is administered by artificial means when the patient is unable to obtain adequate amounts from the atmosphere to supply the needs of the body. If the patient requires supplementary oxygen, it is delivered to the respiratory tract under pressure. When the flow rate is high, the oxygen is humidified to prevent excessive drying of the mucous membranes. This can be done by passing the oxygen through distilled water, because it is only slightly soluble in water. The procedure for moisturizing oxygen varies somewhat from one institution to another, but often the receptacle for distilled water is attached at the wall outlet, and the oxygen passes through the water and then into the delivery system.

In most hospitals, oxygen is piped into patient rooms, postanesthesia areas, emergency suites, and the diagnostic imaging department. Wall outlets make it readily available. Oxygen supplied in this fashion comes through pipes from a central source at 60 to 80 pounds of pressure per square inch. A flowmeter is attached to each wall outlet to regulate flow (Fig. 6–12).

If oxygen is not piped in through wall outlets, it is available compressed and dispensed in tanks of varying sizes. A full tank contains 2,000 pounds per square inch of pressure. These tanks have two regulator valves—one valve indicates how much oxygen is in the tank, and the other valve measures the rate of oxygen flow through the delivery tubing. If you must use this type of system, take care not to allow the tank to fall or the regulator to become cracked (Fig. 6–13). If this were to happen, the buildup of pressure within the tank may cause the regulator to act as a dangerous projectile.

Twenty-one percent of the air we breathe normally is composed of oxygen, often abbreviated as FiO_2. This percentage of oxygen may need to be increased if a patient is in respiratory distress and unable to inspire enough room air to fulfill his body's oxygen needs.

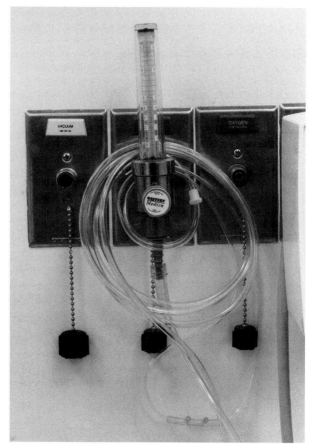

Figure 6–12. A wall oxygen outlet with flow meter and nasal cannula and tubing attached.

There are many types of oxygen delivery systems that transport oxygen from wall outlets or tanks. The more complex systems deliver a controlled amount of premixed room air and oxygen. The simpler systems deliver a prescribed amount of oxygen mixed with room air, but the concentration varies as the patient's rate of respiration varies because they are not closed systems. The physician determines the amount of oxygen that the patient needs and the type of delivery device needed. The flow rate of oxygen is measured in liters per minute (LPM). The systems that you will be dealing with most commonly deliver low to moderate concentrations of oxygen. They are discussed in the following text.

Nasal Cannula

The nasal cannula is a disposable plastic device with two hollow prongs that deliver oxygen into the nostrils (Fig. 6–14). The other end of the cannula is attached to the oxygen supply, which may or may not pass through a humidifier, and it has a flow meter attached. The cannula is held in place by an elastic strap that fits over the patient's ears and behind the head. This device is the most commonly seen delivery

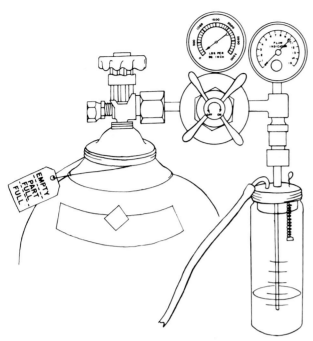

Figure 6–13. An oxygen tank. The regulator valve on the top of the tank allows the oxygen to flow out of the tank. The valve to the right of the tank regulates the flow. The gauge on the left indicates the amount of oxygen in the tank; the gauge on the right indicates the rate of flow. The container to the right of the tank is a humidifier.

system in the diagnostic imaging department. Patients on long-term oxygen delivery have a nasal cannula because of the comfort and convenience of the cannula.

The concentration of oxygen delivered by nasal cannula varies from 21% to 60%, according to the amount of room air inspired by the patient. Oxygen delivery by nasal cannula is indicated for patients whose breathing rate and depth are normal and even. With this method, 1 to 4 LPM of oxygen is usually prescribed for adults. For children, the rate is much lower (1/4 to 1/2 LPM). Rates at higher levels dry the nasal mucosa because of the position of the tubes against the skin of the nostrils.

Remember to have the oxygen turned on and flowing at the desired rate before placing any low-flow device on a patient. This prevents a sudden burst of oxygen into the patient's nostrils when the regulator is first turned on. The nasal prongs must be kept in place in both nostrils.

Nasal Catheter

A nasal catheter is another means of low-flow delivery of oxygen. In this system, a French-tipped catheter is inserted into one nostril until it reaches the oral pharynx. This type of catheter is used to deliver a moderate to high concentration of oxygen. As with the nasal cannula, the other end of the French-tipped catheter is attached to the oxygen supply with a flow meter attached. The prescribed flow rate for this method of delivery is usually 1 to 5 LPM. Oxygen delivered by this method does have associated hazards. For example, oxygen may be misdirected into the stomach, causing gastric distention; or, the mucous membranes may become dry, causing a sore throat. This method of oxygen delivery is not routinely used.

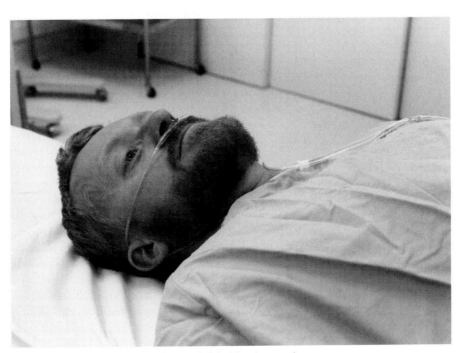

Figure 6–14. Nasal cannula.

FACE MASK

A simple face mask is used to deliver oxygen for short periods of time. It, too, is attached to an oxygen supply and a flow meter. The mask is placed over the nose and mouth and attached over the ears and behind the head with an elastic band (Fig. 6–15). A mask is uncomfortable for long periods because the patient is unable to eat, drink, or talk with it in place. Moreover, the percentage of oxygen is so variable with the face mask that it is not the method of choice for long periods. Because the mask does not fit tightly against the face, the concentration of oxygen delivered varies from 30% to 50%.

When the face mask is used, it should be run at no less than 5 LPM. This rate is needed to flush the CO_2 from the mask. Other face masks are usually used to administer more precise concentrations of oxygen. Several types of face mask delivery systems are available at present, and the physician will prescribe the one best suited to the patient's needs.

The different types of mask include a *nonrebreathing mask*, which, if correctly used, may supply 100% oxygen. This high-flow system has a reservoir bag attached. The bag fills with oxygen to provide a constant supply of oxygen. A valve prevents the

exhaled gases from entering the reservoir bag and prevents rebreathing of exhaled gases. A *partial rebreathing mask*, which delivers 60% to 90% oxygen, operates similarly to the nonrebreather mask. The rebreather mask does not have a valve between the mask and the bag; therefore, exhaled air flows into the reservoir bag and allows the patient to breathe a mixture of oxygen and carbon dioxide. Two other types of face mask delivery systems include a *Venturi mask*, which limits oxygen to 24% to 50% by mixing room air and the oxygen in specific percentages; and an *aerosol mask*, which provides 60% to 80% oxygen mixed with particles of water.

Other Oxygen Delivery Systems

Persons who must have continuous oxygen therapy for long periods of time may have a *transtracheal delivery system*. This system has a catheter that is inserted into the trachea and tubing that is connected to a portable tank.

Patients in acute respiratory failure are often placed on *mechanical ventilators* (also known as respirators), which control or partially control inspiration and expiration and FiO_2. You will usually encounter these patients in the critical care units of the hospital while you are performing mobile radiography. These patients are generally unable to breathe on their own accord. The rate of oxygen flow is determined by many factors and is regulated by the equipment. Because the ventilator tubing is generally over the patient during the performance of the procedure, you must get help to move the patient and place the image receptor.

Before working with any patient who is on high-flow oxygen therapy or a mechanical ventilator, you need to consult with the nurse in charge of the patient and plan your work carefully before beginning.

OXYGEN TENT

Oxygen tents are used when there is a need for humidity and a higher concentration of oxygen than is present in the natural environment of the patient (Fig. 6–16). This method of delivery is rarely used for adults, but you may be called to the pediatric unit to attend a child in a tent. If so, you may request that the oxygen be turned off for brief periods while you make the required exposures. When you are finished, replace the tent, raise the side rails, and request that the nurse restart the oxygen and mist at the required concentrations. The hazard of fire is especially great with an oxygen tent. Smoking is not permitted, nor is the use of any equipment that might generate sparks.

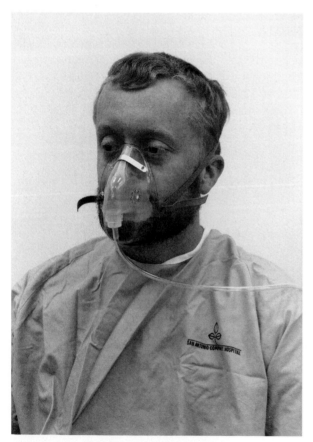

Figure 6–15. Simple oxygen face mask.

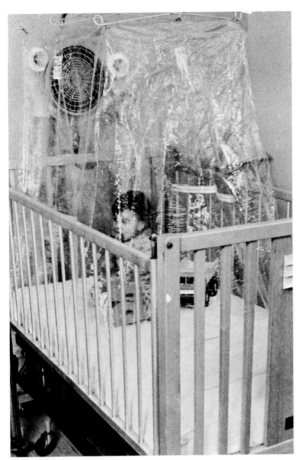

Figure 6-16. Oxygen tent.

Home Oxygen Delivery Systems

As the radiographer, you are sometimes assigned to take radiographs in the home of a patient who is unable to be transported to a health care facility. These patients are often using oxygen, and the oxygen may be delivered as a liquid, as compressed gas, or by means of an oxygen concentrator.

Compressed oxygen comes in tanks, which are usually smaller than the tanks used in the hospital; however, the principles of delivery are similar. Pure oxygen may be delivered by this method.

Liquid oxygen is a liquefied gas that concentrates oxygen into a lightweight container the size of a thermos bottle. It is conveniently portable and lasts longer than other forms of oxygen. It is used by people who must take oxygen with them when they leave home. This is an expensive method, chiefly because the oxygen evaporates quickly.

The oxygen concentrator is economical and is an excellent source of oxygen. Oxygen is concentrated by means of an electric machine that removes the nitrogen, water vapor, and hydrocarbons from room air. Oxygen is delivered at 90% by this means.

Oxygen Delivery Equipment for the Imaging Department

The following is a list of equipment that you will need to have on hand for oxygen administration in your diagnostic imaging department:

1. An oxygen source, either a piped-in source or a tank. If the source of oxygen is a tank, the tank must be checked daily to make certain that it is filled. Tanks should be stored on their side and not in the upright position if standard carriers are not available.

2. A sterile nasal cannula or simple face mask that is packaged and has not been used. These are disposable items.

3. Connecting tubing and an adapter to fit into a wall unit or tank.

4. A humidifier, if indicated. Humidifiers are not always used for short-term oxygen administration.

5. A flow meter.

6. A "no smoking" sign.

Radiographic Examinations of the Chest

Normal lung tissue is radiolucent; therefore, pathological conditions that produce densities may be detected by radiographic imaging techniques (Fig. 6-17).

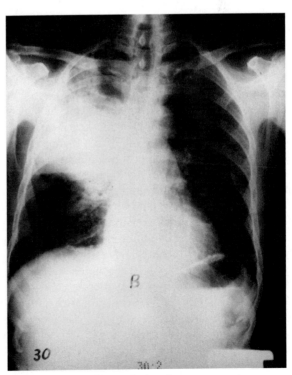

Figure 6-17. Radiograph showing pneumonia.

Posterior/anterior and lateral radiographs are frequently ordered to diagnose pulmonary pathology and to determine placement of endotracheal tubes and hemodynamic devices. These radiographs are frequently taken at the patient's bedside because he or she is too ill to be moved. If this is the case, you must confer with the nurse in charge of the patient's care before beginning your assignment. Remember that the patient in respiratory distress has difficulty complying with your needs and requests. You will need critical thinking and problem-solving skills to accomplish your task in a safe and efficient manner.

Before taking the radiograph, you need to assess the oxygen delivery system, the oxygen monitoring equipment, and the placement of associated tubing to prevent repeat exposures. Transporting patients or moving patients from a wheelchair or stretcher to the table or to the upright position can pull on oxygen tubes and cause pain to the patient.

Summary

Body temperature is a physiologic balance between heat produced in body tissues and heat lost to the environment. Fever indicates a disturbance in the heat-regulating centers of the body. It can be detected by an elevation in body temperature, which can be measured by oral, tympanic, rectal, and axillary methods. The site and device selected to measure body temperature depend on the patient's age, as well as the mental and physical status. The reading varies depending on the site used for measurement. The body temperature of a normal adult man or woman is 97.6°F (36.7°C) axillary, 98.6°F (37°C) oral, and 99.6°F (38°C) rectal. These readings vary somewhat in infants and children. Time of day, age, exercise, environmental temperature, and disease also alter body temperature.

The pulse is a reflection of the heartbeat, which sends blood to the arteries and causes them to throb. The areas where pulse can be measured best are at the radial artery (radial pulse), the temporal artery (temporal pulse), the carotid artery (carotid pulse), the femoral artery (femoral pulse), the apex of the heart (apical pulse), the dorsalis pedis artery (pedal pulse), the posterior tibial artery (posterior tibial pulse), and the popliteal artery (popliteal pulse). The apical pulse is measured by listening to it through a stethoscope. The average adult man or woman has a pulse rate of 60 to 90 beats/min. This rate varies in infants and children. The rate changes with age, exercise, time, and physiologic disturbances.

The exchange of oxygen and carbon dioxide between the atmosphere and the circulating blood is accomplished by respiration, which involves the inspiration of air containing oxygen and the expiration of air containing carbon dioxide. The rate of respiration for a normal adult male or female is from 15 to 20 breaths/min. This varies in infants and small children. Exercise, medication, age, or disease may change the respiratory rate.

Blood pressure is exerted by the blood on the walls of the blood vessels during the expulsion of blood from the heart and during the resting phase of the heart. It is measured with a sphygmomanometer and a stethoscope or with an electronic device. The most practical place to measure blood pressure is at the brachial artery, located at the center of the anterior elbow.

To record blood pressure, two or three readings are noted. The systolic reading is the highest point of pressure reached during a heart contraction. The diastolic reading is the lowest point to which the pressure drops during the relaxation of the ventricles and indicates the minimal pressure exerted against the arterial walls continuously. The diastolic reading is heard first as a softening and then as a disappearance of sound, in which case both readings are recorded. Blood pressure readings are influenced by age, exercise, medication, disease, and time of day.

To determine critical changes in a patient's vital signs, as a radiographer you must know what the patient's usual or baseline vital sign readings are. If these are not available, you have to rely on established norms to detect critical changes in the patient's vital signs.

Life cannot continue without oxygen; yet oxygen cannot be stored in the human body. When a patient has a disease that prevents the body from taking in enough oxygen, the necessary oxygen must be supplied to the patient by artificial means. Oxygen may be administered in the diagnostic imaging department in emergency situations and is frequently administered on hospital wards. Pure oxygen is a hazardous substance to be used only when prescribed by a physician. It supports combustion, so all health care workers need to take precautions when it is in use. No flames or machinery that might produce sparks may be used when oxygen therapy is in progress. Oxygen may also be toxic to lung tissues and may produce other harmful physiologic effects if not used cautiously. You should not make any radiographic exposures without first consulting the nurse in charge of the patient if a patient is receiving oxygen.

There are many types of oxygen delivery systems, including nasal cannulas, catheters, face masks, nonrebreather masks, partial rebreather masks, rebreather masks, Venturi masks, aerosol mask, and oxygen tents and ventilators.

The rebreather masks deliver a controlled amount of oxygen mixed with room air. Patients who need continuous oxygen for long periods of time may have a transtracheal delivery system, whereas patients in acute respiratory failure may receive oxygen by means of mechanical ventilators.

The most commonly seen type of delivery system is the nasal cannula; the most infrequently seen system is the nasal catheter. Oxygen tents are generally reserved for pediatric patients. The face mask is used for short-term administration of oxygen because it is uncomfortable for the patient to wear. Nasal cannulas are used for long-term administration because they allow the patient to speak and eat with little difficulty.

You may be responsible for assisting with oxygen administration or for monitoring vital signs in emergency situations in the diagnostic imaging department. You must become proficient in these skills, and you must make sure that the equipment needed for these purposes is present at all times.

Chapter 6 Test

_____ 1. An essential part of the initial assessment of a patient who is in the diagnostic imaging department for an invasive procedure is measuring vital signs. Why is this important?
   a. It establishes a baseline for further assessments.
   b. It allows the radiographer to become acquainted with the patient.
   c. It allows the radiographer to know whether the patient is hypertensive.
   d. It assists the physician.

_____ 2. Systolic blood pressure can be defined as
   a. The lowest point to which the blood pressure drops during relaxation of the ventricles
   b. The highest point reached during contraction of the left ventricle
   c. The difference between the systolic and diastolic blood pressure
   d. The pressure in the pulmonary vein

_____ 3. What range of breaths/min is the normal adult respiratory rate?
   a. 8 to 10
   b. 10 to 20
   c. 20 to 30
   d. 80 to 90

_____ 4. An adult patient is considered to be hypertensive or to have hypertension if the systolic blood pressure and diastolic blood pressure are consistently greater than
   a. 100 systolic and 60 diastolic
   b. 120 systolic and 80 diastolic
   c. 130 systolic and 86 diastolic
   d. 140 systolic and 90 diastolic

_____ 5. Oxygen can be toxic to patients if it is incorrectly used. What must you remember as the radiographer?
   a. Oxygen can be administered as the occasion requires.
   b. Oxygen administration must be ordered by the patient's physician.
   c. Oxygen is a vasodilator.
   d. Oxygen is inflammable.

_____ 6. A patient may be considered to have tachycardia if the pulse rate is higher than
   a. 60 beats/min
   b. 80 beats/min
   c. 90 beats/min
   d. 100 beats/min

_____ **7.** You must be certain that the following items are in your department, readily available, and in working order at all times.

1. Catheterization sets	a. 1 and 2
2. Suture removal sets	b. 2 and 4
3. Oxygen delivery equipment	c. 3 only
4. Blood pressure monitoring equipment	d. 3 and 4

_____ **8.** The normal oral body temperature of an adult is
   a. 96.6°F
   b. 99.6°F or 38°C
   c. 98.6°F or 37°C
   d. 97.6°F or 37.7°C

9. Match the following:
   1. Sphygmomanometer   _____
   2. Clinical thermometer   _____
   3. Stethoscope   _____
   4. Brachial artery   _____
   5. Radial artery   _____
      a. Point where the blood pressure is most often measured
      b. Measures apical pulse
      c. Measures blood pressure
      d. Measures body temperature
      e. Point where the pulse is most often measured

10. List the various sites of the body where a pulse can be counted. Which site is used most often?

11. List four devices that might be used to deliver oxygen by the low-flow method.

12. List two hazards that you as the radiographer must be aware of when assisting with oxygen administration.

13. Explain why the pulse rate goes up when the blood pressure drops.

14. List the sites available for measurement of body temperature.

_____ **15.** A stethoscope is needed to locate the pulse at which site?
   a. Radial
   b. Femoral
   c. Carotid
   d. Apical

7

Medical Emergencies in Diagnostic Imaging

Objectives

After studying this chapter, you will be able to:

1. Assess the basic levels of neurologic and cognitive functioning.

2. List the three classifications of shock, and describe the shock continuum.

3. Define distributive shock; list and define the three types of distributive shock.

4. Explain your role as a radiographer in recognizing and responding to the patient's immediate medical needs in the various categories of shock.

5. List the clinical manifestations of pulmonary embolus, and describe what your response should be if these symptoms appear in a patient in your care.

6. Differentiate among hypoglycemia, ketoacidosis, and hyperosmolar nonketotic syndrome, and explain the actions that you must take if the symptoms of each appear while you are caring for a patient.

7. List the clinical manifestations of a cerebral vascular accident and your role if these symptoms appear in a patient who is in your care.

8. List the clinical manifestations of cardiac and respiratory failure, and describe the action that you must take in each of these emergencies.

9. Explain the symptoms of mechanical airway obstruction and the emergency intervention necessary if this is suspected.

10. Describe the action that you as the radiographer must take if a patient faints or has a seizure while in your care.

11. List and describe the three basic categories of pain, and explain its harmful effects.

12. Explain your role as the radiographer in responding to a patient's complaint of pain or sudden alteration in his or her condition.

Glossary

Angioneurotic edema or angioedema: An allergic reaction characterized by rapid development of an edematous area of skin

Bradycardia: An abnormal circulatory condition in which the heart beats in a regular pattern but at a rate of less than 60 beats per minute

Bronchospasm: Contraction of smooth muscles in the walls of the bronchi and bronchioles causing narrowing of the lumen

Diaphoresis: Profuse sweating; heavy perspiration

Glucagon: A hormone secreted by islets of Langerhans in response to hypoglycemia or stimulation of growth hormone

Hemiparesis: Paralysis affecting one side of the body

Hypercoagulable: Characterized by abnormally increased coagulation

Periorbital: Relating to the periosteum of the orbit, usually of the eye

Tachycardia: An abnormal condition in which the myocardium contracts at a rate greater than 100 beats per minute

Ventricular: Relating to the ventricle in any sense; example: ventricular tachycardia

Many patients come to the radiographic imaging department in poor physical condition. This may be due to illness, injury, or a lengthy preparation for a diagnostic examination. When a person is in a weakened physical condition, physiologic reactions may not be as expected. Many abnormal physiologic reactions occur quickly and without warning and may be life-threatening if not recognized and treated immediately.

The non–trauma-related medical emergencies that are most likely to occur while the patient is undergoing radiographic imaging are shock, anaphylaxis (a type of shock), pulmonary embolus, reactions related to diabetes mellitus, cerebral vascular accident, cardiac and respiratory failure, syncope, and seizures. As the radiographer, you may be the first member of the health care team to observe these reactions; therefore, you must be able to recognize the symptoms and initiate the correct treatment.

You must be able to assess the behaviors that determine a patient's level of neurologic and cognitive functioning on admission for a radiographic procedure. If this initial assessment is performed, you will be able to recognize changes in the patient's mental status if they occur while the patient is under you care.

In most cases, the first action that you should take in a life-threatening emergency is to call the hospital emergency team, the physician conducting the procedure, and a co-worker for assistance. You must learn the correct procedure for calling the hospital emergency team in the institution in which you work. In many health care institutions, this procedure is dubbed "calling a code" or CODE. Memorize the emergency team number, and be prepared to explain the exact location of the emergency and the problem that has occurred.

All radiographic imaging departments have an emergency cart that contains the medications and equipment that are needed when a patient's condition suddenly becomes critical. This is often called a "crash cart." You must know where to obtain this cart quickly, and you must know who is responsible for maintaining the cart and all its equipment and supplies in working order. You must be familiar with the oxygen administration equipment so that you can assist with its use quickly.

Although you are not the health care worker who is responsible for a patient's pain management during most of his or her medical care, you must be sensitive to complaints of pain and discomfort while the patient is in your care. You must also be aware of your responsibilities if your patient complains of pain or has a change in his or her condition during an imaging procedure.

Assessment of Levels of Neurologic and Cognitive Functioning

As the radiographer assigned to care for a patient, you must be able to quickly assess the patient's neurologic functioning. This is important so that if the patient's condition deteriorates, you can quickly recognize this based on changes in the initial assessment data. Neurologic assessment can be highly technical and complex and is not within the scope of your practice. However, a rapid neurologic assessment tool that is used frequently in health care institutions is the Glasgow Coma Scale. This scale addresses the three areas of neurologic functioning and quickly gives an overview of the patient's level of responsiveness. It is simple, reliable, and convenient to use.

You can readily observe the three areas—eyes opening, motor response, and verbal response. (Display 7–1). A patient can be rated a maximum of 15 points for neurologic functioning. If the patient's score

DISPLAY 7–1
Glasgow Coma Scale

Eyes Open		Extension	2
Spontaneously	4	No response	1
To voice	3	**Verbal Response**	
To painful stimuli	2	Oriented	5
No response	1	Confused speech	4
Motor Response		Inappropriate words	3
Obeys commands	6	Incomprehensible sounds	2
Localizes pain	5	None	1
Withdraws from painful stimuli	4	Total points possible	15
Abnormal flexion	3		

begins to drop after your initial assessment, notify the physician in charge of the patient immediately.

Another indicator that a patient's condition is deteriorating is a change in the level of consciousness (LOC). These changes can be subtle but must not be ignored as you care for the patient. The LOC can be assessed quickly as follows:

1. Ask the patient to state his or her name, date, address, and the reason for coming to the radiographic imaging department. *If the patient gives these responses readily and correctly, you learn that the patient responds to verbal stimuli and that he or she is oriented to person, place, time, and situation. Note any undue need to repeat questions and any slow response, difficulty with choice of words, or unusual irritability.*

2. As you instruct the patient in positioning for your examinations, note his or her ability to follow directions. Also take note of any movement that causes pain or other difficulty in movement, as well as any alterations in behavior or lack of response. Report these to the physician in charge of caring for the patient. *These measures provide a baseline against which changes in the patient's mental and neurologic status can be assessed.*

3. Assess the patient's vital signs at this time if current readings are not on the chart. *You must have baseline readings against which to note changes if they occur!* An increasing systolic blood pressure or widening of the pulse pressure may indicate increasing intracranial pressure. Slowing of the pulse may also indicate increasing intracranial pressure. As compression of the brain increases, the vital signs change. Respirations increase, blood pressure decreases, and the pulse rate decreases further. A rapid rise in body temperature or a decrease in body temperature are also ominous signs.

If the patient has no complaints on initial assessment, note this. If the patient begins to complain of a headache, becomes restless or unusually quiet, or develops slurred speech or a change in the level of orientation as a procedure progresses, report this to the physician immediately. Stop the procedure, stay with the patient, and summon assistance, which includes ordering the emergency cart to be brought to the patient. Then, prepare the patient for oxygen and intravenous fluid administration.

CALL OUT!

Changes in a patient's neurologic status or LOC must never be ignored! Stop your work and notify the physician of these changes.

Shock

Shock is the body's pathological reaction to illness, trauma, or severe physiologic or emotional stress. It may be caused by body fluid loss, cardiac failure, decreased tone of the blood vessels, or obstruction of blood flow to the vital body organs. Shock is a life-threatening condition that may occur rapidly and without warning. It may be reversible if it is not allowed to progress. You may be the first health care worker to observe the initial symptoms of shock; therefore, you must be able to recognize them and begin the interventions that will halt its progress.

The Shock Continuum

The vital organs of the body depend on oxygen and other nutrients supplied by the blood for their survival. When this supply is diminished, adverse effects on normal physiologic functions occur. The shock syndrome may progress as a continuum in the patient's struggle to survive and return to a normal physiologic state.

At the onset of the shock continuum, the changes in physiologic function are in the cells of the body and are not clinically detectable except for a possible increase in heart rate. As the condition progresses, blood is shunted away from the lungs, skin, kidneys, and gastrointestinal tract to accommodate the brain's and the heart's critical need for oxygen. At this stage, called the *compensatory* stage, a host of symptoms are noticeable.

Compensatory Stage

1. Skin is cold and clammy.

2. Urine output decreases.

3. Respirations increase.

4. Bowel sounds are hypoactive.

5. Blood pressure is normal.

6. Anxiety level increases; patient may begin to be uncooperative.

If shock is allowed to progress beyond the compensatory stage, the mean arterial pressure (the average pressure at which blood moves through the vasculature of the body; abbreviated MAP) falls. All body systems are inadequately perfused, including the heart, which begins to pump inadequately.

The peripheral circulation reacts to the chemical mediators released by the body in this state, and fluid leaks from the capillaries, further decreasing the amount of fluid in circulation. The patient has acute renal failure, and the liver, gastrointestinal, and hematologic systems begin to fail. This stage in the shock syndrome is called the *progressive* stage. Progressive-stage symptoms are as follows:

Progressive Stage

1. Blood pressure falls.

2. Respirations are rapid and shallow.

3. Severe pulmonary edema results from leakage of fluid from the pulmonary capillaries. This is referred to as *acute respiration distress syndrome or shock lung.*

4. Tachycardia results and may be as rapid as 150 beats per minute.

5. The patient complains of chest pain.

6. Mental status changes beginning with subtle behavior alterations such as confusion with progression to lethargy and loss of consciousness.

7. Renal, hepatic, gastrointestinal, and hematologic problems occur.

If shock progresses beyond this point, it is called the *irreversible* stage. The organ systems of the body suffer irreparable damage, and recovery is unlikely.

Irreversible Stage

1. Blood pressure remains low.

2. Renal and liver failure result.

3. There is a release of necrotic tissue toxins and an overwhelming lactic acidosis.

Shock may be classified in several ways. For your purposes, it can be classified as hypovolemic, cardiogenic, and distributive or vasogenic shock. Descriptions of these classifications follow.

HYPOVOLEMIC SHOCK

Body fluids are contained within the cells of the body and in the extracellular compartments. The extracellular fluid is further distributed to the blood vessels (intravascular) and into the surrounding body tissues (interstitial). Approximately three or four times more body fluid is within the interstitial spaces than is within the vasculature of the body. When the amount of intravascular fluid decreases by 15 to 25 percent or by a loss of 750 to 1,300 milliliters, hypovolemic shock occurs. This decrease in volume may be due to internal or external hemorrhage; loss of plasma from burns; or fluid loss from prolonged vomiting, diarrhea, or medications.

CLINICAL MANIFESTATIONS

The signs and symptoms of hypovolemic shock may be placed into classes as follows:

- Class I: A blood loss of 15%
  Blood pressure is within normal limits.
  Heart rate is less than 100 beats per minute.
  The patient is slightly anxious.
  Respiration ranges from 14 to 20 per minute.
  Urine output is within normal limits.

- Class II: A blood loss of 15% to 30%
  Blood pressure is within normal limits.
  Heart rate is greater than 100 beats per minute.
  The patient is increasingly anxious.
  Respiration ranges from 20 to 30 per minute.
  Urine output begins to decrease.

- Class III: A blood loss of 30% to 40%
  Blood pressure begins to decrease to below-normal limits.
  Heart rate is greater than 120 beats per minute.
  The patient is anxious and confused.
  Respiration increases to 30 to 40 per minute.
  Urine output is greatly decreased.

- Class IV: A blood loss of more than 40%
  Systolic blood pressure decreases from 90 to 60 mm Hg.
  Heart rate is greater than 140 beats per minute, with weak and thready pulse.
  The patient is confused and lethargic.
  Respiration is greater than 40 per minute.
  Urine output further diminishes or ceases.

The patient may become excessively thirsty as a result of the fluid loss from hypovolemic shock. The extremities are cold; the skin is cold and clammy with cyanosis starting at the lips and nails. If the patient is dark-skinned, observe for cyanosis by pressing lightly on the fingernails or earlobes. If the patient is cyanotic, the color will not return to the compressed area in the usual 1-second interval. A bluish discoloration of the tongue and soft palate of the mouth is also indicative of cyanosis. If this condition is allowed to continue, cardiac and respiratory failure follows.

RADIOGRAPHER'S RESPONSE

1. Stop the ongoing radiographic imaging procedure; place the patient in a supine position with legs elevated 30 degrees (unless there is a head or spinal cord injury). Do not place the patient in Trendelenburg position.

2. Notify the physician in charge of the patient, and call for emergency assistance.

3. Make certain that the patient is able to breathe without obstruction caused by positioning or blood or mucus in the airway.

4. If the patient has blood loss from an open wound, don gloves and apply pressure directly to the wound with several thicknesses of dry, sterile dressing.

5. Have the emergency cart brought to the patient' side.

6. Prepare to assist with oxygen, intravenous fluids, and medications. Have large-gauge intravenous catheters on hand.

7. Keep the patient warm and dry. Do not overheat the patient; to do so will increase body metabolism and increase the need for oxygen.

8. Assess pulse, respirations, and blood pressure every 5 minutes until the emergency team assumes this role.

9. Do not leave the patient unattended. Inform him or her as appropriate of what is happening to alleviate anxiety.

10. Do not offer fluids to the patient, even if requested. Explain that he or she may need examinations or treatment that requires an empty stomach.

Cardiogenic Shock

Cardiogenic shock is caused by a failure of the heart to pump an adequate amount of blood to the vital organs. The onset of cardiogenic shock may occur over a period of time or it may be sudden. The patient who has been hospitalized by myocardial infarction, cardiac tamponade, dysrhythmias, or other cardiac pathology is most vulnerable.

CLINICAL MANIFESTATIONS

- Complaint of chest pain that may radiate to jaws and arms

- Dizziness and respiratory distress

- Cyanosis

- Restlessness and anxiety

- Rapid change in level of consciousness

- Pulse may be irregular and slow; may have tachycardia and tachypnea

- Difficult-to-find carotid pulse indicates decreased stroke volume of the heart

- Decreasing blood pressure

- Decreasing urinary output

- Cool, clammy skin

RADIOGRAPHER'S RESPONSE

1. Summon the emergency team and have the emergency cart placed at the patient's side.

2. Notify the physician in charge of the patient.

3. Place the patient in semi-Fowler's position or in another position that will facilitate respiration.

4. Prepare to assist with oxygen, intravenous fluid, and medication administration. Chest pain must be controlled.

5. Do not leave the patient alone; offer an explanation of treatment as appropriate; alleviate the patient's anxiety.

6. Assess pulse, respiration, and blood pressure every 5 minutes until the emergency team arrives.

7. Do not offer fluids.

8. Be prepared to administer cardiopulmonary resuscitation (CPR), if indicated.

Distributive Shock

Distributive shock occurs when a pooling of blood in the peripheral blood vessels results in decreased venous return of blood to the heart, decreased blood pressure, and decreased tissue perfusion. This may be the result of loss of sympathetic tone. Distributive shock is characterized by the blood vessels' inability to constrict and their resultant inability to assist in the return of the blood to the heart. It may also occur when chemicals released by the cells cause vasodilatation and capillary permeability, which in turn prompt a large portion of the blood volume to pool peripherally. There are three types of distributive shock: neurogenic, septic, and anaphylactic. Each is discussed in the following text.

Neurogenic Shock

Neurogenic shock results from loss of sympathetic tone causing vasodilation of peripheral vessels. It can be caused by spinal cord injury, severe pain, neurologic damage, the depressant action of medication, lack of glucose (as in insulin reaction or shock), or the adverse effects of anesthesia.

CLINICAL MANIFESTATIONS

- Hypotension
- Bradycardia
- Warm, dry skin
- Initial alertness if not unconscious because of head injury
- Cool extremities and diminishing peripheral pulses

RADIOGRAPHER'S RESPONSE

1. Summon emergency assistance.
2. Notify the physician in charge of the patient.
3. Keep the patient in supine position; legs may be elevated with physician's orders.
4. Have emergency cart brought to the patient's side.
5. If spinal cord injury is possible, do not move the patient.
6. Stay with the patient and offer support.
7. Monitor pulse, respiration, and blood pressure every 5 minutes.
8. Prepare to assist with oxygen, intravenous fluids, and medications.

Septic Shock

Septic shock is the least likely to be observed by you as the radiographer in the radiographic imaging department. However, you must be able recognize septic shock. You may also be called to the intensive care unit or emergency room to take portable radiographs of a patient in septic shock. In spite of the wide availability and use of antibiotics in recent years, the incidence of septic shock has risen and has a 40% to 50% mortality rate for its victims.

Gram-negative bacteria are the most common causative organisms in septic shock; however, gram-positive bacteria and viruses can also be the cause. When invaded by bacteria, the body begins its immune response by releasing chemicals that increase capillary permeability and vasodilatation, leading to the shock syndrome. The clinical manifestations of septic shock are divided into two phases.

CLINICAL MANIFESTATIONS

First Phase

- Hot, dry, and flushed skin
- Increase in heart rate and respiratory rate

- Fever, but possibly not in the elderly patient
- Nausea, vomiting, and diarrhea
- Normal-to-excessive urine output
- Possible confusion, most commonly in the elderly patient

Second Phase

- Cool, pale skin
- Normal or subnormal temperature
- Drop in blood pressure
- Rapid heart rate and respiratory rate
- Oliguria or anuria
- Seizures and organ failure if syndrome is not reversed

RADIOGRAPHER'S RESPONSE

The radiographer is rarely the person who initiates action if septic shock is present. However, if you care for a patient in septic shock, remember to keep the patient from becoming chilled because shivering increases the body's oxygen consumption.
If you are first on the scene, you should do the following:

1. Stop the procedure; notify the physician in charge of the patient.
2. Notify the emergency team and have the emergency cart available.
3. Place the patient in a supine position.
4. Keep the patient as quiet and calm as possible.
5. Do not leave the patient unattended.
6. If the skin is very warm, cover the patient with a lightweight blanket.
7. Monitor vital signs every 5 minutes.
8. Prepare for oxygen, intravenous fluid, and medication administration.
9. Keep the patient as comfortable as possible.

Anaphylactic Shock

Because some imaging procedures use contrast agents that contain iodine, to which some people are allergic, this is the most frequently seen type of shock in radiographic imaging. You must be able to recognize it at its onset to prevent life-threatening consequences.

Anaphylactic shock (anaphylaxis) is the result of an exaggerated hypersensitivity reaction (allergic reaction) to re-exposure to an antigen that was previously encountered by the body's immune system. When this occurs, histamine and bradykinin are released, causing widespread vasodilatation, which results in peripheral pooling of blood. This response is accompanied by contraction of nonvascular smooth muscles, particularly the smooth muscles of the respiratory tract. This combined reaction produces shock, respiratory failure, and death within minutes after exposure to the allergen. Usually, the more abrupt the onset of anaphylaxis, the more severe the reaction.

The most common causes of anaphylaxis are medications, iodinated contrast agents, and insect venoms. The path of entry may be through the skin, respiratory tract, or gastrointestinal tract, or through injection.

You have the responsibility as a radiographer of caring for the patient who is to receive a contrast agent while in your care. You must take a careful history of previous allergic responses that a patient may have had to any medication or food, including previous incidents when receiving contrast agents in imaging. If any of these responses is reported, you must inform the radiologist before injecting the contrast agent.

When iodinated contrast agents are being used for diagnostic procedures, observe the patient continuously for signs of allergic reaction. If early symptoms of anaphylactic shock are observed, you must act quickly to halt the progression of symptoms.

CLINICAL MANIFESTATIONS

The signs of anaphylactic shock may be classified as mild, moderate, or severe as follows:

Mild Systemic Reaction

- Symptoms beginning within 2 hours of exposure to the antigen
- Nasal congestion, periorbital swelling, itching, sneezing, and tearing of eyes
- Peripheral tingling or itching at the site of injection
- Feeling of fullness or tightness of the chest, mouth, or throat

Moderate Systemic Reaction

- All symptoms listed above with rapid onset
- Flushing, feeling of warmth, itching, and urticaria
- Anxiety
- Bronchospasm and edema of the airways or larynx
- Dyspnea, cough, and wheezing

Severe Systemic Reaction

- All symptoms listed in previous reactions with an abrupt onset
- Decreasing blood pressure; weak, thready pulse either rapid or shallow

- Rapid progression to bronchospasm, laryngeal edema, severe dyspnea, and cyanosis
- Dysphasia, abdominal cramping, vomiting, and diarrhea
- Seizures, respiratory and cardiac arrest

RADIOGRAPHER'S RESPONSE

1. Before beginning a procedure that requires administration of an iodinated contrast agent, make certain that the emergency cart has been monitored and that all emergency medications and equipment are up-to-date and in working order.

2. Before starting any procedure that involves the use of iodinated contrast medium, ask the patient the following questions:
   "Are you allergic to any food or medicine? Which ones?"
   "Do you have asthma or hay fever?"
   "Have you ever had hives or other allergic skin reactions?"
   "Have you ever had an x-ray examination that involved the use of a contrast medium? If so, did you have a reaction during or following that examination?"

3. Do not leave the patient who is receiving an iodinated contrast agent alone. Stop the infusion or injection immediately, and notify the radiologist if any of the following occurs: the patient complains of itching, redness, or swelling of the skin, or the patient seems unduly anxious.

4. If the patient complains of respiratory distress or has any of the later symptoms listed previously, call the emergency team.

5. Place the patient in semi-Fowler's position or in a sitting position to facilitate respiration.

6. Monitor pulse, respiration, and blood pressure every 5 minutes until the emergency team arrives to assume responsibility.

7. Prepare to assist with oxygen, intravenous fluid, and medication administration. Have large-gauge venous catheters available.

8. Prepare to administer CPR.

The medications usually given for anaphylactic shock are epinephrine, diphenhydramine, hydrocortisone, and aminophylline.

Many radiographic imaging departments have a standardized procedure form that must be completed before the administration of contrast agents. This form may request the information shown in Display 7–2.

Information Requested Before Administration of Contrast Agents

Name
Age
Date
Have you had the study that you are having today at any other time?
If the answer is yes, did you have any allergic or unusual reactions?
Are you allergic to any foods, medications, or any other substance? If you are, please specify.
Recent laboratory tests performed and results
Blood urea nitrogen (BUN) and creatinine

Have you had any protein in your urine? If so to what degree: +1, +2, +3, +4?
Do you have heart disease?
Hypertension?
Diabetes mellitus?
Sickle cell anemia?
Asthma?
Have you had any procedures such as a cystogram that involved use of contrast agents? If so, please explain.

After the examination, the physician completes a report indicating the type of contrast agent used and any unusual responses. If the patient has an anaphylactic reaction, the nature of the reaction should be written on the patient's film jacket in bold colors. Documentation of the reaction must also be made in the patient's chart by the physician performing the injection and examination.

A copy of this report is kept in the patient's diagnostic imaging department file, and a copy is also kept by the senior radiographer. If these precautions in documentation are taken, the history of the patient's previous problem will be on record, and the correct decisions can be made subsequently.

Patients who have received contrast agents as part of the diagnostic imaging procedure should remain in the department for 30 minutes for observation if they are not patients in the hospital. If they are having no problems after 30 minutes, they may be allowed to return home, accompanied by another person. They should be clearly instructed in the signs and symptoms of an anaphylactic reaction and told to return to the hospital emergency department immediately if any of these symptoms appears. A patient who has had even a mild allergic reaction during a diagnostic procedure that involves the use of a contrast agent should be instructed to report this if he or she is ever to receive iodinated contrast media in the future. If the reaction was severe, the patient may need to wear an alert bracelet to prevent further exposure to antigens of this sort.

CALL OUT!

A meticulous history is urgent when a patient is to receive a contrast agent!

Obstructive Shock

Obstructive shock results from pathological conditions that interfere with the normal pumping action of the heart; however, the heart itself may be free of pathologic conditions. The cause of obstructive shock may be pulmonary embolism, pulmonary hypertension, arterial stenosis, constrictive pericarditis, or tumors that interfere with blood flow through the heart. Because pulmonary embolism is the only condition mentioned here that may have an impact on you as the radiographer in the care of your patients, it is the only condition discussed in this chapter.

Pulmonary Embolus

A pulmonary embolus is an occlusion of one or more pulmonary arteries by a thrombus or thrombi. The thrombus originates in the venous circulation or in the right side of the heart and is carried through the vessels to the lungs, where it blocks one or more pulmonary arteries. This is a common medical emergency, which results in more than 50,000 deaths each year. The onset is sudden and requires immediate action to prevent severe consequences.

Pulmonary embolus is associated with trauma, orthopedic and abdominal surgical procedures, pregnancy, congestive heart failure, prolonged immobility, and hypercoagulable sites. Emboli may also be the result of air, fat, amniotic fluid, or sepsis. The severity of symptoms depends on the size or number of emboli that disturb the pulmonary circulation. The end result is arterial hypoxemia, which may be a life-threatening emergency.

When you are working with postoperative patients and patients who have suffered traumatic events affecting the long bones of the body, you must be aware of the complication of pulmonary embolism and be prepared to initiate emergency action if it occurs.

CLINICAL MANIFESTATIONS

- Rapid, weak pulse
- Hyperventilation
- Dyspnea and tachypnea
- Tachycardia
- Apprehension
- Cough and hemoptysis
- Diaphoresis
- Syncope
- Hypotension
- Cyanosis
- Rapidly changing levels of consciousness
- Coma; sudden death may result

RADIOGRAPHER'S RESPONSE

1. Stop the procedure immediately, and call for emergency assistance.

2. Notify the physician, and bring the emergency cart to the patient's side.

3. Monitor vital signs.

4. Do not leave the patient alone; reassure the patient.

5. Prepare to assist with oxygen administration, administration of intravenous medication, and fluid.

Diabetic Emergencies

Diabetes mellitus is now recognized as a group of metabolic diseases resulting from a chronic disorder of carbohydrate metabolism. It is caused by either insufficient production of insulin or inadequate utilization of insulin by the cells of the body. The result is an abnormal amount of glucose in the blood (hyperglycemia). The underlying cause of this disease process is a disturbance in the production, action, or utilization of insulin. Insulin is a hormone normally secreted by the islets of Langerhans located in the pancreas. In diabetes mellitus, the cells either stop responding to insulin or the pancreas ceases to produce insulin. In either case, the result is hyperglycemia, which leads to a series of metabolic complications. These complications may be diabetic

ketoacidosis or hyperglycemic hyperosmolar nonketotic syndrome complications. The structure and function of blood vessels and other organs of the body are adversely affected by these disease processes.

There are a series of emergencies that may result from diabetes. You may be the first health care worker to observe these emergencies, and you must be aware of the patient who has a medical diagnosis of diabetes mellitus and be able to recognize the symptoms of a pending emergency so that you can take appropriate action if these symptoms occur.

There are four major types of diabetes mellitus. The causes are not identical, and the course of the disease process and the treatment vary according to the type presenting. They are as follows:

1. *Type 1 diabetes mellitus.* Usually occurs in persons younger than 30 years of age and has an abrupt onset. The insulin-producing pancreatic beta cells are destroyed by an autoimmune process, and the affected person must receive insulin by injection to control blood glucose levels in the body and prevent ketoacidosis.

2. *Type 2 diabetes mellitus.* Usually occurs in persons older than 40 years of age and has a gradual onset. It results either from an impaired sensitivity to insulin or from a decreased production of insulin. This disease may be controlled by weight loss, dietary control, and exercise. However, if these measures do not control the problem, the person affected must take oral hypoglycemic agents to prevent hyperglycemia. Diabetic ketoacidosis does not occur in type 2 diabetes because there is enough insulin present in the body to prevent the breakdown of fat. However, a syndrome called hyperosmolar nonketotic syndrome may result and present an acute problem.

3. *Diabetes mellitus associated with or produced by other medical conditions or syndromes.*

4. *Gestational diabetes.* A diabetic condition that occurs in the later months of pregnancy. It is caused by hormones secreted by the placenta that prevent the action of insulin. This condition is usually treated with diet, but insulin may be prescribed to maintain blood glucose levels.

There are other conditions or physiologic problems that result in impairment of glucose tolerance that are not discussed in this text because they do not usually result in the need for emergency care. You must remember that persons who have diabetes mellitus are extremely susceptible to infections and therefore require extra skin care and infection-control precautions.

Acute Complications of Diabetes Mellitus

There are three complications of diabetes mellitus that may occur as you are caring for the patient: hypoglycemia, diabetic ketoacidosis, and hyperosmolar nonketotic syndrome (also called hyperosmolar nonketotic coma). The description and radiographer's responses follow.

Hypoglycemia

Hypoglycemia occurs when persons who have diabetes mellitus have an excess amount of insulin or oral hypoglycemic drug in their bloodstream, an increased metabolism of glucose, or an inadequate food intake with which to utilize the insulin.

When the blood glucose level falls below 50 to 60 mg/dL, hypoglycemia may result. A patient who has diabetes mellitus may come to the diagnostic imaging department after taking insulin or another hypoglycemic agent, but before having had sufficient food intake to use the insulin. The result may be a hypoglycemic reaction. The onset of symptoms is rapid, and immediate action is necessary to prevent coma.

CLINICAL MANIFESTATIONS

- *Mild reaction:* mild tremor, sweating, complaint of hunger, tachycardia, nervousness, and irritability
- *Moderate reaction:* dizziness, headache, and numbness of lips or tongue; confusion; profuse perspiration; cold, clammy skin; blurred or double vision; incoordination; irrational behavior; slurred speech
- *Severe reaction:* disorientation; difficulty arousing from sleep; impaired motor function; diminishing level of consciousness; seizures and rapid lapse into coma

RADIOGRAPHER'S RESPONSE

1. If the patient is conscious and complains of any early or moderate symptoms or says that he or she is a diabetic, has not eaten, and feels shaky or weak, notify the physician and administer some type of sugar immediately.

2. If there is nothing else available, the packets of sugar kept in most coffee rooms are acceptable. If the patient is carrying glucose tablets, 2 to 4 commercially prepared glucose tablets should be taken. If orange juice is available, you may offer it. Hard candy or 6 to 10 Lifesaver-type hard candies are also acceptable.

3. If the patient complains of any of the latter symptoms, check the chart or look for a bracelet that identifies the patient as a diabetic.

4. If the patient is having trouble swallowing or is unconscious, place 2 teaspoons of granulated sugar, corn syrup, or jelly into his mouth under his tongue. It will be absorbed through the mucous membranes.

5. Stop the diagnostic imaging procedure immediately, and call for emergency assistance.

6. Do not leave the patient unattended.

7. Monitor vital signs every 5 minutes.

8. Prepare to assist with administration of oxygen, intravenous medications, and fluids.

9. Glucagon, 1 mg intramuscularly or subcutaneously may be given, or 20 to 50 mL of 50% glucose in solution may be administered intravenously.

Hypoglycemia must be treated immediately because it interferes with the oxygen supply to the brain and may quickly result in cerebral damage or death.

Diabetic Ketoacidosis

When the body has insufficient insulin, the amount of glucose entering body cells decreases, and the liver begins to produce more glucose, which results in hyperglycemia. The kidneys attempt to compensate for this by excreting glucose with water and electrolytes. There is excessive urination (polyuria) with an outcome of dehydration and electrolyte imbalance in the body.

Another physiologic reaction to insulin deficiency in the body is the breakdown of fat into free fatty acids and glycerol. The liver in turn converts these free fatty acids into ketone bodies (ketosis) because insulin is not present to prevent this from occurring. Ketone bodies in the bloodstream result in metabolic acidosis. If this condition is not corrected quickly, the patient will become comatose and may die. Ketoacidosis occurs more slowly than hypoglycemia, but may result from a diabetic patient being detained for so long in the diagnostic imaging department that he or she misses a dose of insulin or hypoglycemic agent. Other possible causes of diabetic ketoacidosis are infection, illness, and undiagnosed or untreated type 1 diabetes mellitus.

CLINICAL MANIFESTATIONS

- Weakness, drowsiness, headache, blurred vision, abdominal pain, nausea, and vomiting
- Sweet odor to the breath and orthostatic hypotension
- Warm, dry skin; parched tongue; dry mucous membranes; extreme thirst (polydipsia); and polyuria
- General weakness, lethargy, and fatigue
- Flushed face; deep and rapid respirations
- Tachycardia; weak, thready pulse; and coma

RADIOGRAPHER'S RESPONSE

1. Check patient chart or look for a bracelet identifying the patient as a diabetic. Remember that patients with this condition may not be identified as diabetic.
2. Stop treatment and notify the physician.
3. Call for emergency assistance.
4. Do not leave patient unattended.
5. Monitor vital signs.
6. Prepare to assist with administration of intravenous fluids, medications, and oxygen.

Hyperglycemic Hyperosmolar Nonketotic Syndrome

Hyperglycemic hyperosmolar nonketotic syndrome or coma may be a complication of mild type 2 diabetes mellitus, or it may occur in an elderly person with no known history of diabetes mellitus. The patient with the symptoms of this condition is usually first seen in the emergency department and not in the diagnostic imaging department.

Frequently, the patient is perceived as being inebriated or having had a stroke, but it is, however, an extremely serious, life-threatening condition. Factors that precipitate this reaction are acute illness; therapeutic procedures such as dialysis; and diagnostic procedures that require changes in diet, especially a procedure requiring the patient to have nothing by mouth for 12 hours. There is a loss of effective insulin, leading to diuresis and loss of fluid and electrolytes. The blood glucose level in patients with this problem is often greater than 600 mg/dL; there is little or no ketosis and plasma is hyperosmolar.

CLINICAL MANIFESTATIONS

- Extreme dehydration; dry skin, sunken eyes
- Hypotension, tachycardia, increased body temperature

- Extreme thirst; muscle twitching; difficult, slurred speech
- Mental confusion, seizures, hemiparesis, coma

RADIOGRAPHER'S RESPONSE

1. Call for emergency assistance; do not leave patient unattended.
2. Notify the physician in charge of the patient, and stop the diagnostic procedure.
3. Monitor vital signs; prepare to administer intravenous fluids, medication, and oxygen.

Cerebral Vascular Accident (Stroke)

Cerebral vascular accidents (CVAs) are caused by occlusion of the blood supply to the brain, rupture of the blood supply to the brain, or rupture of a cerebral artery, resulting in hemorrhage directly into the brain tissue or into the spaces surrounding the brain. Strokes vary in severity from mild transient ischemic attacks to severe, life-threatening situations. CVAs occur most frequently with little or no warning and may possibly occur in the radiographic imaging department during a stressful procedure.

Strokes are now being termed "brain attacks." A stroke is now recognized as an event that is as great a medical crisis as a heart attack. It is extremely important that the stroke victim receive immediate emergency evaluation, because being started on fibrinolytic therapy reduces the neurologic damage from an ischemic stroke. You must be familiar with the warning signs and symptoms of this medical crisis and be prepared to initiate emergency care.

CLINICAL MANIFESTATIONS

- Possible severe headache
- Numbness
- Muscle weakness or flaccidity of face or extremities, usually one-sided
- Eye deviation, usually one-sided; possible loss of vision
- Confusion
- Dizziness or stupor
- Difficult speech (dysphasia) or no speech (aphasia)
- Ataxia
- May complain of stiff neck

- Nausea or vomiting may occur
- Loss of consciousness

Cardiac and Respiratory Emergencies

Respiratory failure, cardiac failure (also called cardiac arrest), or an airway obstruction may occur in the diagnostic imaging department without warning and when least expected. You may be the first health care worker to witness this event and thus will be the person to call the code and initiate emergency action. The human brain can survive without oxygen for only 2 to 4 minutes. This means that there is little time to ponder the situation before acting.

All health care staff must be prepared to perform basic CPR and the abdominal thrust maneuver. New basic life support guidelines have recently made early cardiac defibrillation a high-priority goal and the ability to use an automated external defibrillator (AED) a basic life support skill. All health care workers are expected to have this skill included in their basic life support classes.

Many health care facilities have classes for their employees on a regular basis to teach them and keep them current in these procedures. Other health care facilities require the employee to obtain this training at classes offered in the community. The American Red Cross and the American Heart Association provide basic life support classes regularly for the general public. The techniques must be demonstrated by a licensed instructor, and return demonstrations must be given by the student until proficient.

You must understand that there are frequent changes in basic life support methods, and it will be your responsibility to keep abreast of the changes and rules in your particular institution concerning your responsibility if you need to respond to a cardiac or respiratory type of emergency. The brief descriptions of CPR, the use of the AED, and the abdominal thrust maneuver do not prepare you to administer these techniques. Complete explanations and directions are not within the scope of this text. You must take an authorized class and successfully achieve its goals before using these skills. Basic life support for an infant or small child requires special consideration and is addressed only briefly in this text.

To protect yourself from communicable diseases contracted through exposure to blood and body fluids, you must wear clean gloves when clearing a patient's airway if the need arises. A disposable mask with a one-way valve is recommended when performing CPR (Fig. 7–1). This type of mask should be available in every diagnostic imaging room. A manual resuscita-

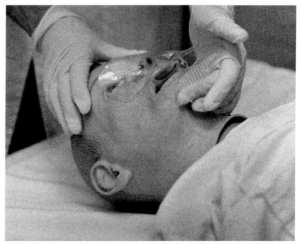

Figure 7–1. Disposable mask with a one-way valve.

tion bag may be used if available, and you should be instructed in its use. AEDs must also be made available and ready for use for a health care worker who is competent to use them.

Cardiac Arrest

When the heart ceases to beat effectively, the blood can no longer circulate throughout the body, and the person no longer has an effective pulse. There are a number of possible causes of this type of event. The electrical activity of the heart may be disrupted, causing the heart to beat too rapidly, as in ventricular fibrillation or ventricular tachycardia. The heart may beat too slowly, as in bradycardia or atrioventricular block. Pulseless electrical activity may also result from hypovolemic shock, cardiac tamponade, hypothermia, or a pulmonary embolism. In addition, drug overdoses, severe acidosis, or a severe myocardial infarction may cause this to occur. Irreversible brain damage and death result within minutes of a cardiac event, depending on the person's age and health status before the arrest.

CLINICAL MANIFESTATIONS OF CARDIAC ARREST

- Loss of consciousness, pulse, and blood pressure
- Dilation of the pupils within seconds
- Possibility of seizures

Respiratory Dysfunction

Respiratory dysfunction may precede respiratory arrest. It can be the result of airway obstruction causes by positioning, the tongue falling backward into the throat of an unresponsive person, a foreign object lodged in the throat, disease, drug overdose, injury, or coma. Whatever the cause, gas exchange is no longer adequate to meet the needs of the body.

CLINICAL MANIFESTATIONS OF A PARTIALLY OBSTRUCTED AIRWAY

- Labored, noisy breathing
- Wheezing
- Use of accessory muscles of the neck, abdomen, or chest on inspiration
- Neck vein distention
- Diaphoresis
- Anxiety
- Cyanosis of the lips and nailbeds
- Possibly a productive cough with pink-tinged frothy sputum

RADIOGRAPHER'S RESPONSE TO A PATIENT WITH A PARTIALLY OBSTRUCTED AIRWAY

1. Call for assistance; do not leave the patient alone.
2. Assist the patient to a sitting or semi-Fowler's position.
3. Attempt to relieve the patient's anxiety.
4. Prepare to administer oxygen.
5. Prepare to use the emergency cart.

Respiratory Arrest

CLINICAL MANIFESTATIONS

- The patient stops responding.
- The pulse continues to beat briefly and quickly becomes weak and stops.
- Chest movement stops and no air is detectable moving through the patient's mouth.

RADIOGRAPHER'S RESPONSE TO CARDIAC AND RESPIRATORY ARREST

1. If the patient is an adult and is found to be unresponsive, shake the patient and ask, "Are you all right?" If no response, call immediately for emergency medical services. In a hospital, this would be calling a CODE. If you are not near a telephone, shout for help, stating your location. "I need help STAT in Room 102." Do not leave the patient.

2. Assess the carotid pulse of an adult patient. Do not waste time taking the blood pressure or listening for a heartbeat! Do not assess the electrocardiogram contact if one is in place.

3. If the patient is pulseless and an adult and the emergency medical team has been summoned, place the patient in a supine position on a hard surface. A backboard is available for use in hospital rooms. In the diagnostic imaging area, the tables have a hard surface and this may not be an issue.

4. If a neck or spinal cord injury is suspected, the patient must be log rolled into a supine position.

BEGIN CARDIOPULMONARY RESUSCITATION IN THE CLINICAL AREA

1. Open the airway. Don gloves; remove any obvious material in the mouth or throat. If the patient has dentures that are loose, remove them. Avoid pushing a foreign object farther back in the mouth or throat. Do not perform blind fingersweeps! Direct the chin up and back. Never sweep the mouth of an infant or small child unless the object is clearly visible!

2. If you suspect a neck injury, use the jaw thrust maneuver. Do not extend the neck (Fig. 7–2).

3. Look, listen, and feel for airway movement. If you don't feel or hear air or see movement of breathing, tightly place the bag- or mouth-mask over the patient's mouth and nose. Take a deep breath and slowly, over 2 full seconds, with the least amount of your breath needed to make the chest rise, exhale into the mouth-mask. Allow the patient to exhale as you take in another deep breath and repeat this maneuver. The rationale for this sequence is to reduce the amount of air that enters the stomach of the patient to prevent the complication of regurgitation, aspiration, and pneumonia.

4. If the patient is not breathing and initial ventilation attempts are not successful, assess for foreign body in airway. If you are unable to administer successful rescue ventilations and if you suspect airway obstruction, use abdominal thrusts to remove obstruction (as explained later in this section). Recheck for breathing.

5. If patient is breathing, place him or her in a recovery position (Fig. 7–3).

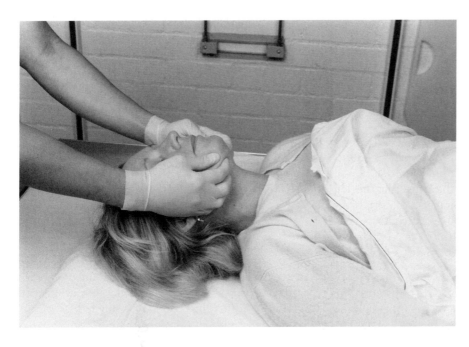

Figure 7–2. Direct the chin up and back. Do not extend the neck.

6. Assess for signs of circulation by checking carotid pulse, and evaluate for coughing, movement, and breathing.

7. If no signs of circulation or breathing are present, the AED is not readily available, and the emergency team has not arrived, begin chest compressions.

Defibrillation

Cardiac arrest may precede or follow respiratory arrest. It may also occur when the electrical activity of the heart is present but not effective in delivering oxygenated blood to vital organs. When cardiac arrest occurs and the patient is being monitored or is immediately placed on a monitor, use the quick-look paddles found on most defibrillators to determine the presence of ventricular tachycardia or ventricular fibrillation. If these are not available, apply the AED as quickly as possible to analyze the patient's heart rhythm. For every minute that defibrillation is delayed, the patient's chances for survival decline by 10 percent. The AED procedure is briefly described below; however, you must be properly instructed in this procedure in a certified class with clinical practice.

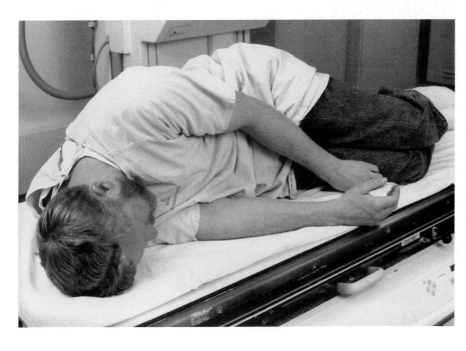

Figure 7–3. Patient in recovery position.

RADIOGRAPHER'S RESPONSE

1. Place the AED pack near the patient's left ear and open it. Turn on the power if it does not come on automatically. (This will initiate voice instruction from the pack.) CPR may be continued until it is time to attach the electrodes.

2. Attach the electrodes onto the patient's anterior chest: one at the right upper sternal border below the clavicle and the other on the left chest lateral to the left nipple (Fig. 7–4). If the patient's chest is extremely hairy, you may need to remove some of the hair to make adequate contact with the skin. If the chest is very moist, dry it first with a towel.

3. When the electrodes are correctly attached, press the analyze button to assess the need for defibrillation. The machine will tell you whether defibrillation shock is required.

4. If a shock is required, all persons must be totally clear of the bed or table and any contact with the patient. The machine will dictate a "clear" order.

5. Then, press the shock button when the AED dictates the order. Do not press the shock button before the order.

6. If the AED states that no shock is indicated and the patient remains pulseless, resume CPR.

7. Analysis of heart activity may be repeated in 1 or 2 minutes or until the CODE team arrives.

When the patient is a child, the cause of the arrest is frequently respiratory in nature. Because of this, calling the emergency medical team should take place after CPR is administered for 1 minute unless another person is present who can call the code while you administer CPR. The procedure is much the same for infants and children; however, there are some variations, which are listed in Display 7–3.

You may also use a one-way mask on the infant or child to protect you or any other member of the health care team. If you are adequately trained in the use of a breather bag, you may use it. The equipment must be of a size to adequately fit the patient (Fig. 7–5).

External cardiac compression is effective only if the patient is lying on a firm surface. If the patient is on a radiographic table, you must kneel on the table beside the patient. If the patient is lying on a soft surface, you

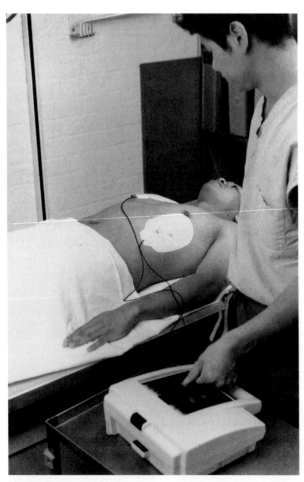

Figure 7–4. Attach electrodes at right upper sternal border below the clavicle and the other on the left chest lateral to the left nipple.

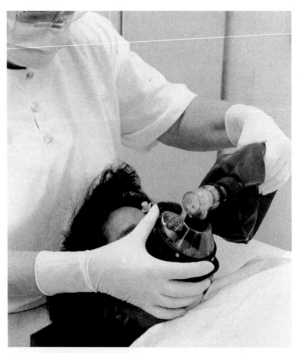

Figure 7–5. Rescue breathing with breather bag.

DISPLAY 7–3

Variations in CPR Techniques for Infants and Children

Neonate

- Head-tilt, chin-lift, or jaw thrust if trauma is present.
- 2 effective breaths at 1 second per breath, then 30 to 60 breaths per minute.
- Back blows or chest thrusts; no abdominal thrusts!
- Umbilical pulse check.
- The compression landmark is the lower half of the sternum, 1 fingerwidth below the intermammary line.
- Use 2 fingers for compression at approximately 1/2 inch at about 120 compressions per minute or 90 compressions to 30 breaths.

Infant under age 1 year

- Head-tilt, chin-lift or jaw thrust if trauma is present.
- 2 effective breaths at 1 to 1 1/2 seconds per breath, then 20 breaths per minute.
- Back blows or chest thrusts. Do not use abdominal thrusts on a baby!

- Brachial pulse checked.
- The compression landmark is the lower half of the sternum, 1 fingerwidth below the intermammary line.
- Use 2 thumbs or 2 fingers at 1/2 to 1 inch compression at a rate of at least 100 compressions per minute.

Child ages 1 to 8 years

- Head-tilt, chin-lift or jaw thrust if trauma is present.
- 2 effective breaths at 1 1/2 seconds per breath, then 20 breaths per minute.
- Abdominal thrusts or chest thrusts.

The carotid pulse is checked. The compression landmark is the lower half of the sternum with the heel of the hand. The compression depth of the chest is about 1 to 1 1/2 inches at the rate of 100 per minute or 5 compressions to 1 ventilation.

From American Heart Association, Guidelines 2000 for Cardiopulmonary Resuscitation.

---

may place a cardiac board under his or her chest. If none is available, the patient must be moved to the floor.

Take an adequate amount of time to determine pulselessness (5 to 10 seconds). Performing cardiac compressions on a person whose heart is functioning is extremely dangerous to the patient. Once cardiac compressions have been started, they should not be interrupted for more than 7 seconds at a time. (Two-person CPR is not discussed in this text because it demands actual demonstration and return demonstration to be successful.)

Be certain that your hands are positioned correctly to prevent internal injury while the cardiac compressions are being performed. Do this in the following manner:

1. Move your fingers up the lower margin of the patient's rib cage to the area where the ribs and sternum meet. When you have located this area, place your index finger above it, and place the heel of your hand beside the index finger with your second hand on top of it.

2. Your hands should be located 1.5 inches from the tip of the xiphoid process toward the patient's head. Your fingers should not touch the chest wall. Use the weight of your body for compression of the chest wall, and keep your elbows straight (Fig. 7–6).

3. Compress the sternum 1.5 to 2 inches directly downward; then release the compression completely.

4. Keeping your elbows straight, give 15 compressions in a smooth, even rhythm.

5. Inflate the patient's lungs two more times.

6. Reassess the patient's carotid pulse and respiratory status. If the patient has no pulse or respiration, continue with 15 compressions followed by 2 inflations until the emergency team arrives.

7. Allow them to take over at a time specified for the change.

Radiographers and all health care personnel must guard against becoming infected by a communicable disease while performing lifesaving procedures by wearing disposable gloves and by learning to use a manual resuscitation bag or a one-way face mask. Education in the use of this equipment must be obtained before it can be used effectively; such education should be a part of CPR training.

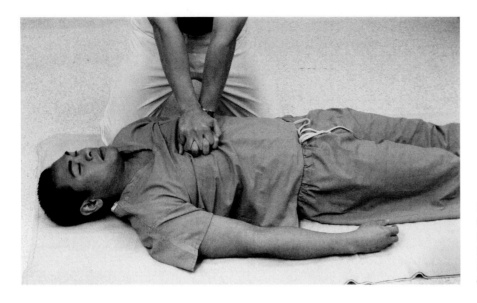

Figure 7–6. Position for one-man cardiac compression. Place heel of hand beside the index finger with second hand on top of it. Keep elbows straight.

Airway Obstruction

A foreign body such as a piece of chewing gum or food may lodge in a patient's throat and produce respiratory arrest. This type of accident occurs most often in the elderly, the very young, or the intoxicated while eating. However, you must consider this possibility in any case of respiratory arrest.

When airway obstruction caused by a foreign object occurs, the patient usually appears to be quite normal, then suddenly begins to choke. The patient grabs the throat and is unable to speak. If no one is present to observe this, the patient eventually loses consciousness. Unless the early signs are observed, it is impossible to know the cause of the unconscious state. Airway obstruction may occur with the patient sitting, standing, or lying down and must be dealt with initially in that position.

RADIOGRAPHER'S RESPONSE

1. If the patient does not respond and breathlessness is established as described in the preceding paragraphs, seal the patient's nose and mouth, and ventilate him or her as in the initial steps of CPR.

2. If you see the patient's chest rise and fall, proceed as for basic CPR.

3. If the patient's chest does not rise and fall, reposition the head using the head tilt, chin lift, or jaw thrust as indicated. Then attempt to ventilate again.

4. If this is unsuccessful, assume that the airway is obstructed and use the abdominal thrust to attempt to remove the obstruction.

Abdominal Thrust: Patient Standing or Sitting

Stand behind he patient and grasp with both hands above the patient's umbilicus and below the xiphoid process of the sternum. Position your lower hand with the thumb inward; your other hand firmly grips the lower hand. Then make a rapid upward movement that forces the abdomen inward and thrusts upward against the diaphragm (Fig. 7–7). This maneuver forces air up through the trachea and dislodges the foreign object. Never attempt to practice this maneuver on a person who is not in distress because you may cause serious injury. Be sure to place your hands so that you avoid the patient's xiphoid process to prevent internal injury.

Abdominal Thrust: Patient in Supine Position

Place the patient in a supine position with face up. Kneel astride the patient's thighs and place the heel of one hand against the patient's abdomen above the navel and below the tip of the xiphoid process. Place your other hand over the first and quickly press the abdomen upward. You must be certain to direct the thrust directly up and not to deviate to the left or right (Fig. 7–8). This maneuver acts in the same way for the patient who is sitting or standing.

Chest Thrust: Patient Sitting or Standing

The chest thrust is used to dislodge a foreign object only if the patient is in advanced stages of pregnancy

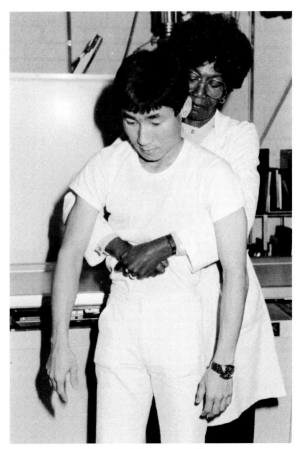

Figure 7–7. Abdominal thrust, standing.

or is excessively obese and the abdominal thrust cannot be used effectively.

Stand behind the patient and put your arms under the patient's armpits and around the chest. Place the thumb side of your fist in the middle of the sternum, avoiding the xiphoid process and the margins of the rig cage. Place your other hand on top and thrust backward. Repeat this maneuver until the object is dislodged.

If the patient is an infant and you suspect an obstructed airway, place the patient face down over your forearm with the infant's legs straddling your elbow. Your hand should support the patient's head and neck between your thumb and index finger with the patient's head lower than the chest but not straight down. Deliver five sharp blows to the patient's back between the shoulder blades (Fig. 7–9). If this is not successful, perform chest thrusts with two or three fingers on the midsternum about one per second.

The method of dealing with foreign body airway obstruction for infants and children also varies with their weight, age, and size.

Chest Thrust: Patient Pregnant or Excessively Obese/Unconscious

After determining breathlessness in the prescribed manner, attempt ventilation. If this is not successful and the patient is in the advanced stages of pregnancy or is excessively obese, you may use the chest thrust to attempt to dislodge the foreign object.

Kneel beside the patient and place your hands in the same position as with thrust for external cardiac compression. Make sure thrusts are slow and firm and performed as many times as is necessary to relieve the obstruction.

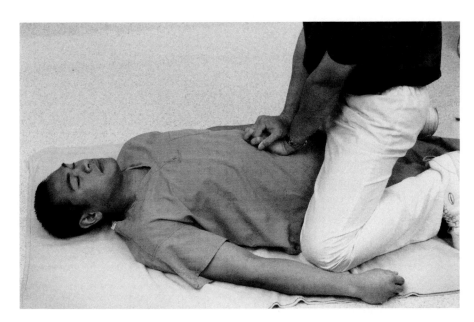

Figure 7–8. Abdominal thrust; patient in supine position.

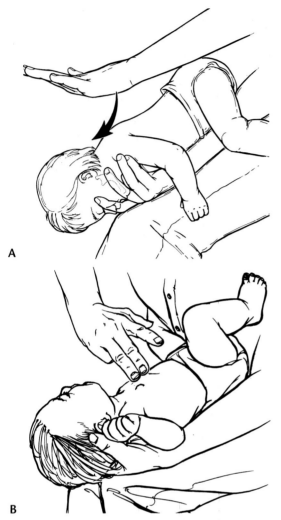

A

B

Figure 7–9. Back blows (**A**) and chest compression (**B**) to relieve complete foreign body airway obstruction in an infant. (American Heart Association: Pediatric basic life support. *Journal of the American Medical Association* 269;2251-2261, 19xx.).

CALL OUT!

REMINDER: The methods described in this text to remove airway obstructions for adult, child, or infant patients are taught in basic CPR classes, and all radiography students must have formal instruction in this type of treatment. The foregoing descriptions do not render the radiographer competent to perform these maneuvers.

Seizures

A seizure is an unsystematic discharge of neurons of the cerebrum that results in an abrupt alteration in brain function. It usually begins with little or no warning and may last only seconds or for several minutes. A seizure is accompanied by a change in the level of consciousness.

Seizures are a syndrome or symptom of a disease, not a disease in themselves. They may be caused by infectious disease, especially those that are accompanied by high fever. They may also be caused by extreme stress, head trauma, brain tumors, structural abnormalities of the cerebral cortex, genetic defects (epilepsy), birth trauma, vascular disease, congenital malformations, or postnatal trauma. Odors and flashing lights can cause a seizure in a person who is seizure-prone.

There are basically two types of seizure: generalized and partial.

Finger Sweep

Use the finger sweep maneuver only on an unconscious patient with the patient lying in a supine position, face up. Open the patient's mouth by grasping the tongue and lower jaw between your thumb and fingers. Then lift the mandible. This is done to move the tongue away from a foreign body that may be lodged behind it. Next insert the index finger of the other hand along the base of the tongue using a hooking motion to dislodge and remove the object (Fig. 7–10). This must be done with extreme care so that a foreign object is not forced farther into the airway. For infants and small children, this must not be done if the object is not clearly visible in the mouth.

After the obstruction is expelled, log roll the patient to his or her side for recovery.

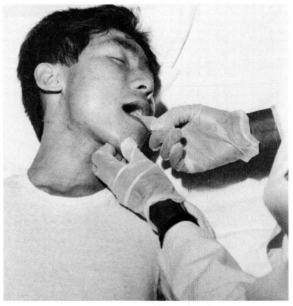

Figure 7–10. Finger sweep.

Generalized Seizures

CLINICAL MANIFESTATIONS

- May utter a sharp cry as air is rapidly exhaled
- Muscles become rigid, and eyes open wide (tonic phase)
- May exhibit jerky body movements and rapid, irregular respirations (clonic phase)
- May vomit
- May froth and have blood-streaked saliva caused by biting the lips or tongue
- May exhibit urinary or fecal incontinence
- Usually falls into a deep sleep after the seizure

RADIOGRAPHER'S RESPONSE

1. Stay with the patient and gently secure him or her to prevent injury.
2. Call for assistance.
3. Do not attempt to insert hard objects into the patient's mouth because you may damage tissues or teeth.
4. Do not put your fingers in the patient's mouth; they may be bitten.
5. Remove dentures and foreign objects from patient's mouth if possible, but do not finger sweep.
6. Place a blanket or pillow under the patient's head to protect it from injury.
7. Do not restrain the arms or legs, but protect them from injury.
8. Do not attempt to move the patient to the floor if he or she has not fallen there; if on a radiographic table, do not allow the patient to fall to the floor.
9. Observe the patient carefully, and keep track of the time of the seizure to record later.
10. Provide patient privacy.
11. After the seizure has ceased, position the patient to prevent aspiration of secretions and vomitus. Turn the patient to a Sims' position and put the face downward so that secretions may drain from his or her mouth (Fig. 7–11).

Partial Seizures: Complex and Simple

The seizure activity depends on the area of the brain involved. The clinical manifestations of the patient during a complex partial seizure are as follows:

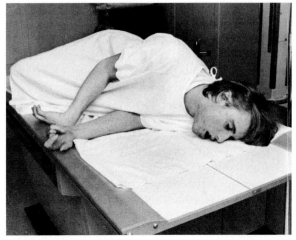

Figure 7–11. Position the patient with head and face downward so secretions may drain from the mouth.

CLINICAL MANIFESTATIONS OF A COMPLEX PARTIAL SEIZURE

- The person may remain motionless or may experience an excessive emotional outburst of fear, crying, or anger.
- The person may manifest facial grimacing, lip smacking, swallowing movements, or panting.
- The person will be confused for several minutes after the episode with no memory of the incident.

CLINICAL MANIFESTATIONS OF A SIMPLE PARTIAL SEIZURE

The clinical manifestations of the patient during a simple partial seizure are as follows:

- Only a finger or a hand may shake.
- The person may speak unintelligibly.
- The person may be dizzy.
- The person may experience smelling strange odors, tastes, or hearing sounds.
- The person will not lose consciousness.

Syncope

Syncope, or fainting, is a transient loss of consciousness, which usually results from an insufficient blood supply to the brain. Heart disease, hunger, poor ventilation, extreme fatigue, and emotional trauma all are possible causes. The elderly patient who is asked to change positions from lying to standing too quickly may also have a syncopal reaction owing to orthostatic hypotension. Orthostatic hypotension is an abnormally low blood pressure occurring when a person stands up before the blood pooled in the extremities has time to circulate to the upper body.

Patients are frequently instructed not to eat breakfast before coming to the diagnostic imaging department from their homes or hospital rooms. Often they are ill and lack of nourishment may increase the likelihood of fainting. The patient cannot choose the "proper" place in which to faint, so he or she may fall and cause injury to him- or herself. You must be able to recognize and watch for the symptoms that a patient is about to faint.

If you suspect that the patient is in a weakened condition because of a recent traumatic injury or illness, you must not request that the patient stand for a diagnostic film and then leave the patient to support him- or herself; the patient is likely to fall. Consider other methods of obtaining the exposure, or have an assistant stand beside the patient to support him or her, if necessary.

If you are caring for an elderly patient, allow the patient time to sit for several minutes before requesting that he or she stand or walk. You must always be at the patient's side to protect him or her from falling.

CLINICAL MANIFESTATIONS

- Pallor, complaints of dizziness and nausea
- Hyperpnea, tachycardia
- Cold, clammy skin

RADIOGRAPHER'S RESPONSE

1. If the patient complains of feeling dizzy or appears to be confused, have the patient lie down.

2. If the patient has actually fainted, place him or her in a prone position with legs elevated.

3. If the patient begins to fall, do not try to keep him or her standing. Support and assist the patient to the floor in a manner that prevents injury. Place your knee behind the patient's and your arm around the waist and assist the patient to the floor (Fig. 7–12).

4. When the patient is in a safe position, summon medical assistance.

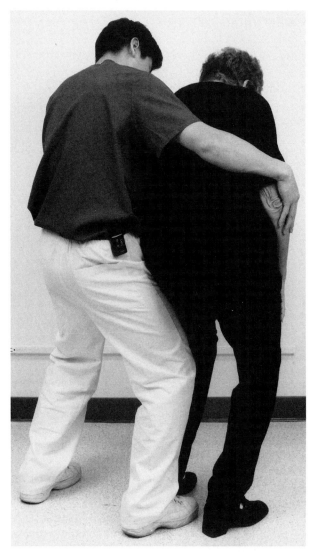

Figure 7–12. Place your knee behind the patient's knee to support her.

The Radiographer's Response to the Patient in Pain

Although you are not the health care worker who will be responsible for many aspects of pain management, you need to be sensitive to the patient's need for pain control while in your care. In recent years, pain management has become a recognized health care problem that must be dealt with adequately and not left to the subjective judgment of health care workers as in the past. In 1999, the Joint Commission on Accreditation of Healthcare Organizations (JCAHO) established standards for pain management for all patients. Pain control practice must be in compliance with those standards. Hospitals, long-term care facilities, home health care agencies, outpatient clinics, and managed care organizations must be knowledgeable in pain assessment and management. They must also have policies and procedures in place concerning use of analgesics and pain control therapies. You must be instructed in the pain control policies of your department as well as of the institution in which you are employed. To ignore a patient's complaint of pain can result in extreme suffering for that patient and may jeopardize your license.

According to a noted pain theorist, Margo McCaffery, "Pain is whatever the experiencing person says it is, existing whenever he says it does" (McCaffery, 1968). All pain is real and must not be ignored by the health care worker. Many factors affect pain and the patient's response to pain. The age of the patient is significant. Children do not understand pain and become frightened when the sensation of pain occurs. The elderly patient often misinterprets the symptoms of pain and may ignore them or attribute them to other problems. The gender of the patient is also significant. Men tend to be more stoic than woman when in pain. Culture also has a strong influence on the manner in which a patient perceives and reacts to pain. In some cultures, people are expected to endure pain without response, whereas in other cultures, an emotional response is expected. The patient's mental status also affects pain receptors. Increased anxiety tends to increase the level of pain perception. Fatigue may also intensify the reaction to pain. A patient who has had many experiences with pain may accept more pain stimuli before responding than one who has had no previous experience with pain. Personal coping styles also influence the manner in which a patient reacts to pain as well as his or her social support system. An emotional person may respond to pain more quickly than a person with a stoic-type personality. A person who feels little significant family or social support also may have a more difficult time dealing with pain.

There are three basic categories of pain. They are listed and defined in Table 7–1.

All accredited health care facilities must have a pain assessment tool with which to rate the degree of pain the patient is feeling. This tool must differ according to the patient's age, cultural background, and medical condition so that each patient can easily understand it. The scales used often are numerical in nature: that is, a scale from 1 to 10, with 10 being the most excruciating pain. Other facilities use faces that smile, which change ultimately to tears for the most intolerable pain. When you begin to assess a patient, you may use the scale that is preferred in your institution as a guide.

You must make sure that your patient remains as comfortable as possible while in your care, and you must never ignore a patient's complaint of pain. You can achieve this by using your critical thinking skills when planning the patient's care. Your plan to manage pain control and maintain comfort and safety must include the following:

1. Carefully assessing the patient's physical and emotional condition preceding the diagnostic imaging procedure

2. Educating the patient concerning all aspects of the examination and what the patient expects of them during the examination

3. Instructing the patient to inform you if he or she feels any pain or abrupt changes in the general condition while the procedure is in progress

4. Stopping the procedure and immediately notifying the physician if the patient complains of sudden pain or change in his or her condition during the procedure

5. Conferring with the patient's physician if the patient comes to the department in pain and, if possible, having the patient receive analgesic medication before you work with the patient

TABLE 7-1 **Categories of Pain**	
CATEGORY	**DESCRIPTION**
Acute pain	Lasting from seconds to 6 months; indicates that damage or injury has occurred. Acute pain draws attention to the fact that the situation causing the pain should be avoided. If treated, acute pain will heal or may heal spontaneously.
Chronic (nonmalignant) pain	Lasting constantly or intermittently for a long period of time; more than 6 months. Chronic pain may not have a defining cause or may persist beyond the healing time of an injury or illness. It is not well defined and may become a major disorder.
Cancer-related pain	May be acute or chronic and is directly related either to the disease process, the treatment of the cancer, or the trauma related to the disease. After the fear of death response, cancer-related pain is the most feared aspect of the disease; 70 percent of persons afflicted with cancer experience pain.

Summary

Medical emergencies occur frequently in the radiographic imaging department. You may be the first or only person present at the onset of symptoms in a patient, so it is important that you learn how to recognize an emergency situation and take the appropriate action if one occurs.

You must assess your patient's levels of neurologic and cognitive functioning as you prepare him or her for the assigned procedure. You will then be able to identify changes in the patient's level of consciousness and mental status if they occur while you work with the patient.

Shock is a common medical emergency. There are many causes of physiologic shock. Blood loss, infection, and cardiac failure are among the most common. Anaphylactic shock is caused by an allergic reaction and is the type that you are most likely to see in your work as a radiographer. This is because iodinated contrast agents that are used for some radiographic imaging procedures and examinations may produce this reaction. Early symptoms of an anaphylactic reaction are nasal congestion, periorbital swelling, itching, dyspnea, tearing of eyes, peripheral tingling, followed by flushing, urticaria, anxiety, and bronchospasm. If early symptoms of an anaphylactic reaction are suspected, you must not wait; you must stop the administration of the contrast agent immediately and initiate emergency action. If symptoms are not relieved, the patient may have seizures and respiratory arrest.

Pulmonary embolus is a medical emergency that may occur without warning. If you observe symptoms, you must take emergency action immediately.

Hypoglycemia, ketoacidosis, and hyperosmolar nonketotic syndrome also may be seen in patients who come into the diagnostic imaging department. Patients who have diabetes may come for examinations or procedures after having taken insulin or oral hypoglycemic medication and be without sufficient food intake to use the drug. This may induce a hypoglycemic reaction. Ketoacidosis occurs when a diabetic patient has not had sufficient insulin, and his or her body is not able to metabolize the glucose present. Hyperosmolar nonketotic syndrome occurs most frequently in elderly diabetic patients who have had a recent acute illness, therapeutic procedures such as dialysis, or recent changes in their diet. Any of these reactions constitutes a medical emergency, which, if left untreated, will result in coma and death. Administration of glucose in some form is the treatment for a hypoglycemic reaction. For all diabetes mellitus-related reactions, the physician in charge of the examination or treatment must be notified at once, and you must call for emergency assistance and be prepared for oxygen and intravenous fluid and medication administration.

Cerebral vascular accidents are medical emergencies that must be recognized and dealt with immediately to prevent life-threatening consequences. The early signs and symptoms are often one-sided flaccidity of face and limbs, difficult or absent speech, eye deviation, dizziness, ataxia, possible neck stiffness, nausea, vomiting, and loss of consciousness.

You need to differentiate respiratory failure from cardiac failure. Respiratory failure is recognized by a lack of chest movement, absence of breath sounds, a diminishing pulse rate, and loss of consciousness. Cardiac failure results in an immediate cessation of the pulse and respiration and a loss of consciousness. Both call for immediate action if the patient's life is to be saved.

You should suspect airway obstruction by a foreign object if a patient is feeling well and suddenly begins to demonstrate respiratory distress or is found unconscious and, when ventilation is attempted, the chest cannot be made to rise and fall as it should during resuscitation. The abdominal thrust maneuver must be performed in response to this emergency.

Fainting and convulsive seizures may occur with little or no warning. You should be able to recognize these problems and protect the patient from injuries caused by aspiration of saliva or vomitus, by falls, or by hitting the head or extremities against hard surfaces.

You must be sensitive to the patient's need for pain management and control. You must be able to assess the patient and plan his or her care in such a manner that the patient remains as comfortable and pain-free as possible. If the patient complains of pain or a change in his or her condition, you must stop the procedure and immediately notify the physician in charge of the patient.

As the radiographer, you must know where the emergency cart, oxygen, suction equipment, and other supplies are kept in the diagnostic imaging department. When the physician and the emergency medical personnel have come to the patient's assistance, you should stay close by to offer assistance as needed.

It is your professional obligation to be prepared to administer basic life support procedures to adults and children. Keep your classroom training current by taking a refresher course as recommended by specialists in this care.

Chapter 7 Test

1. List and describe the levels of neurologic functioning according to the Glasgow Coma Scale.

2. Explain the method of assessing mental status.

_____ **3.** General signs and symptoms that you as the radiographer must learn to recognize as probable indicators that your patient is in shock are
   a. Strong, irregular pulse; hypertension; flushed face; noisy respiration
   b. Aggressive behavior, acetone breath, convulsions, and decreased temperature
   c. Decreased temperature; weak, thready pulse; rapid heartbeat; hypotension; and skin pallor
   d. Deep, shallow respirations; hot, flushed skin; confusion; and decreased pulse rate

_____ **4.** Why is anaphylactic shock the most frequently seen type of shock in diagnostic imaging?
   a. Patients who come for diagnostic imaging procedures are weak and debilitated
   b. Iodinated contrast agents are frequently used.
   c. Patients here have more allergies.
   d. X-radiation causes this problem.

_____ **5.** Early signs and symptoms of anaphylactic reaction are
   a. Choking, dyspnea, and cyanosis
   b. Hypertension; pallor; a calm, relaxed facies
   c. Itching, tearing of eyes, and apprehension
   d. Hypotension; weak, rapid pulse; dilated pupils

_____ **6.** Myrtle Maywriter is a 43-year-old female who has come to diagnostic imaging this morning from her home for an upper GI series. After she has been in the room for a short time, she complains of a severe headache. Shortly after that, you notice that she has cold, clammy skin and speaks in a slurred manner. You suspect that Ms. Maywriter is
   a. A diabetic and is having a ketoacidotic reaction
   b. Having a cardiac arrest
   c. An alcoholic and is drunk
   d. An epileptic and is having a seizure
   e. A diabetic and is having a hypoglycemic reaction

_____ **7.** Your immediate emergency treatment of Ms. Maywriter's problem in question 6 would include which of the following action?
   a. Prepare for oxygen administration and call the emergency team.
   b. Check for an identification of the patient as a diabetic, give her some form of concentrated sugar, and notify the physician in charge.
   c. Place the patient in a supine position, keep her warm, and call the emergency team.
   d. Continue with your work, stop the IV, and do not leaving the patient alone.

_____ **8.** Symptoms of a partially obstructed airway may include
   a. Cold, clammy skin; pallor; weakness; anxiety
   b. Flushed, hot skin; hyperactivity; confusion; seizures
   c. Labored, noisy breathing; wheezing; use of neck muscles to assist with breathing
   d. Acetone breath, irregular pulse, noisy respiration, rapid heartbeat, flushed skin

_____ **9.** A 16-year-old patient comes to the diagnostic imaging department for a computed tomography examination. He is lying on the table in a supine position. He suddenly seems to lose consciousness and begins to move violently, with jerking motions. You realize that he is having a generalized seizure. The action that you must take is
   a. Go to the patient immediately and restrain him gently
   b. Call for help, but do not leave the patient
   c. Place the patient on the floor and begin CPR
   d. a and b
   e. a, b, and c

_____ **10.** Mrs. Gertrude Glucose, age 35, had an open reduction of her left femur 3 days earlier and has been transported to the diagnostic imaging department by gurney from her hospital room for radiographs. As you prepare the patient for the film, she suddenly begins to complain of pain in her midchest and appears to be out of breath. You stop your preparation and take her pulse and blood pressure. You find out that her blood pressure is 120/80 and her radial pulse is 120 per minute and is very difficult to palpate because it is so weak and thready. You quickly notify the physician of the problem, and he directs you to call the emergency team. You do this and make other emergency preparations. You believe the this patient may be having
   a. A stroke
   b. A seizure
   c. A pulmonary embolus
   d. Syncope

_____ **11.** Fainting is a common medical emergency in the diagnostic imaging department. If a patient appears to be fainting, the first thing you should do is
   a. Assist the patient to a safe position and then call for help
   b. Give smelling salts
   c. Get the emergency cart
   d. Prepare to administer oxygen

12. Match the following items:
   1. Hypovolemic shock _____
   2. Cerebrovascular accident _____
   3. Airway obstruction _____
   4. Cardiogenic shock _____
   5. Anaphylactic shock _____
      a. Difficult speech; severe headache; one-sided, drooping eye and face; loss of consciousness
      b. Choking, inability to speak, eventual loss of consciousness
      c. Itching of eyes, apprehensiveness, wheezing, choking
      d. Loss of consciousness; decreased blood pressure; weak, rapid pulse
      e. Pallor; thirst; cold, clammy skin; restlessness

13. List the questions that you must ask a patient before the patient receives an iodinated contrast agent.

14. Compare the symptoms of diabetic ketoacidosis, hypersmolar coma, and hypoglycemia.

15. Explain how you will conduct an assessment and plan care to avoid pain and discomfort while caring for a 76-year-old female patient complaining of severe lumbar-sacral pain.

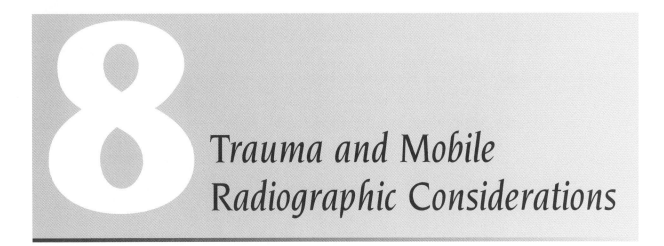

8

Trauma and Mobile Radiographic Considerations

Objectives

After studying this chapter, you will be able to:

1. List the general guidelines for radiographers to follow.
2. List the basic rules in trauma radiography.
3. List the precautions you should take as the radiographer when the patient has a head injury.
4. List the precautions you should take when the patient has facial injuries.
5. List the precautions you should take if the patient may have a spinal cord injury.
6. List the precautions you should take if the patient may have a fracture.
7. List the precautions you should take when the patient has abdominal trauma or is in acute abdominal distress.

Glossary

Abrasion: A scraping or rubbing away of the surface skin by friction

Cervical: Of or pertaining to the neck

Contusion: An injury that does not break the skin; caused by a blow to the body; characterized by swelling, discoloration, and pain

Ecchymosis: An oozing of blood from a vessel into tissues, forming a discolored area on the skin

Ectopic pregnancy: An abnormal pregnancy in which the embryo implants outside the uterine cavity

Gait: Manner of moving or walking

Hemiparesis: Paralysis affecting one side of the body

Hemothorax: Collection of blood in the pleural cavity

Hypovolemic: Abnormally decreased volume of circulating fluid (plasma) in the body

Hypoxia: Decrease in the oxygen supplied to or used by the body

Lucidity: Clearness of mind

Paresthesia: An abnormal sensation such as burning, itching, tickling, or tingling

Pneumothorax: Accumulation of air or gas in the pleural cavity resulting in collapse of the lung on the affected side

Psychosis: A state in which a person's mental capacity to recognize reality, communicate, and relate to others is impaired

Somatic: Pertaining to or characteristic of the body (soma)

Portable or mobile imaging procedures are performed on patients who cannot be transported to the imaging department because of a serious injury, illness, or condition. Therefore, many patients are imaged with the use of mobile radiography equipment in the emergency department, in special care rooms, in the patient's room, or in the operating rooms (Fig. 8–1).

The trauma patient may be strapped to a backboard with a cervical collar and splints in place. These patients commonly have oxygen, intravenous tubing, and life support equipment when you are to perform mobile radiography. You must adapt your skills to achieve diagnostic images according to the patient's condition and needs, since these patients cannot be transported to radiology. Specifically, you need to adapt positioning and technical considerations during the course of performing trauma and mobile radiography. In addition, you must analyze each patient situation in relation to the procedures requested by the physician while at the same time keeping in mind general radiation protection measures. Pre-planning is essential for achieving diagnostic outcome images under trauma or mobile circumstances. This chapter introduces additional information that is needed in trauma and mobile radiography.

Traumatic Injuries

Traumatic injuries are caused by external force or violence. Injury (trauma) is the leading cause of death among all age groups under the age of 44. The injuries may be the result of:

- Motor vehicle accidents
- Pedestrian accidents
- Motor cycle accidents
- Falls from heights
- Assaults (stabbings and gunshot wounds)
- Blunt trauma
- Choking
- Industrial accidents
- Suicides
- Drowning
- Smoke inhalation
- Sports injuries

The trauma patient presents a wide variety of challenges for you as a radiographer. The nature of the injury to the patient and the patient's condition require you to be a knowledgeable radiographer. Technical knowledge combined with creativity is required to provide the physician(s) with the necessary diagnostic information to treat the patient. In some cases, trauma radiographs are obtained rapidly to screen for life-threatening injuries.

As the radiographer, you are one of the first members of the health care team to see the patient admitted to the emergency room after traumatic injury or acute illness. Trauma patients can have a single injury or multiple injuries. When you are called to the emergency room to take diagnostic radiographs, you must assume that you will be exposed to the patient's blood or body fluids. To avoid infecting yourself or the patient, always maintain standard precautions by having clean disposable gloves available before beginning the procedure. Wear gloves, mask, goggles, and a protective gown or apron when caring for a patient who is hemorrhaging or who is nauseated and vomiting. If it is necessary to touch an open wound, you must wear sterile gloves.

Many patients admitted to the emergency room are in severe pain. You will be required to assist in diagnosing the extent of injuries or illness by taking a series of radiographs, depending on the injuries. This requires patience and skill. You need to accomplish the procedure without extending present injuries or increasing the patient's discomfort. Usually, time for achieving the goal is brief, since the patient's life is at risk. In trauma radiography, general radiation safety measures must be combined with speed and accuracy.

If the injured or acutely ill patient is transferred from the emergency room to the diagnostic imaging department for radiographs, observe the patient for symptoms of shock. You must assess the patient's neurologic status and level of consciousness before beginning any procedure and then reassess every 5 to 10 minutes while the patient is in the department. If you observe any changes in the patient's condition, you must quickly alert the physician and the emergency team and prepare to assist with emergency measures as outlined in Chapter 7.

General Guidelines

General guidelines for you to follow when caring for a patient who has traumatic injuries are as follows:

1. Do not remove dressings or splints.

2. Do not move patients who are on a stretcher or backboard until ordered to do so by the physician in charge of the patient.

3. When performing an initial cross-table lateral cervical spine radiograph, never move the patient's head or neck or remove the cervical collar. The physician must interpret the radiograph and "clear" the cervical spine for injury before removing the collar or moving the patient.

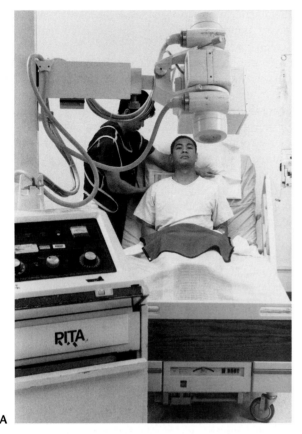

A

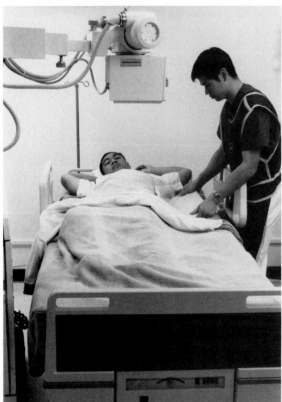

B

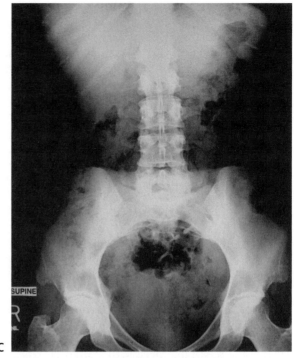

C

Figure 8–1. (**A**) Setting up for a portable AP chest semi-erect procedure. (**B**) Setting up for a portable radiograph of the abdomen. (**C**) AP supine radiograph of the abdomen.

4. Request direction from the emergency room team when planning moves, and assemble adequate assistance to move the patient safely and as painlessly as possible.

5. Do not disturb impaled objects. Support them so that they do not move as you image the patient.

6. Do not remove pneumatic antishock garments.

7. Have oxygen, suction equipment, and an emesis basin ready for use.

8. Work quickly, efficiently, and accurately to minimize repeat radiographs.

Basic Rules for Trauma Radiography

Basic rules for trauma radiography for you to follow are:

*   Assess the situation and develop an action plan for the imaging procedure.
*   Determine patient mobility, and explain the procedure to the patient.
*   Predetermine equipment and accessories needed for the procedure.
*   Take at least two radiographs at 90-degree angles to one another for each body part (Fig. 8–2).

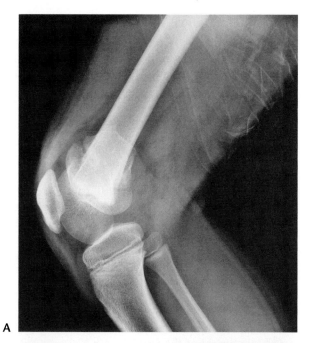

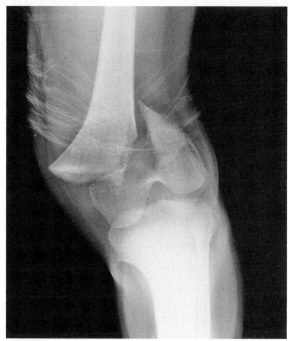

Figure 8–2 (A) Lateral knee radiograph. **(B)** Second projection 90 degrees from lateral knee.

- Make sure the central ray and image receptor alignment approaches routine positioning applications, adapting to the patient's condition.
- Include all anatomy of interest.
- For long bone radiography, always include the joint nearest the trauma; if possible, also include the joint farthest from the trauma.
- Provide protective apparel for anyone who needs to be in the room caring for the injured patient.

A cooperative environment with all personnel involved in the emergency procedure will facilitate the proper care of the patient.

The Patient With a Head Injury

Injuries to the head are exceedingly common. Each year approximately 10 million head injuries are predicted to occur in the United States. The term head injury may refer to any injury of the skull, brain, or both that requires medical attention. Radiographers are not called as often as in past years to perform radiographic images, because of the availability of computed tomography. All head injuries are potentially serious because they may involve the brain, which is the seat of consciousness and controls every human action.

The two basic types of head injury are open and closed. With an open injury to the skull or meninges, the brain is vulnerable to damage and infection because its protective casing has been broken. If the injury is closed (also called a *blunt injury*), the brain tissue may swell. The swelling is limited by the confines of the skull, and the resulting pressure may cause extensive brain damage. The brain has little healing power, so any injury to it must be considered potentially permanent and serious.

Fractures at the base of the skull (*basal skull fractures*) often have accompanying fractures of the facial bones. This type of injury may result in a tear in the *dura mater*, the outer membrane surrounding the brain and spinal cord, and a leakage of the cerebrospinal fluid may result.

You must consider all patients with head injuries to have accompanying cervical spinal injuries until it is medically disproved. You must take precautions to alleviate potential extension of these injuries as a matter of routine. It is vital for you as the radiographer to be knowledgeable in understanding the signs and symptoms of patients with a variety of injuries. You must be aware of any change in the patient's status, and report observable changes to the emergency physician and/or team.

CLINICAL MANIFESTATIONS OF HEAD INJURY

Closed Injury

- Varying levels of consciousness, ranging from drowsiness, confusion, irritability, and stupor to coma
- Lucid periods followed by periods of unconsciousness possible
- Loss of reflexes

- Changes in vital signs
- Headache, visual disturbances, dizziness, and giddiness
- Gait abnormalities
- Unequal pupil dilation
- Seizures, vomiting, and hemiparesis

Open Injury

- Abrasions, contusions, or lacerations apparent on the skull
- A break or penetration in the skull or meninges apparent by inspection or on radiographic images
- Basal fractures resulting in leakage of cerebrospinal fluid, as demonstrated by leakage of blood on the sheet or dressing surrounded by a yellowish stain (the halo sign); cerebrospinal fluid may leak from the nose, ears, or as a postnasal drip
- Varying levels of consciousness
- Subconjunctival hemorrhage
- Hearing loss
- Periorbital ecchymosis (raccoon's eyes)
- Facial nerve play

RADIOGRAPHER'S RESPONSE

1. Keep the patient's head and neck immobilized until the physician rules out injury to the spinal cord.

2. If possible, elevate the patient's head 15 to 30 degrees.

3. Do not remove sandbags, collars, or dressings. Take all radiographs with these in place.

4. Do not flex the patient's neck or turn it to either side. Rotation of the head may increase intracranial pressure.

5. Keep the patient's body temperature as normal as possible. Do not allow the patient to become chilled or overheated.

6. Check the patient's pulse and respirations frequently while performing the procedure.

7. Observe for airway obstruction.

8. Apply a sterile pressure dressing if bleeding becomes profuse, and call for emergency assistance.

9. Observe the patient for signs and symptoms of hypoxia and changes in level of consciousness. If a patient who is initially alert and cooperative suddenly appears to be drowsy or slow to respond, immediately notify the physician in charge of the patient.

10. Be prepared to assist with oxygen administration and other emergency treatment. Patients with head injuries must not be suctioned through nasal passages.

The Patient With a Facial Injury

Injuries to the facial bones are usually associated with injury to the soft tissues of the face. Often these injuries do not seem serious, but all are potentially disfiguring. Treat all patients who have serious facial injuries as if they also have basal skull fractures and injuries of the cervical spine.

CLINICAL MANIFESTATIONS

- Misalignment of the face or teeth
- Pain at the site of injury
- Ecchymosis of the floor of mouth and buccal mucosal
- Distortion of facial symmetry
- Inability to close the jaw
- Edema
- Abnormal movement of face or jaw
- Flatness of the cheek
- Loss of sensation on the side of injury
- Diplopia (double vision)
- Blindness caused by detached retina
- Nosebleed (epistaxis)
- Conjunctival hemorrhage
- Paresthesia
- Halo sign (indicates base skull fracture with leaking cerebrospinal fluid)
- Changes in level of consciousness; unconscious patient may have respiratory distress or failure caused by obstruction of tongue, loose teeth, bleeding, or other body fluids in airway

RADIOGRAPHER'S RESPONSE

1. Observe for airway obstruction. Watch for noisy, labored respiration.

2. Do not remove sandbags, collars, or other supportive devices or move a patient unless supervised by the physician.

3. Apply a sterile pressure dressing if bleeding is profuse, and call for assistance.

4. Patients must not have suction through nasal passages performed on them.

5. Wear sterile gloves if in contact with open wounds.

6. If you find teeth that have fallen out, place them in a container moistened with gauze soaked in sterile water.

7. Be prepared to assist with oxygen and other emergency treatment, if necessary.

8. Observe for symptoms of shock; notify the physician in charge if condition of the patient or level of consciousness changes.

The Patient With a Spinal Cord Injury

The spinal cord carries messages from the brain to the peripheral nervous system. It is housed in the vertebral canal, which extends down the length of the vertebral column. The spinal column is protected by the fluid in the canal and by the vertebrae—the bony structures encircling the canal. Motor function depends on the transmission of messages from the brain to the spinal nerves on either side of the spinal cords. Injury to or severing of the spinal cords causes message transmission to cease. The result is a cessation of motor function and partial or complete cessation of physical function from the level of damage to the cord to all parts below that level.

Most spinal cord injuries occur in the cervical or lumbar areas because these are the most mobile parts of the spinal column. The spinal cord loses its protection when there is injury to the protective vertebrae, and such an injury may result in compression or partial or complete severing of the cord. Spinal cord tissue, like brain tissue, has little healing power; injuries to it usually cause permanent damage.

As the radiographer, you will be among the first of the health care workers to attend the patient with a possible spinal cord injury so that you can assist in making the diagnostic assessment of the injury. If signs or symptoms of cervical spine injury are present, the patient will need a cervical spine series. Take great care in obtaining these radiographs to prevent extending the existing damage to the spinal cord. A portable cross-table lateral radiograph may be taken in the emergency suite without moving the patient or removing the backboard, collar, or sandbags used to immobilize the spine (Fig. 8–3). Remember that any movement can result in bone fragments or unstable vertebrae compressing the spinal cord and extending the injury.

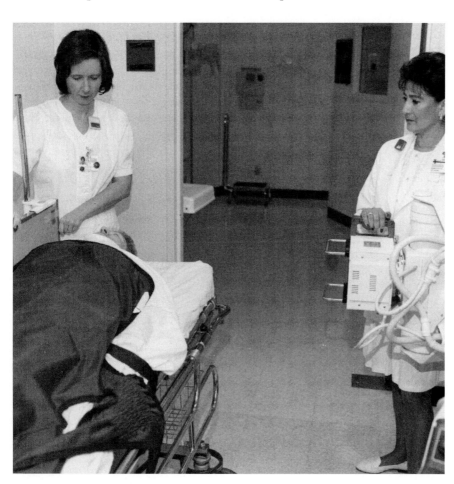

Figure 8–3. If a spinal cord injury is suspected, a cross-table lateral radiograph is taken without moving the patient.

CLINICAL MANIFESTATIONS

Complete Transection of Spinal Cord

- Flaccid paralysis of the skeletal muscles below the level of the injury
- Loss of all sensation (touch, pain, temperature, or pressure) below the level of injury; pain at site of injury possible
- Respiratory distress
- Bradycardia
- Loss of body temperature control
- Absence of somatic and visceral sensations below the site of the injury
- Unstable, lowered blood pressure
- Loss of ability to perspire below the level of injury
- Bowel and bladder incontinence
- Possible priapism in males

Partial Transection of Spinal Cord

- Asymmetrical, flaccid paralysis below the level of injury
- Asymmetrical loss of reflexes
- Some sensory retention: feeling of pain, temperature, pressure, and touch
- Some somatic and visceral sensation
- More stable blood pressure
- Ability to perspire intact unilaterally
- Possible priapism in males

RADIOGRAPHER'S RESPONSE

1. Monitor vital signs.

2. Maintain an open airway. If respirations change, notify the physician at once and call for assistance. If in respiratory failure, use jaw downward. Do not tilt the head.

3. Do not allow or request the patient to move for radiographs. Patient must be log rolled with a synchronized move supervised by the physician.

4. Do not move the patient's head or neck if position is awkward.

5. Do not remove sandbags, collars, antishock garments, backboard, or other supports until diagnosis is confirmed and a physician supervises the removal.

6. Observe for signs and symptoms of shock.

7. Keep the patient warm.

8. If patient is a trauma victim and is unconscious, assume the presence of a spinal cord injury and treat as such until directed to do otherwise by the patient's physician. All patients with head injuries should be assumed to have cervical spine injuries and be treated as such.

Imaging Considerations for the Trauma or Mobile Patient

In the trauma patient, the cross-table lateral cervical spine radiograph, along with a chest radiograph, is commonly obtained immediately on the patient's arrival at the emergency department. The two diagnostic imaging exams are performed to screen for life-threatening injuries. Although injuries are better evaluated with other imaging modalities, the initial lateral cervical spine radiograph can allow early detections and intervention of many serious injuries in the severely injured patient (Fig. 8–4). The lateral projection is considered adequate only when C1 to C7 has been imaged. An image that does not show the upper border of T1 should be supplemented with a swimmer's projection using the Twining method (Fig. 8–5). The radiologist or other physician must carefully assess the image to evaluate the soft tissue structures for swelling, alignment injury, and possible fracture or subluxation. The lateral cervical spine radiograph may also verify proper endotracheal tube position and fracture of the face and skull, since portions of the cranium are included. A sphenoid air-fluid level indicates a skull base fracture.

Before moving the trauma patient, consider that injury to the cervical spine is present until the radiologist or physician has eliminated the possibility of an injury.

1. You must be aware of patient care through observation and analysis of the patient from the onset through the conclusion of the procedure.

2. The knowledgeable radiographer must use creative and accurate radiographic applications in positioning variations, adaptation of the equipment, image receptors, and technical factors to ensure a diagnostic image.

3. You must be prepared to perform exam(s) on patients with speed and have an action plan to facilitate several exams on one patient for the patient's comfort and overall flow of efficient imaging.

4. Practice radiation protection measures, keeping in mind the three cardinal principles of time, distance, and shielding during all trauma or mobile radiography.

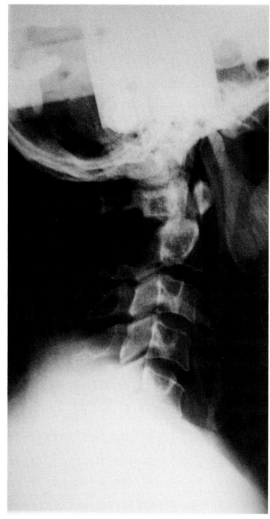

Figure 8–4. Portable cross-table lateral cervical spine radiograph.

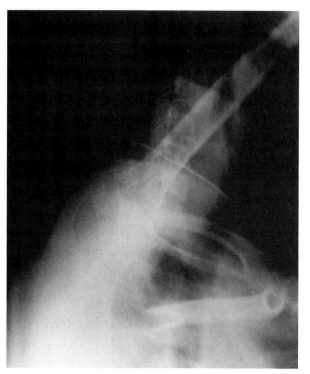

Figure 8–5. Swimmer's projection: cross table lateral radiograph.

RADIOGRAPHER'S RESPONSE

1. Monitor vital signs.

2. Maintain an open airway. If respirations change, notify the physician at once and call for assistance. If the patient is in respiratory failure, use jaw thrust maneuver to move jaw downward. Do not tilt the head.

3. Do not allow or request that the patient move for radiographs. Patient must be log rolled with a synchronized move supervised by the physician.

4. Do not move patient's head or neck if position is awkward.

5. Do not remove sandbags, collars, antishock garments, backboard, or other supports until diagnosis is confirmed and physician supervises the removal.

6. Observe for signs and symptoms of shock.

7. Keep patient warm.

8. If patient is a trauma victim and is unconscious, assume the presence of spinal cord injury and treat as such until directed to do otherwise by the patient's physician. All patients with head injuries should be assumed to have cervical spine injuries and be treated as such.

The Patient With a Fracture

A fracture may be defined as a disturbance in the continuity of a bone. Fractures can be classified simply as open or closed. An open fracture indicates a visible wound that extends between the fracture and the skin surface. The broken bone itself often breaks through the soft tissue, making the fracture clearly visible.

A closed fracture may not be obvious to the untrained eye. Often there is swelling around the injured areas, pain, and deformity of the limb. All or some of these symptoms may be absent, and a closed fracture still may be present.

Internal injuries caused by fractures of the pelvic bones are a leading cause of death after motor vehicle accidents. While caring for trauma patients, always consider the possibility of a fractured pelvis when

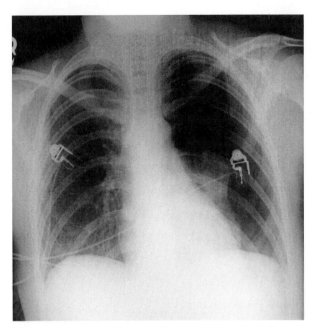

Figure 8–6. Chest radiograph of patient with a left pneumothorax.

caring for patients with multiple traumatic injuries. Use extreme caution when making initial diagnostic radiographs, because the slightest movement may initiate hemorrhage or irreparable damage to a vital organ. Patients with suspected pelvic fractures may be on a backboard or in pneumatic antishock garments. These are radiolucent and must remain in place during initial assessment radiographs. At times, it may be feasible to move the patient to the radiographic table on the backboard that has been placed by the emergency team, since this device allows the patient to remain immobilized.

A large number of trauma deaths result from blunt or penetrating trauma to the thorax. Multiple rib fractures can cause a flail chest, which in turn may result in pneumothorax (air or gas in the pleural space that collapses the lung) (Fig. 8–6) or hemothorax (blood in the pleural space). Fractured ribs are extremely painful and can be life-threatening. Stab and gunshot wounds can also cause fractures to the ribs and hemorrhage into the pleural cavity. When you are working with patients who have suffered this type of trauma, you must work quickly while observing the patient for symptoms of shock due to hemorrhage. You must also avoid causing further pain or extending injuries.

Hip fractures and fractures of the femur are common among elderly patients as a result of bony changes related to age and disease (Fig. 8–7). These fractures are a common result of home accidents in elderly patients, and you must treat these patients with utmost care to prevent extension of the injury.

CLINICAL MANIFESTATIONS

- Pain and swelling
- Functional loss
- Deformity of the limb
- Grating sound or feel or grating (crepitus) if moved
- Discoloration of surrounding tissue caused by hemorrhage within tissue (closed fracture)
- Overt bleeding (open fracture)
- Possible signs and symptoms of shock

In patients with trauma, you may take images to rule out fractures or dislocations with mobile equipment in the emergency department; or, if the patient's condition permits, you may take images in the radiology department.

RADIOGRAPHER'S RESPONSE

1. Keep affected limb or body art immobilized.
2. Any patient movement must be directed by the physician in charge of the patient.
3. Inform the patient of any intended moves and enlist his or her support.
4. Do not remove splints or other supportive devices.
5. In moving a splinted limb, support the joint and support the limb both above and below the fracture. Move the limb with one person at the distal end and one at the proximal end. On a specified signal, move the limb as a single unit (Fig. 8–8).

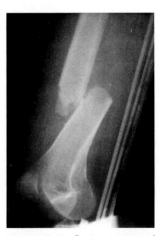

Figure 8–7. Open or comminuted fracture of the distal femur. (Farrell J: *Illustrated Guide to Orthopedic Nursing,* 3rd ed. Philadelphia: JB Lippincott, 1986, p. 44.)

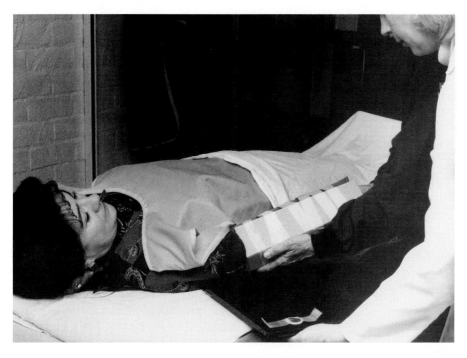

Figure 8–8. To move a patient with a splinted limb, the limb must be moved as a single unit.

6. If the patient has an open fracture, wear sterile gloves if in contact with the wound, and use standard precautions measures.

7. Observe the patient for signs and symptoms of shock, and be prepared to act if such an emergency occurs.

Follow-up studies ordered on patients following the initial exam are usually performed in the radiology department, but may also be performed as a portable procedure. In some cases, the patient may require surgery after initial exam. Therefore, you will be required to go to surgery during various procedures. In addition to the conventional portable mobile x-ray equipment, you must be prepared to use the C-arm fluoroscopic mobile unit for a wide variety of procedures as part of the health care team in the operating room. Your role during operating room procedures is to provide the physician or physicians with images of the site of interest for determining the exact location, position, and alignment for the appropriate fixation or approach for the patient treatment and care.

The Patient With Abdominal Trauma or Acute Abdominal Distress

There are a number of causes of acute abdominal distress, many of which are life-threatening. Among them are blunt or penetrating trauma, resulting in internal and possibly external hemorrhage, appendici-

tis, bleeding ulcers, ectopic pregnancy, cholecystitis, pancreatitis, and bowel obstruction (Fig. 8–9). Whatever the cause of the distress, the symptoms are somewhat similar and, for the radiographer's purpose, may be grouped together. It will be your responsibility to take the diagnostic radiographs as quickly as possible and with the least possible discomfort to the patient. An assistant may be needed to help position

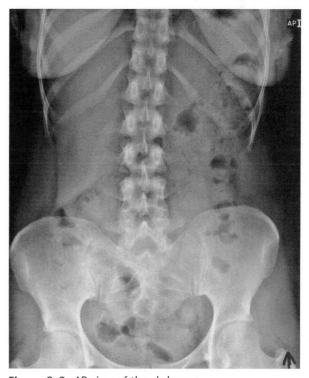

Figure 8–9. AP view of the abdomen.

and move the patient who is too ill to assist. Patients in acute abdominal distress are frequently sent to the operating room for a surgical procedure following diagnosis.

CLINICAL MANIFESTATIONS

- Possible abrasions, lacerations, entry and exit bullet wounds, seatbelt contusions
- A rigid abdomen
- Severe abdominal pain
- Nausea and vomiting
- Extreme thirst
- Possible symptoms of hypovolemic shock

RADIOGRAPHER'S RESPONSE

1. Do not remove antishock garments.

2. If the patient has open wounds, wear gloves; sterile gloves are indicated if in direct contact with the wound.

3. Call for assistance if the patient is too ill to help you move him or her.

4. If the patient is unable to stand for upright exposures or maintain the position on a tilt table, use other means of obtaining necessary radiographic images.

5. Transport the patient by gurney.

6. Have an emesis basin and tissues prepared in case the patient vomits.

7. Do not give the patient anything to drink or eat.

8. Observe for symptoms of shock, and be prepared to call the emergency team.

The Agitated or Confused Patient

Patients with emotional problems may come to the emergency suite for treatment that requires diagnostic radiographs, or patients who are hospitalized in mental health units may require diagnostic imaging procedures. These patients are frequently agitated or confused and may become combative.

Patients who react in a combative or aggressive manner usually do so because they are frightened or feel that they have no control over what is happening to them. They resort to violent behavior as a means of self-protection. This behavior may be caused by chemical abuse or by psychosis of varying causes. At times, the confused elderly patient forgets that he or she is not at home and mistakes you for an intruder. Whatever the cause, you must take precautions to protect yourself and the patient when threatened with this type of behavior.

Patients whom you can predict will demonstrate combative behavior are those who have a history of such outbursts or a history of growing confusion and disorientation. Other warning signals are increasing agitation demonstrated by rapid pacing back and forth across the room; a patient in animated and increasingly noisy conversation with a person who is not present; a demonstration of illogical thought processes; refusal to cooperate; distrust of you as the radiographer and your explanation of a procedure; and examination of the diagnostic imaging room or equipment unnecessarily. Patients who are combative occasionally display no emotion at all, or they may display irrational fear of a procedure.

Before approaching a patient who is not reacting in a rational manner, discuss the case with nursing personnel or with the patient's physician. If the patient is behaving in a combative manner or has a history of combativeness, you should request assistance with the examination. It is wise to trust first instincts about a patient's behavior. You should not isolate yourself with a potentially assaultive patient. Always leave a door open, and clear a direct path so that you are able to leave the room, if necessary. If the patient is apt to become violent, you should not begin the procedure without assistance from a person who can protect you and the patient, if necessary. A person often chosen to assist in these situations is a security officer.

At times, patients who are agitated or confused react more favorably to persons of a specific sex. If this seems to be the case, having a radiographer of the preferred sex conduct the procedure will be helpful.

It is best to approach a patient who is agitated or confused from the side, not face to face. Never touch a confused or agitated patient without first asking permission and explaining what you are planning to do. Use simple, concise statements to explain the purpose of your visit. You should call the person by name. Give an angry person the opportunity to express the anger. Make no attempt to defend or try to reason with the patient.

If a patient is speaking in a delusional or irrational manner, it is important for you not to become involved in the conversation. To do so might increase the patient's agitation. If the patient refuses to proceed, simply stop what you are doing and return the patient to his or her quarters. Explain that you will complete the examination at a later time. To continue to work with an agitated and confused person who is belligerent may cause injury to you or to the patient.

If the radiograph is essential to the patient's treatment, the patient will have to be restrained and supervised by persons in the hospital who are educated to care for such patients. Use of immobilizers is explained in Chapter 4.

If the situation escalates beyond control and the patient is actually prepared to strike out at those nearby, you should put as much distance as possible between yourself and the patient. Proceed as follows:

1. Speak in a calm but firm voice to the patient.

2. Let the patient know that you are uneasy, and ask what can be done to appease him or her.

3. Ally yourself with the patient by making statements such as, "You must be really angry at the people here for putting you through all of these tests."

4. If this does not work, get out of the area and summon help. Do not approach the patient or make any effort to take anything out of his or her hands.

The Intoxicated Patient

Patients who are intoxicated are often involved in accidents that result in injuries to themselves and to others. When the intoxicated patient is brought to the emergency unit for care, he or she may be quarrelsome and reluctant to cooperate, may also neglect all rules of safety while being treated, and may inadvertently fall from a gurney or radiographic table.

If you are the radiographer caring for an intoxicated patient, keep the communication simple, direct, and nonjudgmental. You should not become involved in an intoxicated patient's attempts to argue. If the patient refuses treatment or becomes increasingly difficult to manage, you should call for help immediately. Do not attempt to complete your assignment until you have adequate assistance to do so safely. Do not leave the patient alone, and observe him or her at all times to prevent falls. You may need one or two strong persons to assist you while you are taking radiographic films of an intoxicated person.

Often, an intoxicated patient is accompanied by a person who is also intoxicated and belligerent. The companion may become aggressive and combative. If you assess such a situation, do not allow the intoxicated companion to come into the examining room with the patient. Simply inform the companion that it is against the rules of radiation safety to be present and that he or she must wait outside. If the companion debates this request, stop the assignment and call for assistance. Note that under no circumstances should an intoxicated patient be allowed to leave the health care facility accompanied by an intoxicated companion. If necessary, notify the police to prevent this.

The Patient at Home

The home is rapidly becoming one of the major areas for health care. As the cost of hospital care increases, the patient is being discharged from the hospital, in many instances, while still acutely ill. This change requires members of the health care team to go to the patient in the home to continue care. Therefore, you may be required on occasion to go to a patient's home to take portable radiographs.

For a patient to be eligible for health care in the home, he or she must be acutely ill, homebound, and in need of skilled nursing care. The cost of home health care is usually paid for by Medicare, Medicaid, or private health care insurance, although it may be paid for by the individual recipient. Most home health care visits are paid by Medicare, since the greatest need for home care is for the elderly patient.

Radiography in the home must be ordered by the patient's physician and, if the patient has private health care insurance, approved by the insurance carrier as well. When you go to a private home, you must expect some differences in methods of delivering care. You must realize that you are a guest in the patient's home and, as such, have little control of the environment in which you work. The cleanliness, organization, and general environment may not be as you would like; however, you must realize that you are not in control of these aspects of the patient's care and that you must work within the limits of each situation. At the same time, you must practice sound medical aseptic technique, patient safety, and radiation safety procedures as you would in your own professional environment. You must also adhere to the rules of patient confidentiality.

Use of therapeutic communication techniques to establish rapport with the patient and the patient's caregivers is the first step toward a successful home visit. You must then prepare the patient for the prescribed radiographs by instructing him or her regarding what is to be done and by planning the procedure with the patient. If the patient is unable to participate in planning the procedure, you can ask the caregiver to assist in planning. You will need to instruct the patient and the caregiver in the requirements for radiation safety. When the assignment is complete, you must be certain that the patient is safe and that the caregiver understands that the visit is over and that the patient's physician will inform the patient and caregiver of the results of the radiographs.

Summary

As a radiographer, you should follow the general precautionary guidelines when assigned to care for patients with traumatic injuries. You must also remember to follow universal blood and body fluid precautions when called to the emergency unit.

Patients with a spinal cord injury must be moved in a specific manner and only with specific directions from the physician in charge. Do not remove supportive devices without physician's orders.

You should treat patients with head injuries and facial injuries as if they also have spinal cord injuries until it is verified that they do not. Also, consider basal skull fractures if the patient has injuries to the facial bones. Patients with these injuries should not be moved for initial diagnostic radiographic films without orders from the physician in charge of their care or without the physician's supervision.

While you are working with trauma patients, observe for changes in the level of consciousness, mental status, hemorrhage, shock, and respiratory distress. Patients with fractured extremities should also be moved with great care and under their physician's supervision so that movement does not increase their pain or extend their injury. If splints or antishock garments are in place, do not remove them. You must use strict aseptic practices for patients with open fractures to prevent infection.

Abdominal trauma and acute abdominal distress also are emergencies. Patients with acute abdominal pain are often very ill and are unable to assist you. Take radiographs as quickly and gently as possible. An assistant should be on hand to help you move the patient who is in severe pain. Some patients may not be able to be placed in an upright position while the exposures are being made. If this is the case, use other methods of obtaining the necessary diagnostic information. These patients should be transported by gurney.

You may have to work with patients who are agitated, confused, and potentially assaultive. The cause may be chemical abuse, psychosis, or confusion due to stress, as is occasionally the case in the elderly patient. You must be cautious in your approach to patients with this type of problem in order to protect yourself and the patient from injury. If the patient refuses treatment, you should immediately comply with this refusal and return the patient to his or her quarters. If the radiographs are essential to the patient's treatment, you should get assistance from personnel who are educated in the care of mentally disturbed patients.

When caring for an intoxicated patient, you must behave in a nonjudgmental manner and address the patient simply and directly. If your safety or that of the patient's is threatened, do not continue your work until adequate personnel are present to complete the assignment safely.

Home health care is increasingly common. You may be assigned to make a home radiography visit. If so, remember that you are a guest in the patient's home and cannot control the environment as you would in your own department. You must, however, adhere to the same rules of radiation safety and medical asepsis that apply in the department.

Chapter 8 Test

_____ 1. When you are the radiographer who is called to the emergency unit, you must expect to need
   a. Gloves
   b. A mask
   c. A protective gown
   d. Goggles
   e. a, b, c, and d

2. List the guidelines that you should follow when caring for a patient with a traumatic injury.

_____ 3. As a radiographer, you must consider that all patients with head injuries may also have
   a. Fractures
   b. Seizures
   c. Shock
   d. Cervical spine injuries
   e. Changes in vital signs

_____ 4. What precaution(s) must you follow when taking radiographic exposures of a patient who has a head injury?
   a. Keep the head and neck immobilized until the physician in charge rules out cervical spine injury.

b. Wear sterile gloves if the patient has open wounds.

c. Check the patient's vital signs frequently.

d. a and b.

e. a, b, and c.

_____ **5.** What precaution(s) must you take when caring for a patient with a fractured extremity?

a. Support the joint above and below the fracture and at the joints if moving a splinted limb.

b. Do not remove splints without the direction of the physician in charge.

c. Inform the patient before you move the fractured limb.

d. None.

e. a, b, and c.

_____ **6.** You have been assigned to radiograph Mr. J. J. He has been transported by the local police to the emergency room of the hospital in which you are employed. He is complaining of severe pain in his right leg. As you approach the patient, you notice that he is walking rapidly up and down the corridor. His head is bent and he is talking rapidly to persons who are not present. He occasionally stops, looks up at the ceiling, and shouts that he has to "get them." Your best manner of dealing with this situation would be to

a. Walk directly up to the patient, introduce yourself, and explain your purpose in being there.

b. Get an assistant, approach the patient from his or her side, stop slightly away from the patient, and explain your purpose.

c. Tell the emergency room nurse to forget it.

d. Have the male orderlies restrain the patient.

7. List three factors that you must consider when caring for the patient with acute abdominal distress.

_____ **8.** If the agitated patient refuses to be radiographed, you should

a. Ask the patient to cooperate for just one more minute

b. Explain what you are going to do in short, concise statements

c. Call for help

d. Stop immediately and return the patient to his or quarters

_____ **9.** Special care is necessary when caring for a patient whose brain or spinal cord might be injured, because

a. Extreme pain may result from the movement

b. This type of injury heals slowly

c. The incidence of infection is high

d. These tissues have very little ability to heal

_____ **10.** What is the leading cause of death for all age groups under 44 years?

a. Cancer

b. Stroke

c. Trauma

d. Drowning

11. List six types of injuries.

12. List the basic rules in trauma radiography.

13. Explain how you should deal with an intoxicated patient when assigned to his or her care.

14. Explain the change in patient care emphasis if the patient is to be radiographed at home.

15. Explain when the cervical collar may be removed on a trauma patient.

Pediatric and Geriatric Radiographic Considerations

Objectives

After studying this chapter, you will be able to:

1. Discuss professional, appropriate, age-effective communication strategies for pediatric patients, parents, and guardians during radiographic procedures.

2. Demonstrate safe methods of immobilizing a pediatric patient.

3. Describe proper radiation protection and safety measures, techniques, and practices used in pediatric radiography (ALARA principle).

4. Discuss your role as the radiographer in a suspected child abuse procedure.

5. Discuss the special considerations while imaging geriatric patients, and describe their special care needs.

6. Explain the precautions you will need to take for a patient who has had an arthroplasty.

7. Discuss your role as a radiographer in a suspected elder abuse procedure.

Glossary

Actinic keratosis: A slow, localized thickening of the outer layers of the skin as a result of chronic, excessive exposure to the sun

Adduct: To draw toward a center, or median, line

Alzheimer's disease: An illness characterized by dementia, confusion, memory failure, disorientation, restlessness, speech disturbances, and an inability to carry out purposeful movements; onset usually occurs in persons aged 55 or older

Arthroplasty: Plastic repair of a joint

Baroreceptor: A sensory nerve terminal that is stimulated by changes in pressure

Biotransformation: The chemical changes that a substance undergoes in the body, usually by the action of enzymes

Dementia: Organic mental syndrome characterized by general loss of intellectual abilities involving impairment of memory, judgment, and abstract thinking

Depression: A morbid sadness, dejection, or melancholy

Dyspnea: Labored or difficult breathing

Geriatrics: The branch of medicine that deals with all aspects of aging, including pathological and social problems

Hallucination: A sensory impression (sight, sound, touch, smell, or taste) that has no basis in external stimulation

Hypothermia: An abnormal and dangerous condition in which the body temperature falls below 95°F.

Kyphosis: An abnormal condition of the vertebral column in which there is increased convexity in the curvature of the thoracic spine

Lentigines: Round, flat, brown, highly pigmented spots on the skin caused by increased deposition of melanin; often occurs on the exposed skin of the elderly

Macule: A small, flat blemish or discoloration that is flush with the skin surface

Neonatal: Newborn, from the time of birth until the 29th day of life

Polypharmacy: Administration of excessive medications or of many drugs together

Prosthesis: An artificial substitute for a missing part

Protocol: An explicit, detailed plan

Urinary incontinence: Inability to control urinary functions

The Pediatric Patient

Pediatric patients range in age from infancy to 15 years. Children in this broadly defined group require special care, depending on their age and ability to comprehend the radiographic procedures. You must use age-appropriate methods of communication and execution of the required procedure according to a child's age to be both sensitive and effective in performing the imaging procedure. Caring for infants and children demands special safety and communication techniques. It also requires a sensitive approach toward the accompanying parents or guardian. Table 9-1 outlines developmental approaches to be taken with children. You may also be required to take mobile radiographic images in the neonatal intensive care nursery. This assignment requires use of infection-control precautions as described in Chapter 3.

Children of all ages respond in a positive manner to honesty and friendliness. A small child may be very frightened when entering the radiographic imaging department and seeing the darkened rooms and massive equipment. If you spend a few moments establishing a rapport with the child and acquaint the child with the new environment, you will save yourself a great deal of time later, and the child will leave the department with a positive attitude.

Most children resist immediate close contact with strangers. Therefore, it is best to talk to the child from a comfortable distance and allow the child to become accustomed to your presence before approaching him or her. You must explain what is going to happen during the procedure to the child who is old enough to understand. You should also give the child an estimate of how long the procedure will last and what will be expected of him or her. The child should be prepared for any discomfort that he or she may feel. If the child is to receive contrast media or medications, you need to explain the method of administration. Explanations to children are most effective if they are brief, simple, and to the point. The child should not be given choices when it is not appropriate, because it may be confusing (Display 9-1).

You should speak to the child face to face even if you must sit or kneel on the floor to do so. To avoid misunderstandings, only one person should explain and direct the child. It may therefore be necessary to reach an agreement with the accompanying adult about who is going to assume this responsibility. Using a soft tone of voice and speaking in terms that are simple and familiar will enhance communication. You must be certain that the child understands what is being said. If the child wishes to carry a toy or security item to the radiographic room, he or she should be allowed to do so if at all possible. If it is not practical,

you may take the toy with you and place it so the child can see it during the procedure and return it immediately after the procedure.

When explaining a procedure to a child, tell him or her what part of the body will be examined, why, and who will be performing the procedure. Also explain how the examination will proceed, what part of the child's body must be touched to accomplish the procedure, and why he or she must hold still during the process.

Some children are very modest. If a child's body must be exposed for an examination, only the necessary part should be exposed. You must guard against allowing the child to become chilled while in your care. This is particularly important for infants, because they lose body heat rapidly and their health can be jeopardized by loss of body heat.

Parents or guardians who accompany the child will feel less anxious if they are given an explanation of the procedure. You can easily enlist their cooperation if you encourage them to explain the child's special needs and sensitivities. If the adult can be allowed to remain with the child during the procedure without jeopardizing the child's safety or the successful completion of the procedure, provide the appropriate protective apparel and other radiation protective measures. Also, you must give parents or guardians specific instructions about what is expected of them during the procedure.

The adult who is holding the child must protect him or her from falling from the x-ray table. If the parents are to put on lead aprons and other protective apparel, you must assist them into these garments. But make sure that the child is not left unattended while this is being done. You must never assume that the parent is watching the child on an x-ray table. You must instruct parents in the exact measures that you wish them to take. For instance:

RADIOGRAPHER: *I would like you to stand on this side of the table with your hands on your child [use child's name] at all times. It will be necessary for you to wear this lead apron while I am x-raying your child, as a radiation protective measure. I will hold the child while you put on the apron. The apron fastens with Velcro attachments on the sides. Now, if you will please keep your hands on the child at all times.*

If the child refuses to follow directions and is emotionally distraught, it may be necessary for you to ask the accompanying adult to leave the room. In this case, the child must be made to understand that the doctor and his or her parents want the examination to be done and that it will be done. Then, repeat the directions and proceed. Do not belittle or criticize the child's behavior; you should remain nonjudgmental and matter-of-fact and accomplish your task as quickly as possible. Display 9-1 summarizes the steps in caring for children during radiographic procedures.

DISPLAY 9–1
Caring for Children During Radiographic Procedures

Infants (Birth–12 Months)
Identify the patient. Educate by explaining the procedure to the parents or guardians. Maintain trust, assess need, maintain safe surroundings, and never leave unattended.

Toddlers (1–3 years)
Identify the patient. Educate by explaining the procedure to the parents and patient, assess needs and level of independence, have concern for privacy, maintain safe surroundings, and never leave unattended.

Preschooler (3–5 years)
Identify the patient. Educate parents and patient, assess needs, support independence, have concern for privacy, maintain safe surroundings, and never leave unattended.

School Age (6–12 years)
Identify the patient. Educate parents and patients, assess needs, and have concern for privacy.

The High-Risk Newborn Infant

Many hospitals have special care units for high-risk newborn infants. In many areas of the United States, infants are transported to such facilities for special care from the hospital in which they were born. Infants may be considered to be at high risk for life-threatening problems if they are of low birth weight or if they have other perinatal problems.

Infants whose lives are at risk require special care considerations in highly specialized neonatal intensive care units (NICU). Here they are protected from threats to their nutritional status, environmental problems such as changes in their body temperature, and infection by being placed in isolettes with environmental and thermal control and by the practice of meticulous infection-control measures.

A surgical scrub or a 2-minute scrub as for medical asepsis is required of all persons entering these nurseries. Protective gowns are worn over uniforms. A sterile gown, gloves, and a mask may be required. You must inquire about the isolation procedure for each infant on an individual basis before beginning your work in the intensive care nursery. You must also be certain that your portable machine is wiped clean with a disinfectant solution and is free of dust before you enter the nursery.

You should consult with the nurse in charge of the infant's care; you will be assisted by that nurse in positioning and immobilizing the infant. Take care to prevent chilling the infant or dislodging any catheters or tubing as you work (Fig. 9–1). You must provide a protective lead apron to the nurse who assists you if that nurse is to hold the infant (Fig. 9–2), and you must provide the infant with gonadal shielding when appropriate.

If you have any sort of respiratory infection or infected cuts on your hands, have another radiographer take the NICU assignment to prevent introduction of infectious microorganisms into the protective environment of the NICU.

The Adolescent or Older Child

The older child or early adolescent is often expected to act as an adult would act under similar circumstances. This is not a fair expectation, since children of this age are not yet adults. When they are threatened

TABLE 9-1
Developmental Approaches by Age

AGE	DEVELOPMENTAL APPROACH
Birth to 6 months	Symbiotic—not fearful of strangers
6 months to 3 years	Separation-individualization—fear of strangers initially, followed by the toddler clinging to the parent
3 to 6 years	Preschool—age of initiative—a period of fantasy play and increasing verbal activity
6 to 12 years	Age of industry—a period of cognitive growth; growing interest in and ability to understand cause and effect
12 to 19 years	Adolescence—age of identity; heightened awareness of the body and its perceived effect on others

From Dixon SD, Stein MT: *Encounters with Children: Pediatric Behavior and Development,* 3rd ed. St. Louis: Mosby-Year Book, 2000.

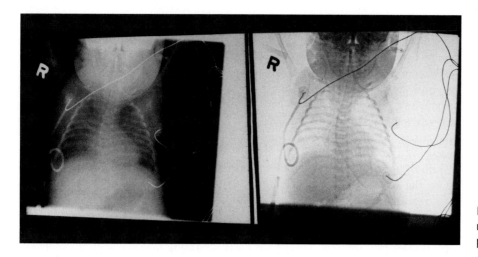

Figure 9–1. Images of newborn infant chest (AP projections).

by illness or injury, they return to the more familiar role of being a child.

The teenager is apt to be perceived as hostile and self-centered. Communication will cease if a health care worker conveys a feeling of disapproval. You can overcome this behavior by conveying a nonjudgmental attitude and using the therapeutic communication technique described in Chapter 2. It is important to:

• Identify the patient

• Educate the patient

• Maintain the patient's concern for privacy

When caring for the older child, you should be as direct and as honest as possible in your explanations of what will occur during the procedure. Use simple terms and allow the patient to ask questions and express fears and apprehension. If the child feels more secure with a parent accompanying him or her, this should be allowed, if it is permitted under hospital policy. If not, the adult may stay close by and be with the child between radiographic images or as often as is appropriate and safe. The child's privacy must be respected. No part of the child's body should be exposed without an explanation of the necessity for doing so. If the patient can be allowed to make choices, let him or her do so. This gives the older child a feeling of having some control of the situation.

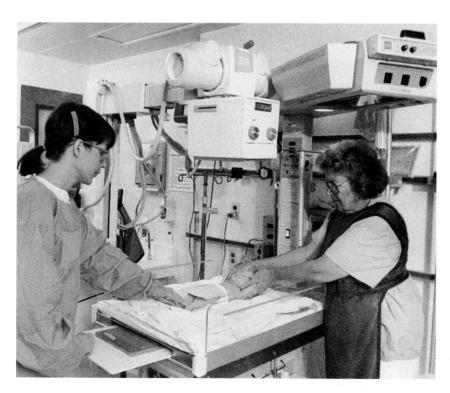

Figure 9–2. Radiograph being taken of an infant in the neonatal intensive care unit.

Transporting Infants and Children

You are responsible for transporting infants and children from place to place in the radiographic imaging department, and you may be responsible for transporting them to the radiology department from hospital rooms. You must take additional safety measures to prevent injuring the very young patient.

Take care to ascertain the identity of the patient, since the patient cannot speak for him or herself. The identity of a patient who comes to the department from outside the hospital must be verified with the adult caretaker. The type of procedure that the child is to receive must also be verified with that person or persons before the child is taken from the adult.

A child who is in the hospital will be wearing an identification band on the wrist or ankle. This band must be checked with the nurse in charge of the patient before the child is taken from the ward and checked again against the patient chart or the requisition for the procedure when the child arrives in the department.

The method of transfer depends on the child's size and the nature of the illness or injury. Under most cir-

cumstances, it is safe to carry infants and very small children for short distances (e.g., from one diagnostic imaging room to another). For longer distances, it is necessary to place the child in a crib with all sides up and locked.

Some cribs come with tops to prevent the active child from climbing over the crib rails. Crib rails must never be placed in a half-raised position because an active child can climb over them and will fall from a greater height than if the rails had not been raised at all.

Older children may be transported on a gurney with the side rails up and locked and a safety belt securely fastened. Some older children may prefer to be transported in a wheelchair. If this means of transportation is appropriate, make sure that the safety belt is securely fastened for the entire time that the child is seated in the wheelchair. Children must never be left alone while in diagnostic imaging. If they are placed on a radiographic table, an attendant must be at their side until the procedure is completed and they are taken from the procedure room. If children must wait in an outside corridor, they must be attended at all times.

Infants or small children must have back support if they are being held or carried. This can be done in a

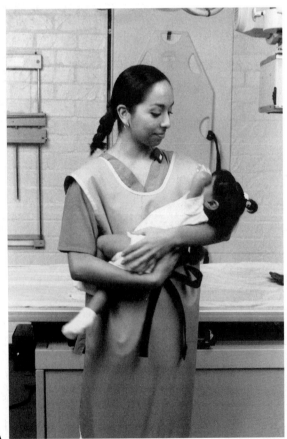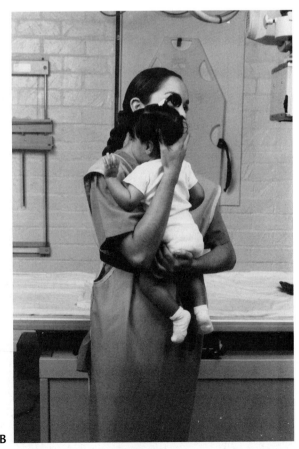

A   B

Figure 9–3. (A) Horizontal hold supporting the infant's back and head. **(B)** Upright hold supporting infant's back and head.

horizontal hold with the child supported against your body and the head supported on your arm at the elbow with your hand grasping the patient's thigh (Fig. 9–3). Another method of holding an infant or small child is holding the child upright with the buttocks resting on your arm with your other arm around the infant supporting the back and neck.

When a child is returned to a hospital room, you must be certain that the side rails of the crib are up, and you must check to be certain that they are locked. The bedside stand should not be at close range to prevent the child from using it as a stepping place to climb out of the crib. No unsafe items or liquids should be within reach of the child's crib. The nurse in charge of the child must be notified that the child has been returned to the room.

Immobilizing the Anxious Child

Occasionally, the very anxious or frightened child is not able to stay quietly in one place long enough for a successful diagnostic procedure to be completed, and the child will have to be immobilized. In other situations, a child may not be able to be held safely in position for an examination and immobilization will be necessary. Immobilizers should be used only when no other means are safe or logical and should be of a quality that will not cause injury to the patient or compromise the outcome of radiographic images.

There are several methods of immobilizing children. An immobilizer can be made by folding a sheet in a specified manner, or by commercial immobilizers. There are several commercial immobilizers that are effective for specific procedures. The child may also be held in position by one or two assistants, provided they are given the proper radiation protective apparel. Whatever type of immobilizer is chosen, the child who is old enough must be made to understand, before the immobilizer is applied, that this is not a method of punishment and that it will be removed as soon as the procedure is completed. The child's parents must also be informed of the use of the immobilizer and the reason for it.

> RADIOGRAPHER: *It is important to immobilize your child [use child's name] during the x-rays. (At this time demonstrate and explain how the child will be immobilized.) By effectively immobilizing your child, we will obtain diagnostic images and eliminate the need for repeat exposures due to motion.*

Ask the parent or guardian if he or she has any questions before proceeding with the immobilization technique.

If a child must be physically restrained by an assistant during the examination, instruct the assistant not to be too forceful and to take care not to pinch or bruise the child's skin or interfere with circulation. It is better to use a sheet or commercial immobilizer than to have the assistant use force, because the former is less frightening to a child. To prevent a small child from rolling his or her head from side to side, the person holding the child should stand at the head of the table and support the child's head between the hands, making sure to exert no pressure on the child's ears or fontanels. Any person who holds a child during a radiographic examination must wear protective lead apparel.

Sheet Immobilizers

Sheet immobilizers are effective and can easily be formed into any size or fashion desired. To make a sheet immobilizer, fold a large sheet. Then place the top of the sheet at the child's shoulders and the bottom at the child's feet. Leave the greater portion of the sheet at one side of the child. Bring the longer side back over the arm and under the body and other arm. Next, bring back the sheet over the exposed arm and under the body again. This method of immobilization keeps the two arms safely and completely immobile and leaves the abdomen exposed (Fig. 9–4).

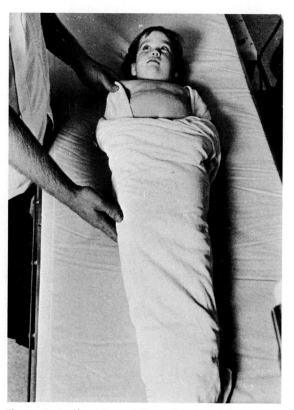

Figure 9–4. Sheet immobilizer allowing abdomen to remain exposed.

Mummy-Style Sheet Immobilizers

Another method of immobilization is the mummy-style sheet immobilizer approach. It is accomplished by folding a sheet or a blanket into a triangle and placing it on the radiographic table. The distance from the fold to the lower corner of the sheet should be twice the length of the child. Then place the child onto the sheet, with the folds slightly above the child's shoulders, making sure that the child's clothes are loosened or removed before being placed on the sheet, if necessary. Bring one corner of the sheet over one arm and under the child's body. If both arms are to be immobilized, turn the sheet and repeat the procedure for the legs (Fig. 9–5). This immobilization method can be used for radiographic imaging procedures of the upper or lower extremities. Kerlix or roller gauze can be used to immobilize an arm or leg of an infant.

Commercial Immobilizers

Several commercial immobilizers are also recommended. The Pigg-o-stat is a mechanical immobilizer that is excellent for holding a child safely in an upright position (Fig. 9–6). It is useful for imaging procedures of the chest or upright abdominal exams. Another immobilizer is a plastic model that has straps to hold the extremities (Fig. 9–7).

Radiation protection is a priority for infants and children because of the radiosensitivity of their rapid and changing cell growth. You are responsible for using effective radiation protective measures during pediatric imaging procedures. The ALARA (As Low As Reasonable Achievable) concept should be your practice in all aspects of the various procedures. Age, gender, and examination-appropriate shielding reduces radiation exposure to the patient. In particular, gonadal shielding, either the contact or the shadow type, reduces patient dose of radiation. The departmental protocol regarding shielding should be implemented for all pediatric procedures. In addition, fast speed imaging systems, short exposure times, and proper collimation greatly reduce the patient's radiation exposure (Fig. 9–8).

Child Abuse

Child abuse is any act of omission or commission that endangers or impairs a child's physical or emotional health and development. Unfortunately, the incidence

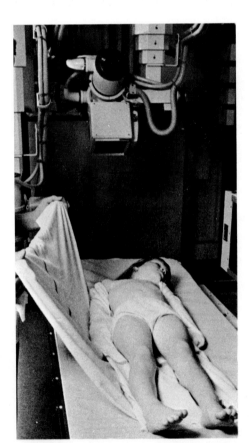
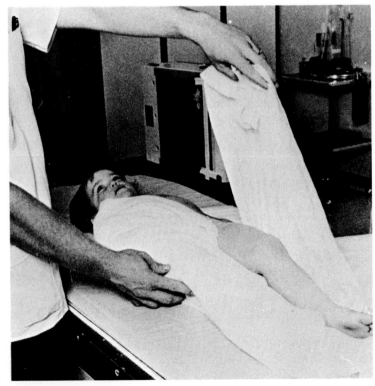

Figure 9–5. Mummy restraint for both limbs and the lower torso.

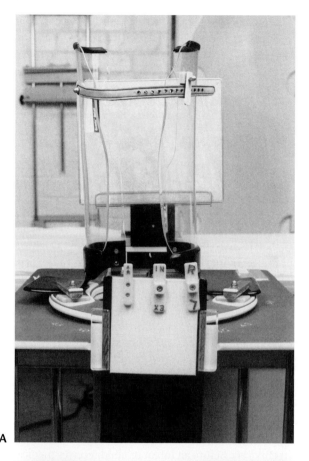

A

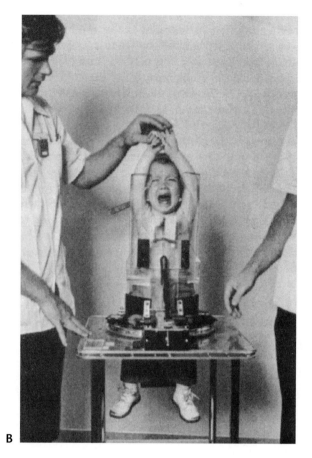

B

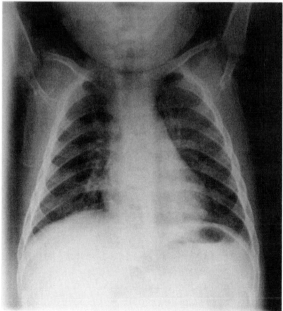

C

Figure 9–6. (**A**) Setting up the Pigg-o-stat for a PA chest radiograph. (**B**) Two radiographers effectively using the Pigg-o-stat for a PA chest radiograph. (**C**) PA chest image performed with a Pigg-o-stat.

of child abuse has increased in recent years. Child abuse includes:

- Physical abuse and neglect
- Emotional abuse

- Sexual abuse

Child abuse usually is not a single act of physical abuse, neglect, or molestation, but is typically a repeated pattern of behavior. A child abuser is most

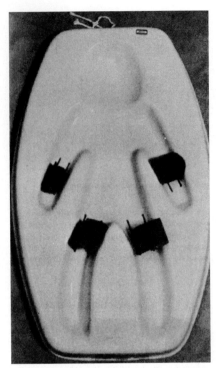

Figure 9–7. Molded immobilizer with Velcro straps for limbs.

often a parent, stepparent, or other caretaker of a child. He or she can be found in all cultural, ethnic, occupational and socioeconomic groups.

You may be the radiographer assigned to radiograph injuries that are the result of child abuse. It will be your ethical and perhaps your legal obligation to report child abuse to the person in your institution who makes the inquiries and reports required in such cases. In some states, all health care personnel are obligated to report suspected cases of child abuse. In other states, designated health care providers are obligated to do so. You must learn the legal parameters of this obligation in the state in which you practice. Each institution also has a protocol that dictates the method of processing suspected cases of child abuse, which you are also obliged to know and use if the situation arises.

Any radiographer assigned to take radiographs of a child's injuries and who notes bruising, burns, or possible fractures that seem out of proportion to the report of how the injury occurred may need to consider abuse.

Perhaps an older child will tell a story about how the injuries occurred that does not correspond to what the caretaker has related. A child may report not having eaten for an inordinately long time because his or her parents have not provided food. Whatever forms the suspected abuse takes; you must report it to the designated person in your workplace. In most states, the health care worker who reports suspected child abuse is protected from legal action if the report proves to be false; however, take care to refrain from false accusations.

Often children misjudge what is a safe action and suffer accidents because of their own mistaken judgment. Display 9-2 outlines common indications of abuse.

Administering Medication to the Pediatric Patient in Radiographic Imaging

Administering medications to children in diagnostic imaging is a sensitive issue. The medical care of children is most frequently the role of physicians and registered nurses who have specialized education in pediatrics. Medicating children can be life threatening and must not be undertaken by the radiographer. However, if a registered nurse is not available to administer medication or a contrast agent to persons under 18 years of age, you must do this. Drug absorption, biotransformation, distribution, use, and elimination are different in infants, children, and early adolescents compared with adults. For this reason, knowledge of pediatric medication administration is required to administer drugs accurately and safely to patients in these age groups.

You must be aware of the potential for overmedication or for an adverse reaction to a drug or contrast agent in children. Before an infant or child receives medication or a contrast agent, you must perform an assessment. Questions for the child's parents or caregiver are:

1. Does the child have allergies to any foods or medicines?

2. How does the child respond to medicines?

3. In what form are medicines administered to the child at home?

4. Will a parent be able to supervise the child after he or she is discharged from this department following this procedure?

5. Are there any unusual circumstances concerning this child and his or her ability to take medicines that the physician should know before administering a drug?

6. Is the parent educated in the action, purpose, and potential side effects of the drug being administered?

After you gather these data, you must pass the information on to the physician who will prescribe the drug and to the nurse who will administer it.

As the radiographer, you must make certain that the child who is receiving drugs or contrast agents in your department is carefully monitored and is not released from the department until there is no risk of complications. The assessment and care of the child is

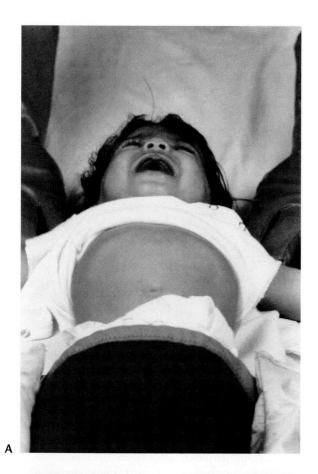

A

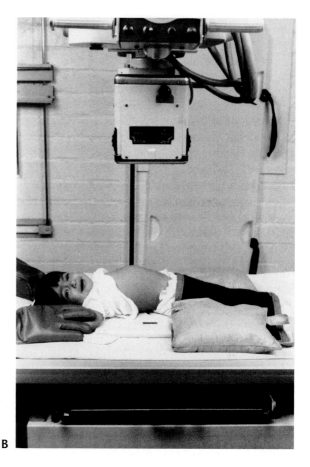

B

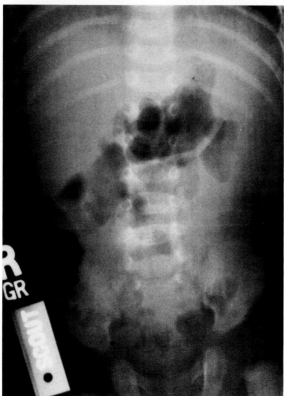

C

Figure 9–8. (A and **B)** Setting up for an abdomen radiograph on an infant. (**C**) Infant abdomen image.

Indicators of Physical Abuse

History

- The child states the injury was caused by abuse.

- Knowledge that a child's injury is unusual for a specific age group.

- Parent is unable to explain the cause of injury.

Behavior Indicators (the following behaviors may result from child abuse)

- Child is excessively passive, compliant, or fearful.

- Child is excessively aggressive or physically violent.

- Child or caretaker attempts to hide injuries.

- Child makes detailed and age-inappropriate comments regarding sexual behavior.

usually done by a registered nurse who works in diagnostic imaging; however, if a nurse is not present, you and the physician must ensure that it is done. Before the child who had received a contrast agent or sedating medication is discharged, he or she must be assessed by a physician and given authorization to leave with a parent or guardian. If the child is sleeping, he or she must remain hospitalized until awakening.

The Geriatric Patient

The number of people aged over 65 in the United States has tripled since 1900. At the present time, one in every eight persons falls into this category. Persons over 85 years of age, constitute one of the fastest-growing portions of the population (Table 9-2). For health care workers, this means that most of their patients will be 65 years of age or older; therefore, they must understand the changes that occur as one ages. As a radiographer, you must understand that age 65 is an arbitrary age that has been designated for convenience as the age at which a person is eligible for Medicare benefits, Social Security benefits, and retirement from many positions. Many persons at this age are still quite youthful and productive; therefore, all persons must be assessed on an individual basis, not merely by their chronological age (Table 9-3).

The human body undergoes normal physiologic and anatomic changes as it ages. These changes do not occur uniformly in all people, so it is not correct to say that all persons begin to demonstrate the changes of age at the same time. Lifestyles, culture, and hereditary factors contribute to the aging process. When you admit an elderly patient to the radiographic imaging department, you must be able to differentiate between

TABLE 9-2 AGING AMERICANS
The Geriatric Patient

Number of people 65 or older	35 million	Percentage of the population 65 or older	13% (2000 projection)
Number of people 85 or older	4 million	Percentage of the population 85 or older	2% (2000 projection)
Life expectancy	% of people age 65 expected to reach age 90: 26%		
Those with moderate or severe memory impairment	Men, 65-69: 5% Women, 65-69: 4% Men, 85 & up: 37% Women, 85 & up: 35%		
Those who consider themselves in good to	65-74: 9% 85 & up: approximately		

Excerpted from the Census Bureau; Centers for Disease Control and Prevention; Federal Interagency Forum on Aging Related Statistics, "Older Americans 2000: Key Indicators of Well-Being"

TABLE 9-3	
Categories of Persons 65 Years and Older	
Young-old	65 to 75 years
Old	75 to 85 years
Old-old	85 to 100 years
Elite old	Over 100 years

the normal changes of aging and deficits resulting from a disease process.

The elderly person is more frequently burdened with major illnesses that are chronic rather than acute in nature. Heart disease, cancer, and strokes are the cause of 80% of deaths in persons over age 65. Hypertension, arthritis, diabetes mellitus, pulmonary disease, and visual and hearing impairments are also common conditions requiring long-term care. These conditions result in a great deal of physical discomfort and a multitude of social and psychological problems.

Large numbers of medications are prescribed and consumed by the elderly. Many of these medications affect the patient's response level. Often, problems attributed to the aging process are the result of multiple medication consumption, which is frequently called polypharmacy.

Depression is a common and debilitating emotional problem of the aged person. The threat of becoming a burden to one's family, the fear of losing one's good health, or the necessity of giving up an independent lifestyle owing to chronic disease result in feelings of helplessness and hopelessness that can give rise to a major depressive episode. Symptoms of depression in the elderly person are often confused with dementia. Symptoms of dementia, including disorientation, confusion, gross memory deficits, paranoid ideation, hallucinations, and depression are not part of the normal aging process. When these symptoms are present in an elderly patient, you must remember that they are indicative of a disease process. Persons with Alzheimer's disease present with symptoms of dementia, which usually occur in persons over age 65, although it may occur at an earlier time. And persons with Alzheimer's disease or other diseases that produce symptoms of dementia are frequently seen for a radiographic imaging examination.

If you are caring for a patient who exhibits symptoms of dementia, remember that the person may not be able to understand or retain directions. You will have to explain to the patient what is to be done and then assist him or her in following the directions. The patient who is confused or has a paranoid ideation may become frightened when confronted by the forbidding atmosphere of the radiographic imaging department. Allowing a familiar person to be present in the examination room to assist the patient may make the patient feel more secure and allow the procedure to be accomplished more effectively.

Persons who are depressed may be so preoccupied that they do not respond to outside stimuli. It may be necessary for you to give the same instructions a number of times to a depressed person and then to assist the patient in following directions.

When an examination of the geriatric patient is complete, you must assist him or her to return to the dressing room or lavatory, because the stress of the procedure may result in forgetfulness. Make certain that the patient is attended before leaving him or her. The elderly patient must not be left alone in the radiographic imaging room, because he or she may become confused and may be in danger of falling from the examining table.

Changes Associated with Aging

Older adults may not have the same symptoms of a disease as a younger adult. They may have nonspecific symptoms such as dizziness, falls for no apparent reason, infections without fever, or urinary incontinence, to name a few. These are symptoms of disease and not a part of the normal aging process. You must be able to differentiate what is normal from what is pathological.

As aging progresses, the body systems change in a gradual manner. A brief overview of how the body systems change with normal aging, as well as the precautions the radiographer must consider because of these changes, follows.

Integumentary System

NORMAL CHANGES OF AGING

- The skin wrinkles, becomes lax, and loses turgor.
- The vascularity of the dermis decreases, and the skin of white people begins to look paler and more opaque.
- Skin on the back of the hands and forearms becomes thin and fragile.
- Areas of skin lose pigment; purple macules and senile purpura may appear as a result of blood leaked through weakened capillaries.
- Brown macules called senile lentigines appear on the backs of the hands, on the forearms, and on the face.
- Seborrheic keratoses and actinic keratoses may develop.
- Nails lose their luster and may yellow and thicken, especially the toenails.

- Hair loses its pigment and begins to gray.
- Hair patterns change, and the hair becomes thin and more brittle.
- There is hair loss on the scalp and other body areas.

Many skin changes listed above occur only in white ethnicities and are not normal in persons of dark-skinned ethnicities.

IMPLICATIONS FOR THE RADIOGRAPHER

The skin of the geriatric patient is more fragile than that of a younger person and is thus more easily traumatized. You must ensure that the skin of the elderly patient is not damaged. The preventive measures listed in Chapter 4 must be followed at all times.

CALL OUT!

Lying on a hard radiographic table may be especially painful for the geriatric patient; place a full table pad.

Changes in the Head and Neck

NORMAL CHANGES OF AGING

- There is mild loss of visual acuity, particularly presbyopia (loss of ability to focus on near objects).
- The light-sensing threshold is affected and adaptation from light to dark and color perception diminishes.
- Tear production is either reduced or increased.
- The skin of the eyelid loosens and the muscle tone decreases.
- Sensory, neural, and conductive changes occur in the ear.
- Hearing loss is common.
- There is loss of muscle mass in the neck.
- There is an accentuated forward upper thoracic curve, which may result in kyphosis.
- The sense of taste and smell decreases.

CALL OUT!

Assess the patient's condition frequently; ask the patient if he or she feels dizzy or feels like falling. Ensure and protect the patient from injury during radiographic examinations.

IMPLICATIONS FOR THE RADIOGRAPHER

Rapid changes in lighting, such as moving from a brightly lighted waiting room into a darkened examining room, may cause the elderly patient momentary blindness. You must offer patients assistance so that they do not fall.

Loss of sense of smell and hearing loss must be considered. You must ascertain that the patient is able to hear your directions and must speak loudly enough for the patient to understand what is being said. Do not assume, however that all older persons have a hearing deficit and need to be spoken to in an abnormally loud voice.

During fluoroscopic examinations, background noise from the equipment may prevent the patient from hearing the instructions. Be especially careful to clearly state instructions and check for understanding.

Pulmonary System

NORMAL CHANGES OF AGING

- Pulmonary function changes with age; lung capacity diminishes owing to stiffening of the chest wall, among other changes.
- The cough reflex becomes less effective.
- The normal respiratory defense mechanisms lose effectiveness.

IMPLICATIONS FOR THE RADIOGRAPHER

The patient becomes breathless and fatigues more easily. Because of the decreasing effectiveness of the cough reflex, the patient is more apt to aspirate fluids when drinking. There will be an increased risk of pulmonary infections resulting from the loss of respiratory defense mechanisms. A patient with chronic pulmonary disease cannot be expected to lie flat for more than brief periods of time, since this position increases dyspnea.

During chest radiographic examination, when possible, ask the geriatric patient to hold his or her breath on the second full inhalation to ensure full lung expansion.

You must instruct the patient to drink slowly to avoid choking when drinking the contrast media for an upper gastrointestinal examination. Position the patient in an upright sitting position to prevent aspiration.

The Cardiovascular System

NORMAL CHANGES OF AGING

- Structural changes occur in the heart as aging progresses.
- The coronary arteries calcify and lose elasticity.

- The aorta and its branches dilate and elongate; the heart valve thickens.
- There is a decline in coronary blood flow.
- The baroreceptors in the aorta and internal carotid arteries become less sensitive to blood volume and pressure changes.

IMPLICATIONS FOR THE RADIOGRAPHER

Owing to normal cardiovascular changes of aging, the elderly patient tires more easily; imaging examinations and procedures should be conducted in as efficient a manner as possible to avoid fatigue. If a procedure is unavoidably lengthy, the patient must be allowed to rest at intervals.

Hypothermia and complaints of feeling cold are common problems for the elderly patient because of decreased circulation; therefore, it is important to avoid chilling.

CALL OUT!

Additional blankets may be helpful to prevent discomfort or, in extreme cases, hypothermia during and between radiographic examinations.

One fourth of people over age 65 have postural hypotension (a drop in systolic blood pressure of 20 to 30 mm Hg) for 1 to 2 minutes after changing from a prone to a standing position. Rapid position changes result in a feeling of dizziness and the patient may fall. You must always assist the elderly patient to a sitting position for a short time before he or she stands and steps off the radiographic table. This allows the patient to adjust to the new position before walking.

The Gastrointestinal System

NORMAL CHANGES OF AGING

- Gastric secretion, absorption, and motility decrease.
- There is a predisposition to dryness of the mouth, and the swallowing reflex becomes less effective.
- The abdominal muscles weaken.
- Absorption of iron, vitamin B12, and folate decreases, with resulting potential for anemia.
- Many elderly patients are edentulous (without teeth), or the teeth present are decayed or gums diseased. Many have full dentures or partial plates.

- Esophageal motility declines.
- The tone of the internal anal sphincter decreases.

IMPLICATIONS FOR THE RADIOGRAPHER

If the patient is required to fast before a diagnostic examination, schedule the examination for the early morning so that the patient can have breakfast close to the usual time.

Medications may not be dissolved and absorbed from the stomach as effectively or as they are meant to be. Therefore, the ability to swallow is also affected. This may impair the elderly patient's ability to drink liquid contrast agents. You must instruct the patient to drink slowly to avoid choking. The patient who must drink liquid in the imaging department must be positioned in an upright sitting position to prevent aspiration.

You must be cautious when dealing with the patient's dentures or partial plates. If they must be removed for some reason, place them in a plastic denture cup and in a secure location where they will not be broken or lost. Return them to the patient as soon as it is possible to do so safely.

The elderly patient may have a difficult time holding barium during a lower gastrointestinal examination because of loss of sphincter control. This potential problem must be considered when planning care.

CALL OUT!

The use of an enema tip with an inflatable cuff will facilitate the lower gastrointestinal examination in patients with loss of sphincter control.

The Hepatic System

NORMAL CHANGES OF AGING

- The liver size decreases.
- Enzyme activity and the synthesis of cholesterol decrease.
- Bile storage is reduced.

IMPLICATIONS FOR THE RADIOGRAPHER

The elderly person has an increased potential for drug toxicity, since most drugs are metabolized in the liver. Be alert for adverse drug reactions in the elderly patient.

The Genitourinary System

NORMAL CHANGES OF AGING: WOMEN

- Muscle tone and bladder capacity decrease.
- Pubic hair becomes sparse.
- Vaginal atrophy occurs.
- Involuntary bladder contractions increases.

NORMAL CHANGES OF AGING: MEN

- The prostate gland enlarges, and the tone of the bladder neck increases.
- The capacity of the urinary bladder is reduced by 500 to 900 mL.
- The size of the penis and testes is decreased, owing to sclerosis of blood vessels.

There is a change in sexual response in men and women, but both can remain sexually active, if they are healthy, into the seventh or eighth decade of life.

IMPLICATIONS FOR THE RADIOGRAPHER

Loss of muscle tone in the female genitourinary system may make the patient more susceptible to urinary incontinence in stressful situations. Both the elderly male and female patient may have a limited bladder capacity and may need to urinate more frequently. Have a bedpan and urinal available for elderly patients in your care who cannot use the lavatory easily.

Musculoskeletal System

NORMAL CHANGES OF AGING

- Bone mass is reduced, and bones become weaker.
- Muscle mass decreases. Muscle cells decrease in number and are replaced by fibrous connective tissue.
- Muscle strength decreases.
- Intervertebral discs shrink and vertebrae collapse, resulting in shortening of the spinal column.
- Articular cartilage erodes.
- The normal lordotic curve of the lower back flattens.
- Flexion and extension of the lower back are diminished.
- Placement of the neck and shaft of the femur change.

- Posture and gait change. In men, the gait narrows and becomes wider based. In women, the legs bow and the gait is somewhat waddling.

IMPLICATIONS FOR THE RADIOGRAPHER

Increased muscular weakness increases a patient's discomfort when he or she is expected to assume positions necessary for imaging procedures. Painful joint and deformities accompanied by decreased tolerance for movement also increase discomfort. You must assist the patient to the required position and then support him or her with positioning sponges to facilitate maintaining that position. The risk of falling is greater when you are caring for elderly patients owing to musculoskeletal changes. It is your obligation to assist patients in positioning and in getting on and off the radiographic table to prevent falls.

The Patient Who Has Had Arthroplastic Surgery

Total joint replacement has become a common procedure in hospitals throughout the United States. The joints of many elderly persons become very painful because of degenerative joint disease, and an operative procedure is done to replace the diseased joint with a prosthesis. Arthroplasty is also indicated for persons with joint diseases such as rheumatoid arthritis or for persons with joint deformities due to injury. Although knee and hip arthroplasty are the most common, almost any joint that is malfunctioning can be replaced (Fig. 9–9).

Radiographs are frequently requested several days after arthroplastic surgery to determine the rate of the healing process and the ability of the patient to return to daily activities (Fig. 9–10). There are restrictions on movement and positioning ordered postoperatively by the patient's surgeon that must be followed by all health care workers involved in the patient's care to prevent damage to the new joint.

The most common complication after hip replacement is dislocation of the prosthesis. Correct positioning following surgery is necessary to prevent this. The affected leg must be prevented from adducting and the operative hip must be kept in extension. A special pillow is sometimes used for this purpose; at other times, a regular, large pillow is used. When the patient is sitting in a chair, the legs must remain uncrossed and the hips must not be flexed more than 90 degrees. Weight bearing on the affected side is restricted for varying lengths of time depending on the type of prosthesis chosen. You must understand the needs of the patient who has had an arthroplasty so that he or she

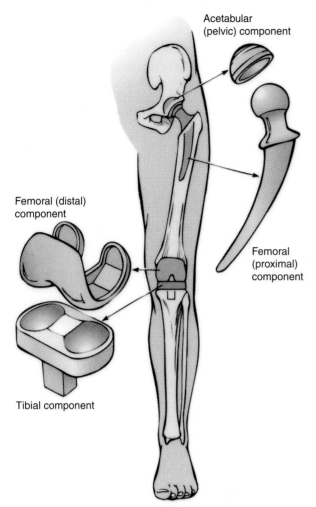

Figure 9–9. Hip and knee replacement. (*Brunner and Suddarth's Textbook of Medical-Surgical Nursing*, 8th ed. Philadelphia: Lippincott-Raven, 1996:1868.)

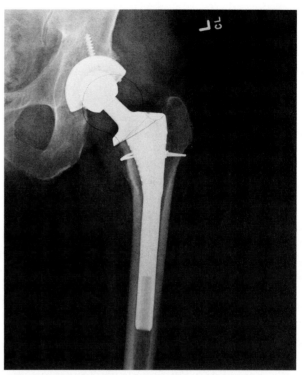

Figure 9–10. Hip prosthesis image: AP projection.

will not be injured while being cared for in radiographic imaging.

After knee arthroplasty, the patient is sometimes placed on a continuous passive motion device. Weight bearing is restricted and restored gradually. The knee should not be hyperflexed and the patient should not kneel. For shoulder and elbow arthroplasty, protocols for postoperative care are variable. Ankle replacement has not achieved widespread use at this time. Whatever the arthroplasty, you must understand the restrictions on weight bearing and movement for each patient and adhere to them to prevent irreparable damage to the joint involved.

RADIOGRAPHER'S RESPONSE

1. When the patient with a recent arthroplasty comes to the radiographic imaging department, you must understand and adhere to the limits that have been placed on the patient's weight bearing and mobility of the restricted joint.

2. Move patients who have had hip, knee, or ankle arthroplasty to and from the department by gurney. They cannot get onto and off the radiographic table without placing weight on the affected limb. Move patients toward their affected side in this situation.

3. After hip arthroplasty, do not allow the patient's affected leg to adduct (move toward the center of the body). Keep a pillow or block between the legs to prevent this.

4. Do not position the patient with weight on the surgical incision site.

5. Do not hyperflex affected joints.

The Neurologic System

NORMAL CHANGES OF AGING

- Brain weight changes, which may be due to reduced size of neurons.

- The ability to store information changes very little in the absence of disease; however, some short-term memory loss occurs.

- Sensorimotor function decreases.
- Reaction time to both simple and complex stimuli decreases.
- The time needed to perform activities increases.
- The lens of the eye thickens, making the pupils of the eye appear smaller.
- There is a decrease in postural stability that is greater in women than in men.
- A decrease in proprioception creates problems with spatial relations.
- There is loss of sensitivity to deep pain.

IMPLICATIONS FOR THE RADIOGRAPHER

Remember that the elderly patient is less responsive to painful stimuli and is not aware of a painful stimulus until an injury has occurred. You must increase awareness of potential for patient injury.

The elderly patient may have visual problems in the dimly lit radiographic imaging rooms. He or she may also need guidance to avoid colliding with objects that are not seen easily. For example, the patient may not see the stool to determine where to place the feet to step down from the radiographic table.

The elderly person processes information and direction in a slower fashion. You must be certain that your patient understands your directions and allow him or her more time to execute moves. You are responsible for preventing accidents.

Culture and Aging

The culture of the patient is reflected in an attitude toward aging, illness and its treatment, pain, death, and dying. Some elderly patients are accepting of whatever treatment the physician and other health care workers offer. Others require a detailed explanation and reassurance at every step. The relationships between the patient and the caregiver also varies with the cultural beliefs of the patient and his or her family. Some caregivers are highly solicitous and anxious concerning the treatment that their relative is to receive. Others leave the patient in the health care worker's hands and attend to other affairs.

You must perform your education plan during and following a procedure with sensitivity to the patient's cultural differences. In some societies, it is understood that the adult child who is the caregiver will attend to every detail of a parent's medical treatment, while in other cultures the patient is expected to know and understand how to conduct his or her own care. If a caregiver is to oversee the patient's care, you should include him or her in the instruction. If this is not the case, the patient will need careful and complete direction appropriately communicated. Whatever the culture of the patient, you must take these differences into consideration with sensitivity. If you do this, the examination or treatment will be more comfortable for the patient and will prevent conflict with the caregivers.

Elder Abuse

Unfortunately, the prevalence and reporting of elder abuse have increased in recent years. There are three categories of elder abuse: (1) domestic elder abuse, (2) institutional elder abuse, and (3) self-neglect or self-abuse. In addition, there are specific types of elder abuse, which include:

- *Physical abuse*: the use of physical force that may result in bodily injury, physical pain, or impairment
- *Sexual abuse*: nonconsensual sexual contact of any kind with an elderly person
- *Emotional or psychological abuse*: the inflicting of anguish, pain, or distress through verbal or nonverbal acts
- *Neglect or self-neglect:* the refusal or failure to fulfill any part of a person's obligations or duties to an elder or self

Display 9-3 lists indications of elder abuse by a caregiver.

Summary

The pediatric patient ranges in age from newborn to 15 years of age. As the radiographer, you must relate to all patients with whom you work in an appropriate and specific manner, regardless of age. The infant is usually accompanied by parents. You should attempt

---

DISPLAY 9-3

Caregiver Indicators of Elder Abuse

- Caregiver responds for the elder, preventing the patient from responding.
- Caregiver is flirtatious in an inappropriate sexual approach to the patient.

- Caregiver lacks affection toward patient.

to ease the parents' anxiety by giving them an explanation of the procedure to be performed and the approximate amount of time it will take.

If it is necessary to immobilize the child, you should explain the reasons for this procedure to the child, if he or she is old enough to understand, as well as to the parents. If it is necessary to immobilize a child, an immobilizer made of soft material such as a sheet may be used. If the child is to be immobilized by being held, it should be done in a firm, safe manner to prevent injury or unnecessary repeat radiographs. You should never place your body over a child as an immobilizer. A sheet immobilizer or one manufactured commercially may be less traumatic for the patient and more effective. Protective apparel and shields should be worn by persons immobilizing a child to prevent exposure to radiation.

You must assess each elderly patient to determine any special needs. You must understand that one cannot generalize concerning the disabilities of aging because they vary in each individual. You must be able to distinguish the physical limitations that are part of the normal aging process from those resulting from a disease process or abuse.

Patients who have had joint replacement surgery have specific postoperative orders for care. As the radiographer, you are obligated to inquire about the patient's restrictions concerning mobility and weight bearing. Patients who have had a knee, hip, or ankle arthroplasty must be transferred to and from the radiographic imaging department by gurney, because they are not able to get on and off the radiographic table without placing weight on the affected joint. Patients who have had hip arthroplasty must not adduct the affected leg and, when sitting, must not flex the hip more than 90 degrees. Patients who have had knee arthroplasty must not flex their affected joint more than 90 degrees.

Chapter 9 Test

1. List four considerations you must incorporate as a radiographer into your communication with a child.

2. Describe the variations in communication you must use in communicating with an adolescent.

3. Describe symptoms that a child may display that may indicate abuse.

4. Describe the normal changes of aging as related to the following body systems:
   a. Integumentary system
   b. Cardiovascular system
   c. Pulmonary system
   d. Hepatic system
   e. Gastrointestinal system
   f. Neurologic system

_____ 5. When caring for a pediatric patient, the best method of transport is always
   a. A gurney
   b. Carrying the child
   c. A crib
   d. Depends on the distance involved and the age of the child

_____ 6. Confusion and other symptoms of dementia are to be expected in an elderly patient, since they are part of the normal aging process.
   a. True
   b. False

_____ 7. Eighty percent of death in persons over age 65 is due to
   a. Trauma, peritonitis, and emphysema
   b. Fractures, chemical abuse, and schizophrenia
   c. Cancer, heart disease, and strokes
   d. Diabetes mellitus, arthritis, and hypertension

_____ **8.** When you must schedule an elderly patient for a difficult diagnostic examination, it is best to schedule the examination for
   a. Evening hours, so that the patient has the day to rest
   b. Early morning hours so that the patient can have breakfast as close to the usual time as possible
   c. In the middle of the day so that traffic is less hectic
   d. At a time that is convenient for you

_____ **9.** When caring for a 6-year-old child, you should
   a. Explain the procedure to the patient in great detail
   b. Tell the patient that there will be no pain or discomfort, regardless of the type of examination
   c. Be friendly, honest, and concise in your explanation to the child
   d. Routinely immobilize the child to be examined

_____ **10.** Physiologic changes that come with aging that you should consider as you work with the elderly patient include
   a. Loss of the sensation of pain
   b. Loss of sensitivity to heat or cold
   c. Diminishing gag reflex
   d. Loss of the sense of humor
   e. a, b, and c

_____ **11.** Assessment of the elderly should include
   a. Ability to see and hear
   b. Ability to move without assistance
   c. Level of understanding
   d. a and b
   e. a, b, and c

12. List six precautions that you must take as a radiographer when a patient who has had an arthroplasty is scheduled to have follow-up radiographs 4 days after surgery.

10

Care of Patients During Imaging Examinations of the Gastrointestinal System

Objectives

After studying this chapter, you will be able to:

1. Differentiate between positive and negative contrast agents.

2. Explain the radiographer's teaching responsibilities before, during, and after radiographic imaging examination of the gastrointestinal (GI) system.

3. List the potential adverse effects of positive contrast agents when they are used in imaging examinations of the GI system.

4. List the potential adverse effects of negative contrast agents when they are used in imaging examinations of the GI system.

5. List the types of cleansing enemas that you may need to instruct the patient to use before and after a GI series.

6. Explain the precautions that you must take during administration of a barium enema or a cleansing enema.

7. Demonstrate the correct method of administering a barium enema and a cleansing enema in the school laboratory.

8. Describe the patient care precautions to be taken when assisting with upper and lower GI series.

9. Describe the patient care considerations for a patient with an ostomy who is having a barium enema.

10. Explain the correct order of scheduling radiographic imaging examinations if multiple examinations are ordered.

Glossary

Adverse effects: The development of undesired side effects or toxicity caused by the administration of drugs

Alimentary canal: The organs of digestion; the digestive tract

Colostomy: An artificial opening (stoma) created in the large intestine and brought to the surface of the abdomen for the purpose of evacuating the bowels

Diverticulitis: Inflammation of a sac or pouch protruding from the walls of the intestines, especially the colon

Electrolyte imbalance: An imbalance in the body of sodium, potassium, calcium, magnesium, and phosphates, the chief conductive ions responsible for nerve and muscle activity and acid-base balance

Enterostomal therapist: A health care worker, usually a registered nurse, who is specially educated to assist patients who have had an ostomy to learn proper methods of caring for their ostomy sites and assist them to adjust to the body change emotionally

Fecal impaction: Accumulation of putty-like or hardened feces in the rectum or sigmoid

Flatus: Gas expelled from the digestive tract through the anus

Fluoroscopic: An instrument for the direct x-ray visualization of the action of the body's joints, organs, and systems

Gallium scans: A nuclear medicine procedure using the radioisotope gallium 67 in the form of gallium citrate

Ileostomy: An artificial opening (stoma) erected in the small intestine (ileum) and brought to the surface for the purpose of evacuating feces

Infusion: A liquid substance introduced into the body by way of a vein for therapeutic purposes

Ostomy: General term for an operation in which an artificial opening is formed

Peritonitis: Inflammation of the serous membrane lining the abdominal cavity and surrounding the abdominal organs

Radioisotope: A radioactive form of an element used in medicine for diagnosis and treatment; the most commonly used are cobalt, gold, iodine, iron, and phosphorus

Radionuclide: A radioactive nuclide; one that disintegrates with the emission of electromagnetic radiation

Stoma: An opening in the body created by bringing a loop of bowel to the skin surface

---

Radiographic imaging procedures of the upper and lower gastrointestinal (GI) system are done in relatively large numbers. As a radiographer, you may consider some of these procedures as routine duties, but you must remember that they are not routine experiences for the patient receiving them. They can be stressful and uncomfortable examinations that may place the patient in physical and emotional jeopardy. This is particularly true for the very young and the very old patient.

Contrast studies that include the use of high-density barium and air are effective methods of detecting conditions of the upper and lower GI system. When imaging of the GI tract using barium is contraindicated, an iodinated contrast agent may be prescribed.

Several methods of imaging the liver, the gallbladder, and the biliary tree are available. These can involve the use of iodinated contrast agents given by the oral or intravenous route. Ultrasound and radionuclide studies are other methods used to visualize particular areas of the GI system. These special methods of imaging are discussed in Chapter 16.

When you are working with contrast medium, you must know the indications and contraindications for their use, the potential adverse reactions of each, safe method of patient care, and the patient teaching that must accompany their use. You must devote an additional amount of time to patient teaching for procedures of this nature because many patients have had no experience with the preparation required for them. Hesitation, and perhaps even revulsion, with the technical aspects of enema administration, dietary restrictions, and medication prescribed before these examinations is not unusual. If you use a matter-of-fact, professional manner when instructing the patient, you will be able to alleviate patient anxiety.

Types of Contrast Media

There are two types of radiographic contrast agents: negative and positive. Negative contrast agents decrease organ density to produce contrast. The most commonly used negative agents are carbon dioxide and air. Positive contrast agents are used to increase organ density and improve radiographic visualization. Positive contrast agents are barium sulfate and iodinated preparations. Contrast agents are discussed in Chapter 12.

Negative Agents

Carbon dioxide and air are the most frequently used negative contrast media. They may be used singly or in combination with a positive contrast medium for studies of the GI system. Complications associated with the use of negative contrast agents can result from inadvertent injection of air into the bloodstream, producing an air embolus. Although the injection of negative contrast agents into the bloodstream during GI procedures is unlikely, it is important to remember the complications associated with this.

Positive Agents

Positive contrast agents create a density difference by attenuating the ionizing radiographic beam. This stops the x-ray beam from hitting the image receptor, thereby creating a white or opaque area on the image. There are two types of positive contrast agents: barium and iodinated contrasts. While barium is relatively nontoxic, iodinated contrasts present a greater danger to the patient. The choice of which positive contrast agent to use is generally the decision of the radiologist, however, as the radiographer you must be familiar with all types of positive contrasts and their use.

CALL OUT!

Both negative and positive contrast agents have potential adverse reactions.

Barium Sulfate

Barium sulfate is the most frequently chosen contrast medium for radiologic examination of the GI tract. It is a white, crystalline powder that is mixed with water to make a suspension. It may be administered by mouth for examination of the upper GI tract, by rectum for examination of the lower GI tract, or by infusion of a thin suspension through a duodenal tube to visualize the jejunum and ileum. The use of high-contrast barium solution in the alimentary canal reveals organ outlines and demonstrates pathologic conditions of the visceral walls. By using double contrast of barium and air, the ability to detect small lesions is improved.

The toxic effects of barium are negligible if the suspension remains within the GI tract; however, if there is a break in the gastric mucosa caused by injury or disease, the barium sulfate may pass into the peritoneal cavity or into the bloodstream and result in adverse reactions. If barium leaks into the peritoneal cavity, peritonitis may result. This possibility increases if the barium is mixed with fecal material. Fibrosis or formation of a barium granuloma may be a further complication. The possibility of leakage of the barium into the venous circulation through a perforation in the gastric mucosa as a result of trauma or disease must also be considered. This would produce an embolus that might be fatal. When perforation of the GI tract is suspected, an absorbable water-soluble iodinated contrast medium is used in place of barium.

Barium sulfate is often constipating. If the patient is not properly instructed following a procedure that involves its use, he or she may ignore the condition rather than have it treated, and fecal impaction or a bowel obstruction may result.

If the patient reports that a previous administration of oral barium suspension produced a sensation of nausea, the radiologist should be notified before it is administered again, because if the patient vomits, aspiration pneumonia can result.

Computed tomography is the imaging technique used most frequently to investigate potential pathologic conditions of the omentum, the retroperitoneum, and the liver. Ultrasound, technetium scans, and gallium scans are other imaging modalities used for evaluation of the GI system and its associated organs.

Barium Studies of the Lower Gastrointestinal Tract

Correct preparation of the patient for barium studies of the lower GI tract is essential and may seem relatively complex to the patient. This preparation varies across health care facilities and with each patient's special needs. Your responsibility as a radiographer is to learn the specific procedure in your place of employment. If the patient is an outpatient, you may be responsible for giving the patient the appointment for the examination and the instruction in its preparation. The following directions generally apply at most institutions, with modifications for particular patients.

If time allows, the patient is instructed to eat foods low in residue for 2 to 3 days before the procedure. A low-residue diet excludes tough meats; raw, cooked, and dried fruits; raw vegetables; juices containing the pulp of fruits or vegetables; whole-grain breads and cereals, especially bran and cracked wheat types; nuts, peanut butter, and coconut; olives, pickles, seeds, and popcorn; and dried peas and beans. The patient should take no more than two cups of milk each day and avoid strong cheeses. The patient should be encouraged to increase fluid intake for 2 to 3 days before the examination to assist in clearing the lower bowel of waste. Water is the recommended fluid.

Twenty-four hours before the examination, a clear liquid diet is usually prescribed. A clear liquid diet may include coffee or tea with sugar but no milk; clear gelatin; and clear broth and carbonated beverages. The patient should be instructed to drink five 8-ounce glasses of water or clear liquids during this 24 hours.

The afternoon preceding the examination, 10 ounces of magnesium citrate or its equivalent is prescribed. The evening before the examination, another laxative may be ordered. Laxatives must never be given to a patient without the physician's order. They can be harmful to persons with bowel obstructions and other pathologic conditions of the GI tract.

Patients with insulin-dependent diabetes mellitus and non-insulin-dependent diabetes mellitus require special pre–examination orders and instruction. You must ascertain the patient's medical status before giving instructions in preparation for any GI series. Patients with diabetes mellitus must also be instructed concerning administration of morning insulin or other antidiabetic medications. Usually these medications are postponed until the examination is complete and the patient is able to eat.

Cleansing enemas are generally prescribed the night before or early in the morning of the examination. Since there are several types and variations of cleansing enemas, you must become familiar with all of them, and you must be able to administer one of them, if necessary. Occasionally, a patient comes to the radiographic imaging department poorly prepared for a radiographic study of the lower bowel, and the radiographer has to complete the preparation in the department by administering an additional cleansing enema. By learning the procedure, you are able to give clear directions to the patient who needs instruction.

The Cleansing Enema

The type of cleansing enema to be used is always ordered by the physician. As the radiographer, you do not decide on the type of enema the patient is to receive, but you may administer a cleansing enema if it is ordered. The most frequently used cleansing enemas include the saline enema, the hypertonic enema, the oil-retention enema, the tap water enema, and the soapsuds enema (SS enema).

Cleansing enemas can influence fluid and electrolyte balance in the body to varying degrees because they each have a different degree of osmolarity, which influences the movement of fluids between the colon and the interstitial spaces beyond the intestinal wall. This means that, in the presence of some cleansing solutions that are instilled into the lower bowel, the bowel extracts fluid from the surrounding interstitial spaces. This happens because the higher osmolarity of the cleansing solution (hyperosmolar) induces the fluid to move across the semipermeable membranes of the intestinal wall. The body fluid that has moved into the large intestine is then excreted from the body along with the enema solution. Dehydration occurs if an excess of body fluid is excreted. This situation can be reversed.

Another situation occurs when an excess of fluid with low osmolarity (hyposmolar) may be instilled into the lower bowel and absorbed into the interstitial spaces surrounding the colon, thus creating a fluid excess in the body. This is called fluid toxicity. These potential hazards must be considered when the physician orders a particular solution for use as a cleansing enema.

CALL OUT!

Hyperosmolar fluids can create dehydration. Hyposmolar fluids can create fluid toxicity.

Saline Enemas

There are two types of saline enemas: normal saline and hypertonic saline. Normal saline is the safest solution to use for a cleansing enema because it has the same osmolarity as that in the interstitial spaces that surround the colon; therefore, it will not change the fluid balance in the body. It is the only safe fluid to use for cleansing enemas for infants and children because they can tolerate very little change in fluid and electrolyte balance. This solution is also used for elderly patients for the same reason.

In hospitals, commercially prepared normal saline is available in containers of varying sizes. For an adult patient, 750 to 1000 mL is the average amount used. The amount of fluid used for infants and children varies with their age and weight. If children are to be given a cleansing enema, a nurse educated in caring for pediatric patients should do it. If commercial preparations of normal saline are not available or are too expensive for the patient to purchase, a normal saline solution can be made by adding 1 teaspoon of table salt per 500 mL of water. If a parent is to administer the cleansing enema to an infant or child, a pediatric nurse or physician should instruct him or her in the procedure.

Hypertonic Enemas

An enema using a hypertonic saline solution or a solution of water and sodium phosphate (Fleet Phospho-Soda) can be administered quickly and easily and is effective for relieving constipation or for eliminating barium sulfate residue after a barium study. It is packaged commercially in a small plastic container with a prelubricated tip. The tip is inserted into the rectum. The patient is asked to retain the fluid for several minutes and then to evacuate it.

Hypertonic solutions pull fluid from the interstitial spaces around the sigmoid colon and fill the bowel with fluid, thereby initiating peristalsis. Only a small amount of solution is required to do this (120 to 180 mL). Hypertonic saline enemas are often available under the name Fleet enema (Fig. 10–1*A*). Hypertonic enemas should not be administered to dehydrated patients or to infants and children.

Oil-Retention Enemas

The oil-retention enema is given for relief of chronic constipation or fecal impaction. It may also be used to eliminate any barium sulfate remaining after a GI series. A small amount of mineral oil or olive oil (120 to 140 mL) is instilled into the rectum, and the patient is requested to retain the oil for as long a time as

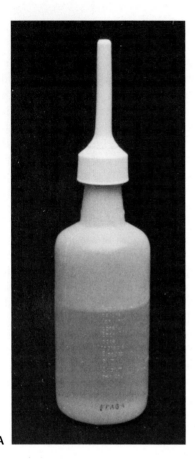

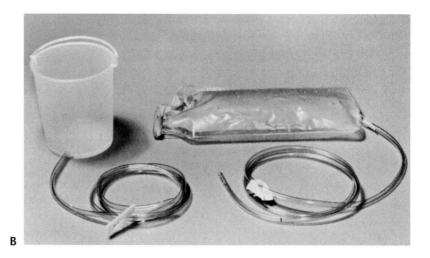

Figure 10–1. (**A**) Hypertonic saline enema set (Fleet enema). (**B**) Two types of cleansing enema sets.

possible, preferably up to 1 hour, and then expel it. The oil lubricates the rectum and colon and softens the fecal material, thereby making it easier to expel.

Although you will probably not be administering this type of enema, you must be knowledgeable about it so that you can discus it as part of your patient-teaching plan. Oil-retention enemas are usually commercially prepared and can be purchased in a container ready for use with a prelubricated tip. The tip is inserted into the rectum, and the oil is slowly instilled into the rectum.

Tap Water Enemas

Tap water may be used to cleanse the bowel preceding diagnostic imaging procedures; however, you must remember that there is a potential for fluid toxicity if this is used. The procedure for administration is the same as for the soapsuds enema, which is described in the following section.

Soap Suds (SS) Enemas

Soap may be added to tap water or to normal saline to increase the irritation of the intestine, thereby promoting peristalsis and defecation. The only soap safe to use for this purpose is a pure castile soap. Detergents and strong soaps may result in intestinal inflammation. For each 1000 mL of liquid, 5 mL of soap is recommended. The SS enema is the cleansing enema most frequently used before barium studies of the lower GI tract. Following is the procedure for administering an SS enema to an adult patient:

1. Ascertain that the treatment is ordered by the patient's physician or the radiologist in charge of performing the procedure. Giving an enema to persons with some GI diseases is contraindicated.

2. Go to the patient and explain that a cleansing enema has been ordered and explain why it has been ordered; also explain the procedure.

3. Wash your hands; then assemble the equipment that is needed for the procedure. This will include:
   a. A plastic container that holds 1000 mL of fluid; this may be a bucket or a plastic bag with an attached plastic tubing
   b. Plastic tubing with a 22- to 26-French lumen (French measurement is discussed in Chapter 14) about 4 feet long with a smooth, perforated tip and a clamping device (see Fig. 10–1*B*)

c. The liquid to be instilled

d. Liquid castile soap (5 mL)

e. Water-soluble lubricant

f. A paper or cloth pad to place under the patient's hips, paper towels to receive the soiled enema tip, and a towel to protect the table where the equipment is placed

g. A bedpan

h. The patient's shoes or slippers and a robe

i. Clean, disposable gloves

j. A drape sheet to cover the patient

4. Attach the tubing to the container if this has not been done, and close the clamp.

5. Go to a utility area that has a sink and hot and cold running water. Prepare the enema solution. The water used should be warmed to 105°F (41°C). Fill the container with 1000 mL of water, place the soap in the container, and mix it.

6. Open the clamp and allow some of the fluid to run through the tubing into the sink to displace the air and to ensure that the enema set is working correctly (Fig. 10–2A).

7. Take the equipment assembled on a tray, if one is available. Place it on a table or stand near the patient. Close the door or otherwise arrange for privacy.

8. Drape the patient with the drape sheet and position him or her in a left Sims' position. Arrange the drape sheet so that only the area of the buttocks that must be exposed for insertion of the enema tip is exposed. Place the towel under the patient's hips to avoid soiling the table or sheet on which the patient is lying (see Fig. 10–2B).

9. Explain to the patient that you are about to begin the instillation of the fluid. Tell the patient that he or she may feel some cramping as the fluid runs in; tell the patient to inform you and that you will stop the instillation until the cramping stops. Also inform the patient to try to retain the fluid for as long as possible. Explain that a bedpan is on hand if he or she is unable to get to the bathroom. If the patient is on a radiographic table, have a stepping stool ready to assist the patient off the table.

10. Tell the patient when you are about to insert the tube, and ask the patient to exhale as you do this.

11. Put on your gloves. Lubricate the tip of the tube if it does not come in a kit with a prelubricated tip.

12. Lift the patient's right buttock with the heel of your hand to expose the anus.

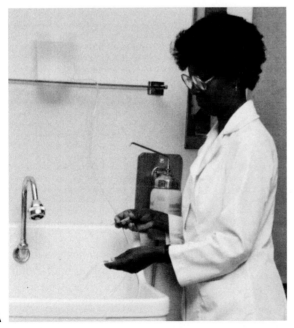
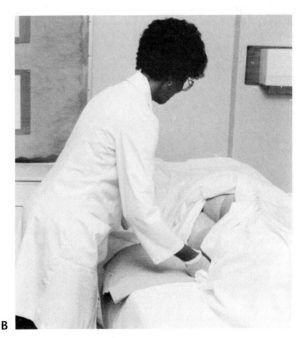

A   B

Figure 10–2. Administering a cleansing enema. **(A)** Allow the air in the tubing to be displaced by the enema solution. **(B)** Place a towel under the patient's hips. **(C)** Insert the enema tip into the rectum toward the umbilicus. **(D)** Insert the tube gently to prevent injury. **(E)** Raise the container of enema fluid 18 inches.

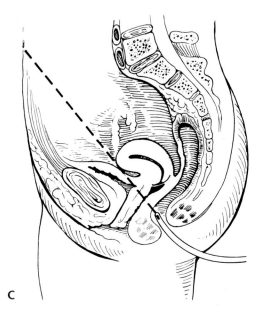

C

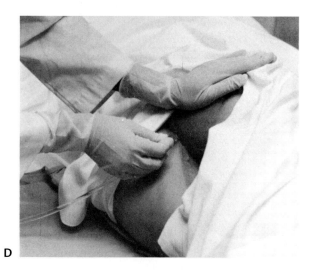

D

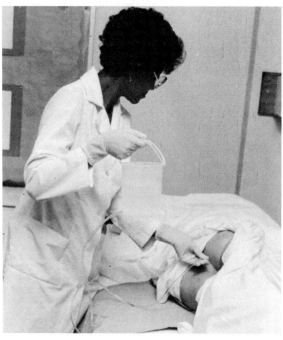

E

Figure 10–2. (Continued)

13. Ask the patient to slowly exhale and gently insert the enema tip into the rectum toward the umbilicus 3 to 4 inches (see Fig. 10–2C). Make certain that you can see the anus as you insert the tip so that you don't injure the patient. Do not insert the tube forcefully, so that you don't damage the mucous membranes (see Fig. 10–2D).

14. When you have inserted the tip, hold it in place with your nondominant hand and release the tube clamp with the other hand. Then raise the container of fluid 18 inches (see Fig. 10–2E).

15. Allow the fluid to run in slowly. It should take about 10 minutes to instill all the fluid. If the physician has ordered the transverse and ascending colon to be cleansed, you may ask the patient to turn onto his or her back and then onto the right side as the fluid is being instilled. The quantity of fluid that a patient can retain varies, but if possible, at least 500 mL of fluid should be instilled. Instruct the patient to tell you when he or she is unable to take more fluid.

16. Clamp the tube before the fluid has reached the bottom of the container so that air does not enter the rectum.

17. Gently remove the enema tip, wrap it in a paper towel, and place it in the enema container.

Dispose of the set in the appropriate receptacle, and remove your gloves according to the rules of medical asepsis.

18. If the patient is able, have him or her rest quietly on the table for as long as possible before going to the lavatory to expel the enema. Stay close by to assist the patient to the bathroom. If the patient cannot go to the lavatory, place him or her on the bedpan; put on gloves to remove the bedpan as discussed in Chapter 4.

You can clean the area and wash your hands as for heavy contamination while the patient is expelling the enema. The patient is instructed not to flush the commode until the expelled material has been assessed for color, quantity, and consistency of the fecal material. Preparation for some barium studies requires a second or even a third enema to be administered so that the bowel is thoroughly cleansed. This process is referred to as giving enemas "until clear" and means that the enema fluid returns with no fecal matter present. Cleansing enemas must not be repeated more than three times because the patient's fluid balance may be jeopardized.

The Self-Administered Cleansing Enema

If a patient is coming from home to the radiographic imaging department for a barium study of the lower bowel, he or she must be taught to self-administer enemas effectively. You must be able to assume this teaching responsibility. Instruct the patient to purchase an enema kit when going to the pharmacy for the laxative medication. The enema prescribed is usually a cleansing enema; the adult patient is required to add 1000 mL water and 20 mL liquid soap. Carefully explain to the patient which type of enema set is needed, because there are many to choose from. The patient should know that, even if the laxative has the desired effect, he or she will not be adequately prepared if not taking the enemas as instructed.

Your instruction to the patient regarding the preparation of the enema proceeds as described earlier.

1. Take the enema on the morning of the examination.

2. If the patient has no one at home to assist, explain that he or she should place a terry towel on the floor near the toilet in the bathroom at home.

3. Instruct him or her to place the enema set with the prelubricated tubing on a low stool or chair nearby so that, when lying down, the solution will be about 18 to 24 inches above hip level.

Since the enema solution must cleanse the entire colon, the patient must not be in a sitting position.

4. The patient may insert the enema tip while lying on the left side. Explain that changing positions from the left side to the back and then to the right side while instilling the enema better ensures that the solution is reaching the entire colon.

5. Instruct the patient to try to relax by taking deep breaths during the procedure so that he or she will be able to hold the solution more easily.

6. If the procedure is unsuccessful the first time or if the patient has been directed to take enemas "until clear," he will have to repeat this procedure.

> **CALL OUT!**
>
> To cleanse the entire colon, the patient must be recumbent.

Barium Enema

Studies performed to diagnose pathological conditions of the lower GI tract use a combination of barium and air or carbon dioxide (double contrast) or barium alone (single contrast). If there is an indication that the patient has a disease entity or injury that would result in a perforation or tear of the lower GI tract, use a water-soluble iodinated contrast agent rather than barium. This is done to protect against barium peritonitis, a condition that results from barium leakage into the peritoneal cavity.

A much larger tubing is required than is used for a cleansing enema to allow the viscous suspension to be instilled into the lower bowel. The tubing may have a plain tip, a tip with an inflatable cuff attached or a tip that is used for double-contrast studies. This type of tip has two lumens—one for the inflatable cuff and one for instillation of air into the patient's bowel (Fig. 10–3). If a tip with an inflatable cuff is selected by the physician for use in the examination, the cuff is inflated after the tip is inserted in the rectum. This holds the enema tip in place and prevents involuntary expulsion of barium. Never inflate the cuff until you are certain that it is positioned beyond the anal sphincter.

Barium is available in a prepared, prepackaged form. Barium comes as either a liquid suspension or as a powder, which must be mixed with water immediately before the procedure. When adding water to the suspension, remember that the consistency should be

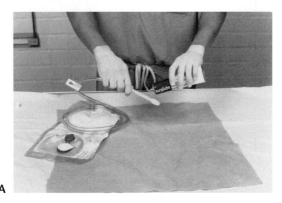
A

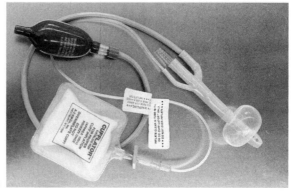
B

Figure 10–3. (**A**) Plain tip for barium enema. (**B**) Double-contrast retention enema tip.

dense so that x-rays are absorbed (Fig. 10–4). After it is mixed with water, barium should remain in suspension for some time before resettling; it should also be able to flow freely. Foam is undesirable in the mixture because, if present, the barium suspension will not coat the mucosal walls evenly, which is necessary for diagnostic purposes.

You should have ready for use a plastic container of barium that has been well mixed (Fig. 10–5). The quantity needed for a single-contrast study of an adult is generally 1500 mL, although it may vary. The amount used for infants or children is much less and depends on their age and size. The correct amount is instilled in the patient by the radiologist in charge of the procedure. A normal saline solution may be mixed

with the barium instead of water to prevent electrolyte imbalance if the patient is an infant, a child, or a frail elderly person. The barium solution is passed through the tubing in the same manner as the solution for a cleansing enema to displace the air in the tubing before insertion of the tip. Premixed preparations of barium should be remixed so that the suspension is uniform, and they should be administered at room temperature.

The bag containing the barium is hung from a metal standard. A clamp on the tubing opens and closes the

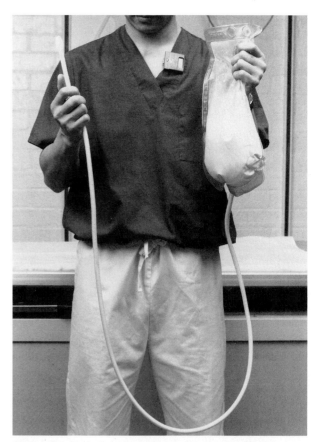

Figure 10–4. Barium in lower bowel (radiograph, lower GI series).

Figure 10–5. Barium must be well mixed and the tubing free of air.

tubing easily. Place the bag about 30 inches higher than the table, You must not begin instillation of barium until the radiologist is present in the room to direct the procedure. However, you may insert the rectal tip before the radiologist is summoned to the room.

This barium enema procedure is much the same as for the cleansing enema. Wash your hands, place the patient in Sims' position, and drape him or her so that only the anal area is exposed. The enema tip should be heavily lubricated. Then don clean, disposable gloves. Instruct the patient to exhale slowly as the tip is inserted 3 to 4 inches or until it passes the anal sphincter. Do not use force to insert the tip because of the potential for laceration of the mucous membranes. If you cannot easily insert the tip, stop the procedure and ask the radiologist to complete the task. The patient may be returned to a supine position after the tip is in place.

When a retention-type tip with an inflatable cuff is used to administer barium, you may inflate the cuff with a hand inflation pump. You must be certain that the cuff is inserted beyond the rectal sphincter before it is inflated. Initially, inflate the cuff with no more than 10 mL of air for an adult patient. If more air is desired, the radiologist may add more. Do not use an inflatable cuff for an infant or a child. Instead, you may tape the tube in place with hypoallergenic tape.

Occasionally, a patient has an allergy to items made of latex (including barium enema tips and many medical products). You must ask the patient before the procedure whether he or she is allergic to latex. If this is the case and another type of tip is not readily available for substitution, you must report the allergy to the radiologist.

Patient Care Considerations During Examinations of the Lower Gastrointestinal Tract

Remember that patients are extremely uncomfortable during this type of procedure and usually highly anxious. They are forfeiting their dignity and comfort to discover the cause of their illness. You must be aware of this and do all that you can to alleviate the patient's discomfort and anxiety.

If the patient cannot hold the barium and cannot tolerate an inflatable cuff, you can place an inflatable bedpan under the patient during the procedure (Fig. 10–6). The patient should be instructed to inform you if he or she is having abdominal cramping during the examination so you can stop administration of barium until the cramping subsides.

An anticholinergic drug or glucagon is often prescribed and administered before or during the examination intravenously to reduce gastric motility, which may help decrease the cramping. If the patient is an insulin-dependent diabetic, glucagon is contraindicated. If the patient receives an anticholinergic drug or glucagon, observe him or her for adverse reactions through the examination and for 30 minutes after the examination. Possible adverse reactions from glucagon include nausea, vomiting, hives, and flushing. Possible adverse reactions from anticholinergic drugs include dry mouth, thirst, tachycardia, urinary retention, and blurred vision. If the patient is to receive these medications, he or she should have another person available to drive home.

Inform the patient that he or she will be moved into several positions to afford maximum visualization while the examination is in progress. You will need to explain that the radiologist will be giving you instructions that the patient may mistakenly think are being addressed to him or her. Tell the patient to ignore single-word commands such as "open," "close," "off," "on." Inform the patient of the approximate amount of barium that will be given. The patient will need to know that any urge to defecate can be relieved when he is taken to the lavatory immediately after the procedure.

Air is often placed into the bowel during this examination. When a double-contrast study is to be performed, the radiologist will limit the amount of barium that is instilled into the patient. The barium is then turned off, and air is instilled into the patient's bowel through a second lumen of the enema tip.

The patient will be extremely uncomfortable during this study. You should remain in close proximity to

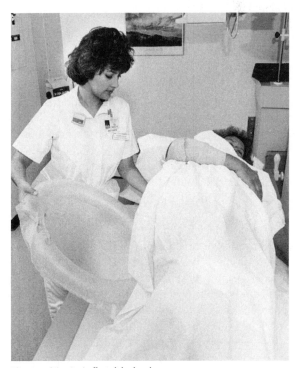

Figure 10–6. Inflatable bedpan.

reassure him or her. Inform the patient that cramping and a feeling of a need to defecate are normal sensations during this examination.

The patient is often requested to move about on the table during the examination, and the table may be positioned at different angles. You must assist the disabled patient to assume the various positions, and you must be certain that the patient is safe while moving or while the table is tilted.

Before removing a rectal enema tip that has an inflatable cuff attached, you must be certain that the cuff is deflated. The barium is sometimes removed by gravity flow before the tip is removed. This is done by placing the barium bag lower than the level of the patient's hips and allowing the barium to flow back into the bag. The air is then permitted to escape from the cuff. After this, gently remove the tip. If there is any resistance, summon the physician to remove it.

> ## CALL OUT!
> Remember to deflate the retention cuff before removing the enema tip.

You must assist the patient to the lavatory after a barium enema. However, the patient may first need to evacuate some of the barium into a bedpan before attempting the trip. Stay with the patient until the problem is resolved because he or she will need assistance and direction.

Instructions After Barium Studies of the Lower Gastrointestinal Tract

A patient must never be dismissed from the radiographic imaging department after a procedure without instruction in postexamination care. This is particularly true for the patient who has received barium because, without adequate care, the barium may be retained, which can cause fecal impaction or intestinal obstruction. The patient may also suffer from extreme dehydration as a result of preparation for the study.

You must explain to the patient that his or her stools will be white or very light-colored until all of barium is expelled. Some physicians regularly prescribe a laxative medication or an enema following barium studies. If the physician in charge of the patient does not do this, tell the patient that if he has not had a bowel movement within 24 hours after the procedure he or she should contact the physician. Stress the importance of eliminating the barium.

It is also extremely important for the patient to increase fluid intake and fiber in the diet for several days if this is not medically contraindicated. The patient should be instructed to rest after the examination. If the patient feels weak or faint; has abdominal pain, constipation, or rectal bleeding; is not passing flatus; or has polyuria, nocturia, or abdominal distention, he or she must contact the physician immediately.

> ## CALL OUT!
> Constipation is a common side effect of barium enemas. Instruct the patient to increase fluid intake to prevent this.

The Patient with an Intestinal Stoma

Several conditions of the lower GI tract require the creation of a stoma through which the contents of the bowel can be eliminated. A stoma is created by bringing a loop of bowel to the skin surface of the abdomen. Some diseases that are treated in this manner are cancer, diverticulitis, and ulcerative colitis. Traumatic injuries of the bowel may also require this type of treatment.

The surgical procedure to repair the bowel and create the ostomy is named by the area of bowel on which the operation is done. For instance, if the opening is from the colon, it is called a colostomy; if it is from the ileum, it is known as an ileostomy (Fig. 10–7). The stoma may be temporary, performed to rest and heal a diseased portion of the bowel; or, it may permanent, done to remove a diseased or traumatized portion of the bowel.

The stoma may have either one or two openings, depending on the type of surgery that was performed. When two openings are surgically created, one opening is located toward the rectum and the other toward the small bowel. One opening, called the proximal stoma, emits fecal material. The other opening, the distal stoma, is relatively nonfunctioning and emits only mucus. Some stoma patients (also called ostomy patients) have had their rectum and lower bowel removed; others have not. A patient who has an ostomy may require barium studies for further diagnosis or further study of the progression of the disease.

You must recognize that an ostomy causes a major change in a patient's body image and that many persons with a new colostomy or ileostomy stoma are going through a grieving process. This is particularly true of younger patients. They may be angry, depressed, in a stage of denial, or just beginning to accept the fact that they must learn to live with this physical change.

Caring for the patient with a new ostomy requires sensitivity and a matter-of-fact attitude. It is suggested that the radiography student who has never seen an

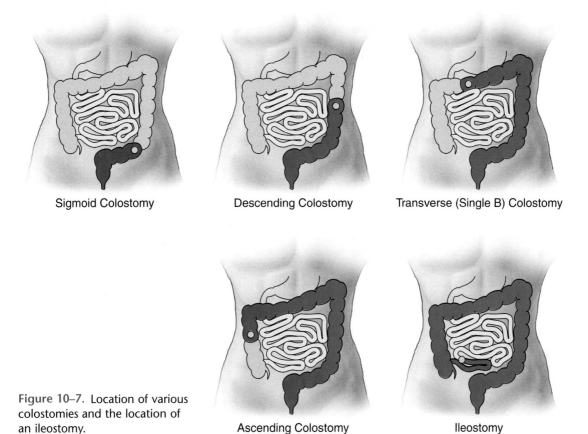

Sigmoid Colostomy   Descending Colostomy   Transverse (Single B) Colostomy

Figure 10–7. Location of various colostomies and the location of an ileostomy.

Ascending Colostomy   Ileostomy

ostomy should observe the diagnostic studies being performed for these patients until he or she can care for them easily.

The ostomy patient will have a dressing or drainage pouch in place over the area of the stoma (Fig. 10–8). Wearing clean gloves, you must remove the dressing, then place it in a plastic bag and dispose of it in a receptacle intended for contaminated waste. Remove the gloves and wash your hands. The procedure for dressing change is discussed in Chapter 5. Remove the drainage pouch, and put aside in a safe place to be reused. You should wear gloves to do this. The patient may want to do this him- or herself or direct you to do it. The pouch must be kept clean and dry.

A patient who has a colostomy or ileostomy and is going to have a barium study of the lower GI tract needs special instructions to be adequately prepared. If the hospital has an enterostomal therapist, the patient should be referred to this person for instruction. If not, the radiologist and the patient's physician should give the instruction before and after the procedure. All ostomy patients should be instructed to bring an extra pouch with them if they are coming from outside the hospital. Dietary, laxative, and cleansing preparations vary depending on the type and location of the ostomy.

Administering a Barium Enema to a Patient with an Ostomy

Ostomy patients have barium studies for diagnostic purposes, and the procedure is somewhat different from that performed on a person with normally functioning bowels. If you are the radiographer assisting with a barium examination for an ostomy patient, you must plan the procedure with the radiologist before

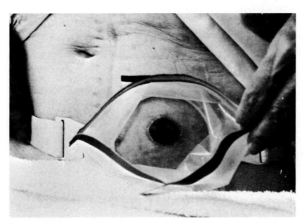

Figure 10–8. A colostomy with a drainage pouch in place.

beginning to ensure the patient's comfort and safety. A cone-shaped tip with a long drainage bag that attaches to it after the procedure is frequently the instillation instrument of choice (Fig. 10–9). Occasionally, a small catheter with an inflatable cuff is used. Other ostomy tips may be used, depending on the patient's situation and the preference of the physician. Examples are the nipple tip and the double-barrel tip. The patient who has had the ostomy for some time may prefer to insert the tip him- or herself.

As the radiographer, you will lubricate the tip of the cone and hand it to the patient for insertion (Fig. 10–10). Then put on clean disposable gloves so that you may assist the patient. However, the radiologist may prefer to insert the tip and tape it in place.

After the cone or tip has been inserted, the procedure is the same as for other patients. The patient may be placed in various positions; however, do not place the patient in a prone position because this may cause injury at the stoma site. Don't begin to instill the barium until the physician who is conducting the examination is present to supervise the procedure. If the patient's rectum and lower bowel are present, barium may be instilled into the ostomy and also into the lower bowel through the rectum. Because these patients have lost portions of their intestines, a considerably smaller amount of barium suspension is needed for them.

CALL OUT!

Never place a patient with a stoma in the prone position because this may cause damage to the patient's ostomy site.

When the examination is complete, you can attach the drainage bag to the cone and drain the barium into it. When the drainage is complete, the patient whose physical condition permits may be taken to the lavatory with the drainage bag still in place; there the drainage bag may be cleansed and the ostomy pouch replaced. You should give the patient as much assistance as needed. Offer the patient a towel, a washcloth, and any other articles he or she may need. Allow the patient privacy if he or she is able to be independent in his care.

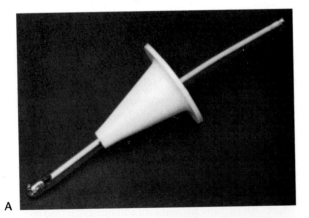

A

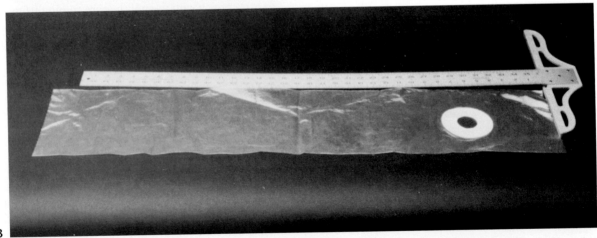

B

Figure 10–9. (**A**) Cone tip for colostomy patients. (**B**) Drainage bag used with cone tip.

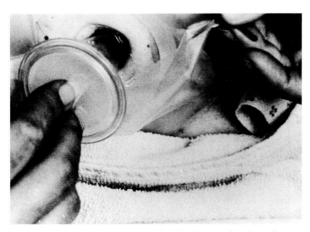

Figure 10–10. The lubricated cone is gently placed over the stoma and is held in place with the hand. (Wolff LV, Weitzel MH, Zornow RA: *Fundamentals of Nursing,* 7th ed. Philadelphia: JB Lippincott, 1987. Reprinted with permission of Hollister Inc.)

Barium Studies of the Upper Gastrointestinal Tract and Small Bowel

Barium examinations of the upper GI tract and small intestine are called an upper GI series and small bowel follow through (SBFT), respectively. They are performed to diagnose pathological conditions of the pharynx, esophagus, stomach, duodenum, and small intestine. The patient is usually instructed to remain on a low-residue diet for 2 to 3 days before the examination and to go on a food fast for 8 hours before the examination. The patient must be instructed not to smoke or chew gum before the examination because this increases gastric secretion, which may cause dilution of the contrast agent. In most instances, medications that the patient routinely takes are restricted for 8 hours before the examination. Enemas are usually not required. The patient must be informed that the examination may take several hours; he or she should be encouraged to bring reading material to pass the time.

Adverse reactions from glucagon may be nausea, vomiting, hives, and flushing. Adverse reactions from anticholinergic drugs may be dry mouth, thirst, tachycardia, urinary retention, and blurred vision. If the patient is to receive these medications, another person should be available to drive home.

The physician will order a water-soluble iodinated contrast agent if the patient has a possible pathological perforation or obstruction of the upper GI tract and if barium is contraindicated. In the event of a perforation or obstruction, barium may intensify the obstruction or pass into the abdominal cavity.

You should inform your patient that he or she will be expected to drink 14 to 16 ounces of flavored barium. For some examinations, a thick suspension of barium is followed by a thin suspension of barium. The solution does not have an unpleasant flavor; however, the chalkiness may be difficult to tolerate. It may be less distasteful for the patient to drink the substance through a straw.

Some examinations of the upper GI tract require passage of a gastric tube before the examination. The use of gastric tubes is discussed in Chapter 11, and complex upper GI examinations are discussed later in this text.

After the barium is swallowed and passes through the digestive tract, fluoroscopic examination outlines peristalsis and the contours of the upper GI tract (Fig. 10–11). Spot films are taken as directed by the radiologist. Double contrast with air is often used; when this is done, the patient should be informed of this and warned that he or she will have a feeling of fullness. The patient must also be informed that during the examination, he or she will be positioned in upright, supine, and side-lying positions while the passage of barium is viewed fluoroscopically. If the passage of barium is delayed or if an SBFT examination is also ordered, the examination will take a much longer time with intervals during which the patient simply waits, lying on the table. Occasionally, changing the patient's position may assist the contrast agent to pass through the upper GI tract.

Instructions After Barium Studies of the Upper Gastrointestinal Tract

If there are no contraindications, you must instruct the patient to increase fluid and fiber intake for several days after the upper GI series using barium. He or she may resume eating immediately after the examination unless another examination is to follow. Also inform the patient that the stools will be light in color and that, if no bowel movement occurs within 24 hours, he or she must notify the physician, who may wish to prescribe a laxative. The patient must be instructed not to allow constipation, because fecal impaction or bowel obstruction may result. If rectal or gastric bleeding occurs, the patient must seek medical treatment immediately.

Scheduling Diagnostic Imaging Examinations

Patients often present for medical treatment with vague symptomatology that requires multiple imaging and direct-view examinations before an

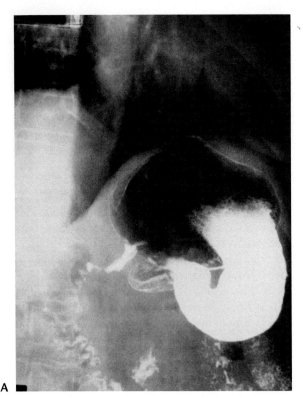
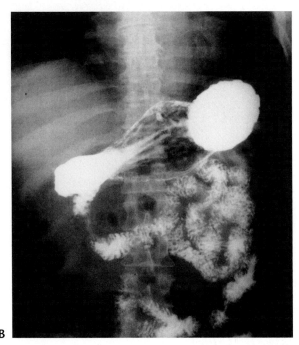

Figure 10–11. (A) Stomach filled with barium (radiograph, upper GI series). **(B)** Barium-filled stomach and small bowel (radiograph, small bowel follow through).

accurate diagnosis can be made. During the medical diagnostic process, one patient may have a series of examinations, some of which are performed in the radiographic imaging department and some elsewhere.

If you are responsible for scheduling radiographic imaging examinations, you must inquire about other examinations that the patient may be expected to undergo. You must understand how to schedule so that all of the examinations may be successfully completed in as little time as possible. This will require critical thinking and thoughtful planning.

When a patient is scheduled for imaging examinations of both upper and lower GI systems with barium as the contrast agent, the lower GI series should be scheduled first, because the barium clears most quickly from the lower bowel.

Some scheduling considerations that you must remember are as follows:

1. All radiographic examinations or procedures that do not involve contrast media should be scheduled first.

2. Ultrasound examinations must be scheduled to precede GI examinations using contrast agents because contrast media in the GI tract will interfere with ultrasound.

3. Radioisotope scans of the liver and spleen must be completed before barium studies.

4. Thyroid scans must be done before any examination using iodinated contrast agents because they will interfere with this test for many weeks.

5. Examinations that involve administration of intravascular contrast agents should precede barium studies because the intravenous agents are less dense than barium.

6. Barium studies of the lower GI tract must precede upper GI examinations.

7. Examinations that require the patient to fast for 8 hours or more should be performed early in the morning. This is especially important when scheduling patients who have diabetes mellitus; pediatric patients, and elderly patients.

Summary

There are two types of contrast agents: positive and negative. The most commonly used positive agents are barium sulfate and iodinated preparations. The most commonly used negative agents are air and carbon dioxide.

Studies using barium and barium in combination with air are frequently conducted in the radiographic imaging department to diagnose pathological conditions of the upper and lower gastrointestinal tracts. Correct preparation for these examinations is essential for a successful outcome. The radiographer's professional responsibility is to teach the patient the correct methods of preparing for barium studies and the care and precautions that he or she must take after these or any diagnostic imaging procedures. Your professional obligation as the radiographer is to instruct other members of the health care team regarding the correct preparation of patients for diagnostic imaging examinations.

The problem-solving process should be used as an outline for your teaching presentations. You can evaluate your teaching plan by requesting the patient to repeat your directions to make certain that he or she has assimilated the instructions and is able to carry them out.

Preparation for examinations of the lower GI tract using barium as a contrast agent usually requires that the bowel be cleansed with enemas. The types of cleansing enemas with which you must be familiar are saline, hypertonic, oil-retention, tap water, and SS enemas. The tap water and SS enemas are the kinds most often prescribed to precede lower GI examinations. You must be able to perform the cleansing enema correctly and to instruct a patient to administer these to himself at home if this is necessary. You must keep in mind the hazards of the enema procedure and take care to prevent serious illness or injury to the patient.

The patient with an ostomy may also require a barium enema. The procedure and the tip used vary for these patients. You must be sensitive in your care of ostomy patients because they are often in the process of grieving over the recent alteration in body image. If you are not accustomed to seeing this type of stoma, you should work with a specially trained technologist or simply observe the procedure until you feel comfortable enough to relate to the ostomy patient in a therapeutic manner.

Barium studies of the upper GI tract are frequently done to diagnose pathological conditions of the pharynx, esophagus, stomach, duodenum, and jejunum. The preparation before and after these studies varies somewhat from that of the lower GI series. You must familiarize yourself with this information so that you can correctly instruct the patient and keep the patient as comfortable and anxiety-free as possible during the procedure.

Scheduling for a series of diagnostic imaging examinations requires careful planning so that the studies can be completed in as brief a time as possible. Imaging examinations must also be scheduled so that they will not conflict with other diagnostic procedures that may be prescribed. You should be knowledgeable concerning which diagnostic imaging examinations will interfere with other tests, and you must schedule in a manner that is safe and efficient for the patient. The very young, the elderly, and the patient with diabetes mellitus must be scheduled to accommodate their dietary restrictions and frailties.

Chapter 10 Test

1. List and differentiate the two types of contrast agents.

_____ **2.** Under which circumstance is barium not the contrast agent of choice?
   a. When the patient has a possible perforation of the GI mucosa
   b. When the patient is a diabetic
   c. When the patient has an emotional problem
   d. When a diagnosis of paralytic ileus is possible

3. Before removing the retention-style enema tip, what is the most important thing to remember?

_____ **4.** Barium is a relatively nontoxic contrast agent; therefore, no special precautions need to be taken.
   a. True
   b. False

_____ **5.** The amount of solution prescribed for a saline or SS cleansing enema before barium studies of the lower GI tract is usually
   a. 10 mL
   b. 1000 mL
   c. 500 mL
   d. 900 mL

_____ **6.** The only safe soap to use for a cleansing enema is
   a. Liquid detergent
   b. Oatmeal soap
   c. Nonperfumed soap
   d. Castile soap
   e. Hypoallergenic soap

_____ **7.** When upper and lower GI series are scheduled, as the radiographer you must schedule the upper GI series first.
   a. True
   b. False

_____ **8.** After a barium study, you must instruct the patient in follow-up care. These instructions will include
   1. Description of the appearance of the stools
   2. Instructions to call the physician if the patient does not have a bowel movement within 24 hours
   3. Need for increased fluid intake and fiber in the diet if not contraindicated
   a. 1 and 2
   b. 1 and 3
   c. 2 and 3
   d. 1, 2, and 3

_____ **9.** You must recognize that the patient with an ostomy has suffered a change in body image and may be going through
   a. The grieving process
   b. The process of self-examination
   c. The aging process
   d. The self-actualization process

_____ **10.** The type of cleansing enema prescribed for a pediatric patient would probably be
   a. An SS enema
   b. A tap water enema
   c. An oil-retention enema
   d. A saline enema

11. Name the side effect that can occur after a barium enema procedure.

_____ **12.** If the patient has the large bowel removed at the sigmoid area and the opening is made on the anterior surface of the abdomen, the patient is said to have:
   a. A colostomy
   b. An ileostomy
   c. A sigmoidostomy
   d. A colonostomy

_____ **13.** When both barium and air are used in a radiographic procedure of the GI system, it is termed
   a. A single-contrast study
   b. A double-contrast study
   c. A pneumogram
   d. There is no special name for this

14. List five preparation criteria that must be included when instructing a patient who is to receive an upper GI series.

11

Caring for Patients Needing Alternative Medical Treatments

Objectives

After studying this chapter, you will be able to:

1. Explain the reasons for nasogastric and nasoenteric intubation and the radiographer's responsibilities when these tubes are in place.

2. Describe the precautions you will need to take as the radiographer in caring for a patient who has a gastrostomy tube in place.

3. Describe the patient care considerations when you are working with a patient who requires parenteral nutrition or has a central venous catheter.

4. Describe the symptoms of a patient who needs suctioning, and explain the action you must take if this situation occurs.

5. Explain the precautions you must take when working with a patient who has a tracheostomy.

6. List the precautions you must take when working with a patient requiring mechanical ventilation.

7. List the patient care precautions you must take for the patient who has a chest tube in place with water-sealed drainage.

8. Describe the patient care considerations for the patient who has a tissue drain in place.

Glossary

Asphyxiation: Severe hypoxia leading to hypoxemia, hypercapnea, loss of consciousness, and death

Barotrauma: Injury due to pressure

Bolus: A concentrated mass of pharmaceutical preparation, such as an opaque contrast medium given intravenously or swallowed

Cannula: A tube used to allow fluids, gases, or other substances into or out of the body

Cystostomy: Surgical opening into the urinary bladder

Dyspneic: Having shortness of breath or difficulty breathing

Fowler's position: Position in which the head of the patient's bed is raised 18 to 20 inches above the level with the knees also elevated

Gastrostomy: Creation of an opening in the stomach to provide food and liquid administration

Hemostat: A clamp-like instrument used to control flow of fluids or blood

Lavage: The process of washing out an organ, usually the stomach, bladder, or bowel

Nasogastric tube: A tube of soft rubber or plastic inserted through the nostril and into the stomach

Saline solution: A solution consisting of a percentage of sodium chloride and distilled water that has the same osmolarity as that of body fluids

Stoma: An artificial opening from the bowel to the body surface

Suspension: Solid particles mixed, but not dissolved, in a fluid or another solid

Suture material: An absorbable or nonabsorbable material used for surgical stitches

Technetium (Tc): A radioactive metallic element

Ulcerative colitis: A chronic episodic inflammatory disease of the large intestine characterized by profuse watery diarrhea, bleeding, and infection

Nasogastric (NG) and nasoenteric (NE) tubes are inserted for therapeutic and diagnostic purposes. These tubes have a hollow lumen through which secretions and air may be evacuated or through which medications, nourishment, or diagnostic contrast agents may be instilled. As the radiographer, you must be able to care for and transport patients with these tubes in place. You must also understand the purposes of gastric suction and be able to attach or discontinue it when the physician's orders require this to be done.

Studies are done in diagnostic imaging that require the passage of NG or NE tubes before the examination. As the radiographer, you will not insert these tubes, but you may be asked to prepare the patient if the tube is to be inserted in the diagnostic imaging department. You must know what type of equipment to assemble and how to assist with the procedure.

Occasionally you will see a patient for a procedure who has a gastrostomy tube in place. These tubes may be required for persons who are gravely debilitated and unable to obtain nutrition in a normal physiologic manner. You must care for these patients safely and with sensitivity.

Patients who are unable to take in nutrients through the gastrointestinal (GI) system, either partially or completely, may be nourished intravenously. This can be accomplished in the short term parenterally by peripheral intravenous means and in the long term by reliance on central venous catheters. To care for a patient with a central venous catheter, you must learn what precautions to take to prevent life-threatening complications.

Occasionally, it is necessary for the patient who has vomited or who has an accumulation of blood or secretions in the mouth or throat to be suctioned while you are caring for him or her. You do not perform the suctioning procedure, but you must be able to assess a patient's need for suctioning and be able to prepare the equipment so that the procedure may be done quickly to prevent aspiration of the fluid into the lungs or respiratory failure.

Patients with the tracheostomy tubes in place may also need diagnostic imaging examinations. You need to give them proper care to prevent injury and to keep them comfortable while the examination is in progress.

Patients who are unable to maintain adequate respiration may require mechanical ventilation to support life. You will frequently be asked to take radiographs of patients who are on mechanical ventilators; therefore, you must understand the precautions to take when working with these patients.

Chest tubes are inserted after surgical procedures, injury, or diseases of the lungs to permit drainage of fluid or air out of the pleural space. If air and fluid become trapped in the pleural space, pressure builds and creates what is called a *tension pneumothorax*. If this condition is not relieved, the resulting respiratory distress may produce a life-threatening situation. You must learn the precautions to take when caring for patients with chest tubes in place with water-sealed drainage.

After surgical procedures, a variety of tissue drains are placed in the areas of the body that poorly tolerate an accumulation of fluid. You must be able to recognize these drains and direct patient care in a manner that prevents dislodging the drains.

Nasogastric and Nasoenteric Tubes

NG tubes are made of polyurethane, silicone, or rubber. They are inserted through the nasopharynx into the stomach, the duodenum, or the jejunum. If a patient has an anatomic or physiologic reason why the nose cannot be used for passage, the tube may be inserted through the mouth over the tongue. NG tubes are used to keep the stomach free of gastric contents and air to assist in the healing process either before or after an operative procedure or during a disease process. NG tubes are also used for diagnostic examinations, for administration of feedings or medications, to treat intestinal obstruction, and to control bleeding (Table 11–1).

NE tubes are made of the same materials as NG tubes and are inserted in much the same way as NG tubes; however, they are allowed to pass into the duodenum and small intestine by means of peristalsis. They are also used for decompression, diagnosis, and treatment purposes (Table 11–2).

Two of the most common NG tubes are the Levin and the sump tube. Other NG tubes often seen are the Nutriflex, the Moss, and the Sengstaken-Blakemore esophageal NG tube. The Levin tube is a single-lumen tube with holes near its tip (Fig. 11–1*A*). The sump tube is a double-lumen tube, which is radiopaque. The opening of the second lumen is a blue extension off the proximal end of the tube (the end that remains outside) called a "pigtail" (see Fig. 11–1*B*). This end is always left open to room air for the purpose of maintaining a continuous flow of atmospheric air into the stomach, thereby controlling the amount of suction pressure that may be placed on the gastric mucosa. This is a means of preventing injury and ulceration of these tissues.

The Nutriflex tube is used primarily for feedings. It has a mercury-weighted tip and is coated with a lubricant that becomes activated when moistened by gastric secretions.

The Moss tube is a more complex triple-lumen tube. One lumen has an inflatable balloon to anchor it in the stomach. The second lumen is used for

TABLE 11-1 _____

Common Nasogastric Tubes

NAMES	NO. OF LUMENS	DESCRIPTION	USE
Levin	1	Plastic tube that is passed through the nose into the stomach	Gastric decompression
Sump	2	Radiopaque tube with a plug pigtail that leaves air flow into the stomach	Drain fluid from the stomach
Nutriflex	1	Mercury-weighted tip; coated with a gastric secretion-activated lubricant	Feedings
Moss	3	Has a balloon to anchor into stomach while 2nd and 3rd lumens are used for aspiration and feeding	Aspiration of fluid; duodenal feeding
Sengstaken-Blakemore	3	Thick catheter with 2 balloons used to exert pressure against walls of esophagus	Control of bleeding from esophageal varices

aspiration of fluid, and the third is for duodenal feeding (Fig. 11–2).

The Sengstaken-Blakemore (S-B) tube is also a triple-lumen tube; two of the lumens have balloons. The balloons are inflated to exert pressure on bleeding esophageal varices. The third lumen is used for lavage and to monitor for hemorrhage. The balloon pressure must be maintained at all times, but if the patient becomes dyspneic, the balloon pressure must be relieved at once by cutting the balloon lumens with scissors. You must not attempt to care for a patient with an S-B tube in place without the patient's nurse on hand. Asphyxiation or aspiration of gastric contents into the lungs is possible without keen and continuous monitoring. The patient with an S-B tube in place is usually cared for in the intensive care unit, and portable radiographic images are ordered.

Three of the most commonly used NE tubes are the Cantor, the Harris, and the Miller-Abbott. The Cantor and Harris tubes have a single lumen (see Fig. 11–1C); the Miller-Abbott tube is a double-lumen tube. One lumen of the Miller-Abbott tube is used for intestinal decompression; the other is for the introduction of mercury after insertion. Some single-lumen tubes are weighted with a metal tip. The progress of the tube may be observed in the diagnostic imaging department

TABLE 11-2 _____

Common Nasoenteric Tubes

NAMES	NO. OF LUMENS	DESCRIPTION	USE
Cantor	1	Long tube with a small mercury-filled bag at the end; contains drainage holes for aspiration	Relieves obstructions in the small intestine
Harris	1	Mercury-weighted tube passed through the nose and carried through the digestive tract by gravity	Gastric and intestinal decompression
Miller-Abbott	2	Long small-caliber catheter; one is a perforated metal tip, and the other has a collapsible balloon; radiopaque tube	Decompression

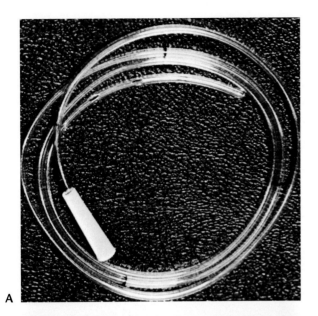

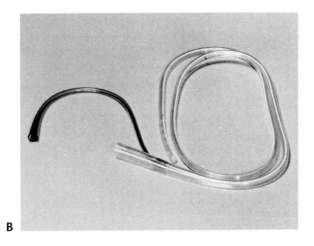

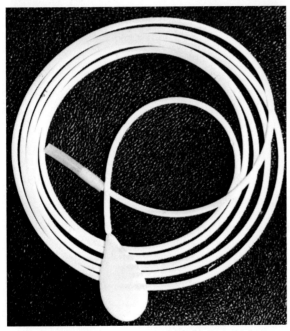

Figure 11–1. (**A**) Levin (NG) tube. (**B**) Sump (Ng) tube. (**C**) Cantor (NE) tube.

fluoroscopically. Radiographs are taken after passage of these tubes to establish correct placement.

Passage of Nasogastric and Nasoenteric Tubes

Radiographers are not responsible for inserting NG or NE tubes. A registered nurse usually inserts an NG tube; a registered nurse or a physician inserts the NE tube. You may be required to assist with the passage of the gastric tube and may often care for patients who have them in place.

The materials needed for passage of an NG or NE tube are the following: a tube of the correct type and size (usually a 14F to 16F lumen for an adult patient); rubber tubes (placed in a basin of ice before insertion to make the rubber more rigid and to facilitate passage); clean, disposable gloves; an emesis basin, a towel, a glass of water, and a drinking straw; a 20- to 50-mL aspirating (bulb) syringe; water-soluble lubricant; wide hypoallergenic tape; a stethoscope; a tongue blade; a safety pin and rubber band; normal saline solution; and a suction machine, if suction is to be used.

Insertion of a tube is an uncomfortable and frightening procedure for the patient, who is often very ill. If this procedure is to take place in the radiographic imaging department, you must explain what is to be done and for what purpose. Assure the patient that if he or she concentrates on swallowing and breathing as

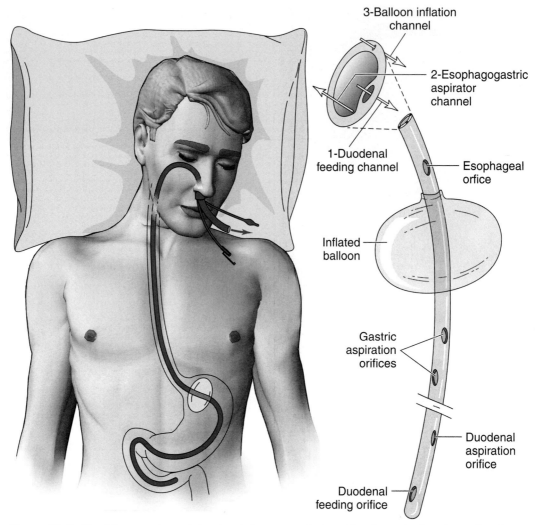

Figure 11–2. The Moss esophageal duodenal decompression and feeding tube has three chambers; the first anchors it in the stomach, the second is for aspiration, and the third for feeding. (Smeltzer SC, Bare BG: *Brunner and Suddarth's Textbook of Medical-Surgical Nursing,* 8th ed. Philadelphia: Lippincott-Raven, 1996.)

the tube is inserted, the procedure will go smoothly and quickly.

The physician may swab the nasal passages and spray the oropharynx with tetracaine (Pontocaine) to promote the patient's comfort by anesthetizing the area and suppressing the gag reflex. A gargle with a liquid anesthetic may also facilitate the procedure.

The patient is placed in a Fowler's position with pillows supporting head and shoulders. Tissues and an emesis basin should be close by for use. The nurse or physician begins the procedure by measuring the distance from the nose to the stomach externally (Fig. 11–3*A*). The Levin tube has black markings that indicate how far the tube has been inserted. When the physician or nurse is ready to insert the tube, the distal end is lubricated with a water-soluble lubricant, and the patient is instructed to swallow as it is passed. A glass of water and a straw may be made available so

that the patient has something to swallow if he or she is permitted to drink fluids. Placing several ice chips in the mouth also facilitates swallowing.

The tube should go down easily and with little force. When the tube is believed to be in the stomach, as shown in Figure 11–3*B*, its position is verified by an initial radiograph. If the tube is to be in place for a considerable length of time, its placement may be verified by attaching the end of the NG tube to a 20- to 30-mL syringe and withdrawing gastric fluid. The fluid is tested with litmus paper, which must test acidic to ensure that the tube is in the correct position.

When it is certain that the tube has reached the stomach, reassure the patient and make him or her comfortable. NG tubes are taped in place, but NE tubes are not taped, because their position is achieved through peristaltic action.

A safe and secure method of taping is the butterfly method. Cut or tear lengthwise a piece of tape approximately 2 inches long, and leave a second 2-inch piece intact. Wrap the intact piece of tape around the tubing. At the front of the tubing, criss-cross the two pieces of tape and place them over the bridge of the nose (see Fig. 11–3C). Another piece of tape may be placed over the first two so that they will remain in place (see Fig. 11–3D).

You must take care to tape the Levin tube securely so that it is not accidentally withdrawn. It should never be necessary to repeat passage of a gastric tube because of careless handling. There should be no pulling pressure on the tube. Patients with gastric tubes in place are not to eat or drink anything unless it is specifically ordered by the physician.

The placement of an NG tube must be ascertained before any medication, food, water, or contrast agent is administered into it. If this is not done, accidental administration of an agent into the pleural cavity may occur with adverse consequences for the patient.

The correct position of an NG or NE tube initially may be determined with a radiographic image or by fluoroscopy. Obviously, a radiograph cannot be used each time it is necessary to know whether the tube is correctly positioned. The other means of determining the correct placement of an NG or NE tube is by aspirating the tube with a syringe. The aspirant is then tested with litmus paper to measure its acidity. Gastric contents are acidic (pH approximately 3). The pH of intestinal secretions is less acidic (pH approximately 6 to 6.5). The pH of respiratory secretions is not acidic (pH 7 or greater). Note that small bowel and respiratory pH levels are similar but are far greater than intestinal secretions. Tubes properly placed in the stomach show a pH in the range from 1 to 4.

If there is any doubt concerning the position of an NG or NE tube, nothing should be administered into it. If instillation of an agent has begun, discontinue it immediately. If the patient seems to have regurgitated gastric contents, you must summon assistance immediately and prepare to assist with suctioning. To reduce the risk of aspiration, the patient with an NG or NE tube should be placed in a semi-Fowler's position during and for 30 minutes after administration of any agent into the tube (Fig. 11–4).

Nasoenteric Feeding Tubes

There are several narrow-lumen tubes that you may see inserted for the purpose of feeding patients. They are used for patients who are unable to obtain nourishment or take oral medications in a natural manner and who are expected to obtain nourishment by this method for some time. Various forms of nutritional supplements may be prescribed depending on the patient's needs. The feedings may be given by continuous gravity drip, by bolus, or by a controlled pump method.

Patients may be discharged from the hospital with these tubes in place, so you may care for them either in the hospital, as outpatients, or in their homes. Your care of persons with feeding tubes in place does not differ from care of persons with NG or other NE tubes in place.

Removing Gastric Tubes

The Levin tube, the sump tube, and other tubes positioned in the stomach are easily removed; however, you must never assume that simply because a radiographic examination that involved its use is complete, it is permissible to remove the tube. Unless you are ordered by the physician to remove the tube, leave the tube in place.

Items needed to remove an NG tube are an emesis basin, tissues, paper towels, an impermeable waste receptacle (a plastic bag is best), clean disposable gloves, a face shield (or a mask and goggles), and a gown. The procedure for removing gastric tubes is as follows:

1. Put on the protective gown.

2. Identify the patient and explain the procedure.

3. Wash your hands. Prepare the disposal bag by folding the large cuff downward.

4. If suction is attached to the tube, turn it off and disconnect it.

5. Gently remove the tape from the tubing.

6. Put on mask, goggles, and gloves. Have paper towels prepared to receive the tube as it is removed.

7. Instruct the patient to take a deep breath.

8. Gently withdraw the tube, wrap it in paper toweling, and place it in the disposal bag.

9. If there is any resistance when the tube is being withdrawn, stop the procedure and call for assistance.

10. Make the patient comfortable, and remove your protective clothing and gloves. Correctly dispose of the contaminated waste.

Do not remove NE tubes. The physician or registered nurse may remove the tube, or it may be passed through the intestinal tract and removed rectally.

CALL OUT!

Although radiographers may remove NG tubes, they may not remove NE tubes.

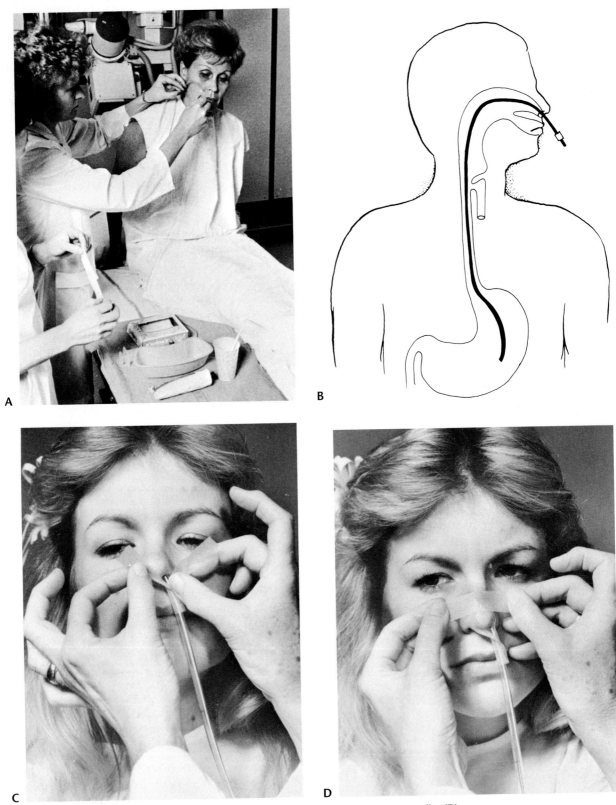

Figure 11–3. (**A**) Measure the distance from the nose to the stomach externally. (**B**) Position of the Levin tube in the stomach. (**C**) Cross the two pieces of tape and place them over the bridge of the nose. (**D**) Add a second piece of tape to reinforce the initial tape.

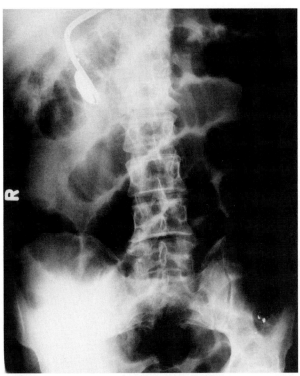

Figure 11–4. Radiograph of a small bowel obstruction with a nasoenteric tube in place.

Transferring Patients with Nasogastric Suction

NG and NE tubes are used before or after surgical procedures that involve the digestive system, for illness of the GI system to keep the stomach and bowel free of gastric contents, and for gastric decompression. The tube may be attached to a suction apparatus that is either portable or piped into the room from a central hospital unit (Fig. 11–5). The suction is maintained either continuously or intermittently, as the patient's needs demand. When you are responsible for transferring a patient who is having either continuous or intermittent gastric suctioning, you must verify the physician's orders before making the transfer. If it is permissible to discontinue the suction, you must know the length of time that it can be interrupted safely. If it is for only a short time, be certain that suction can be reestablished in the diagnostic imaging department. This can be accomplished by taking the patient's portable suction machine with him or her or by using the suction available in the department. You must also know the amount of suction pressure that is required so that you can adjust the pressure accurately. The amount of pressure that is ordered varies, and you can determine the correct level by reading the physician's orders or by asking the nurse in charge of the patient to do this. The maximum amount of suction that can

be used is a pressure equal to 25 mm Hg for an adult patient. More than this can damage the gastric mucosa.

If the suction must be disconnected for a period of time, you may do this. If the tube is a single-lumen tube, you will need the following materials: a pair of clean, disposable gloves, a clamping device, a package of sterile gauze sponges, and two rubber bands. The procedure for discontinuing suction is as follows:

1. Explain the procedure to the patient, then wash your hands, open the package of sponges, and put on the gloves.

2. Turn off the suction; clamp or plug the gastric tube with the clamp or stopper (Fig. 11–6*A*); and place one gauze pad over the end of the tube. Secure it with a rubber band.

3. Cover the connecting end of the suction tubing or the adapter with the other sponge, and secure it with a rubber band. This gauze covering keeps both ends of the tubing clean while not in use (see Fig. 11–6*B*).

4. Secure the suction tubing on the machine so that it will not fall onto the floor, and make certain that the NG or NE tube will not be dislodged during the transfer.

5. Proceed with the transfer by wheelchair or gurney as required.

6. If the suction is to be restarted in the diagnostic imaging department on arrival, set the suction pressure gauge, turn on the suction, and reattach it to the tubing. This procedure is repeated when transferring the patient back to the room.

If the NG tube is a double-lumen tube, never clamp it closed with a hemostat or regular clamping device, because this may cause the lumens to adhere to each other and destroy the double-lumen effect. To prevent leakage from this type of tube, the barrel of a piston syringe may be inserted into the suction-drainage lumen (the blue pigtail); it is then pinned to the gown with the barrel upward to prevent reflux drainage (see Fig. 11–6*C*).

CALL OUT!

Never clamp a double-lumen NG tube because this may destroy the effect.

The Patient with a Gastronomy Tube

A gastrostomy is the surgical creation of an opening into the stomach. Through this opening a tube is placed from the inside of the stomach to the external

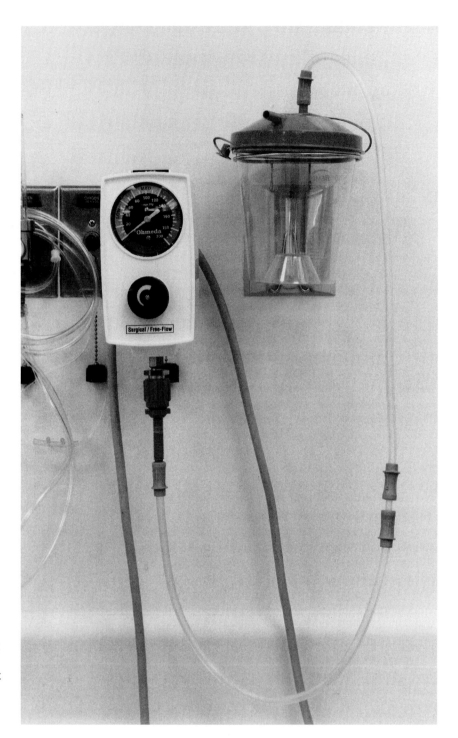

Figure 11–5. Suction equipment is often used in diagnostic imaging. It is piped to the department from a central area in the hospital. The vacuum collecting canister is disposable.

abdominal wall for the purpose of feeding a patient who cannot tolerate oral food intake (Fig. 11–7). This can be a temporary or permanent provision. The tube can be sutured in place or may be held in place with a crossbar that holds the tube against the wall of the stomach.

The patient with a newly applied gastrostomy tube has an unhealed surgical incision and will have a dressing in place. An older gastrostomy may or may not

have a dressing applied. The tube is closed off after feeding with a clamp or a plug-in adapter to prevent leakage of gastric fluid or food. The tube is then coiled and kept in place with tape or a small dressing.

While caring for a person with a gastrostomy tube in place, you must be aware of the potential for infection. If the operative area around the gastrostomy tube is not healed, you must wear sterile gloves if you will have contact with the open area to prevent

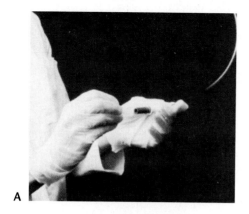

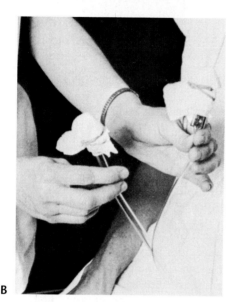

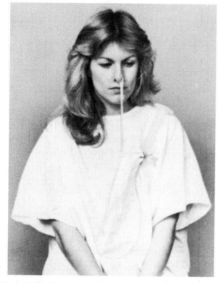

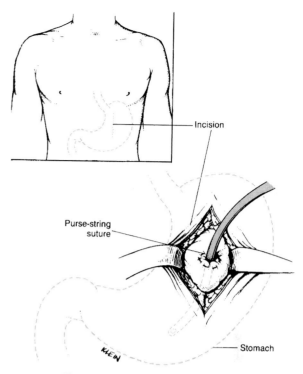

Figure 11–7. A gastrostomy tube.

Figure 11–6. (**A**) Clamping gastric tube with plug. (**B**) Cover the ends of the tubing with gauze pads, and secure the gauze with rubber bands. (**C**) Insert the end of the tubing into the barrel of a piston syringe, and pin the syringe facing upright to the patient's gown. This prevents leakage of gastric fluid.

introduction of microorganisms that may result in infection. The potential for dislodging the tube is also present. Take care to prevent this. There must be no tension placed on the tube.

You must also be sensitive to the feelings of the patient with a gastrostomy. The patient may be grieving owing to the change in his or her body image or because of a chronic illness. You must communicate with the patient in a sensitive and thoughtful manner. The patient who is able should be allowed to direct care of the tube.

The Patient Who Is Receiving Parenteral Nutrition or Has a Central Venous Catheter

Central venous catheters and implanted ports are being used more frequently for patients who must have long-term medication administration, frequent blood transfusions, hyperosmolar solutions, or total parenteral nutrition. You must be aware of their presence and purpose and be familiar with the precautions you must take if they are in place.

When a patient does not have an adequate nutritional intake and cannot tolerate nourishment by means of the GI tract, he or she may be ordered to receive partial or total nutrition by an intravenous route. Partial parenteral nutrition is used when the

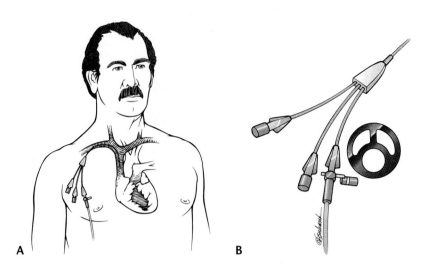

Figure 11–8. Subclavian triple-lumen catheter for total parenteral nutrition and other adjunct therapy. (**A**) The catheter is threaded through the sub-clavian vein and placed in the vena cava. (**B**) Each lumen is an avenue for solution administration; these are secured with Luer-Lok caps when not in use. (Smeltzer SC, Bare BG: *Brunner and Suddarth's Textbook of Medical-Surgical Nursing,* 8th ed. Philadelphia: Lippincott-Raven, 1996.)

patient is able to supply a part of his or her nutritional requirements by natural means. A large-gauge catheter is inserted into a large peripheral vein in the arm, and a parenteral solution containing a combination of lipid emulsion and amino acid/dextrose solution is administered as needed to satisfy the patient's nutritional needs. Vitamins and minerals are often added to these solutions. Care of patients receiving peripheral intravenous therapy is discussed in Chapter 12.

When the patient requires total nutritional support by the parenteral method, it is delivered through a central vein. Total parenteral nutrition (TPN) solutions are hyperosmotic. This means that they are highly concentrated and would damage the intima of a peripheral vein; therefore, a large vein in the central venous system is used. Because fluid imbalance may result if TPN is administered too rapidly, administration is controlled by a pump or an infusion controller. Intravenous pumps are discussed in Chapter 12.

Central venous catheters are used for measuring the central venous pressure (CVP) as well as allowing nutrients and other fluid to be instilled into the patient. To obtain a true CVP measurement, the catheter must be correctly placed in the patient. The best location for a CVP line would be the brachio-cephalic vein at the junction of the superior vena cava (SVC) or actually within the SVC itself. The location of the catheter must be confirmed either by a mobile chest radiograph or by C-arm fluoroscopy during the actual insertion of the catheter. The line should be seen just medial to the anterior border of the first rib on the image.

There are several types of central venous catheters. The tunneled type is inserted into the subclavian or internal jugular vein and then advanced into the superior vena cava or the right atrium. The exit site is on the anterior chest. Most central venous catheters have

more than one lumen and several access ports at the exit site (Fig. 11–8).

The Hickman and Broviac catheters are two commonly used tunnel-type central venous catheters. Two other commonly used central venous catheters are the peripherally inserted central (PIC) and the Groshong. The PIC catheter may be peripherally inserted into the patient's arm and advanced until its tip lies in a central vein. You may be called on to provide C-arm fluoroscopy in the operating suite during the placement of one of these catheters.

Another alternative central venous catheter is an implanted port. These are meant for patients who have long-term illnesses that require frequent intravenous medications or transfusions. The port is made of plastic, titanium, or stainless steel. It is implanted into the subcutaneous tissue, usually in the chest, and sutured in place (see Fig. 11–8). The port is not visible but can be felt as a small, hard surface under the subcutaneous tissue. A catheter from the port is then inserted into the subclavian or internal jugular vein. A needle, called the *Hubur needle,* is inserted to access the central vein through the port.

While caring for a patient with a central venous catheter or port in place, you must use great care to prevent infection at the insertion site. If a dressing around the catheter must be removed, you must receive a physician's order to do so. You must wash your hands for 2 minutes, and put on clean gloves to remove the dressing. If a dressing is to be reapplied, you must use the hospital protocol for applying dressings to central venous catheters. Dressings are usually removed and reapplied with both the health care worker and the patient wearing masks if the insertion site is in the upper thoracic area. If the patient does not wear a mask, he or she must turn away to avoid breathing on the site. The dressing must be removed carefully to avoid dislodging or moving the needle.

Emergency Suctioning

Occasionally an infant, a child, an unconscious patient, or a very weak and debilitated patient is unable to clear emesis, sputum, or other drainage from the nose, mouth, nasopharynx, or oropharynx by coughing or swallowing. While caring for a patient in these circumstances, you must place the conscious person into a semi-Fowler's position and assist him or her to clear the airway. If the patient has a potential spinal cord injury and is in a back brace and a collar and begins to vomit, log roll the patient to the side with face directed downward. No movement of the patient's head or neck should be allowed. If the airway is not cleared quickly, the patient may need to be suctioned. Signs that indicate that a patient may need to receive nasopharyngeal or oropharyngeal suctioning are as follows:

1. Profuse vomiting in a patient who cannot voluntarily change position

2. Audible rattling or gurgling sounds coming from the patient's throat

3. Signs of respiratory distress

Persons with these symptoms may require mechanical suctioning to remove the secretions to prevent aspiration or respiratory arrest.

Suctioning is an emergency procedure. It is not within the scope of your practice to perform suctioning procedures because there are many instances in which suctioning may be contraindicated. The need for suctioning must be determined by a health care professional who has been educated for this and who is familiar with the patient's condition. Some contraindications for suctioning may be head and facial injuries, bleeding esophageal varices, nasal deformities, trauma, cerebral aneurisms, tight wheezing, bronchospasm, and croup.

You must be able to determine whether your patient may need to be suctioned, to call for the physician or the registered nurse to do this if necessary, and to assist with the procedure. You are responsible for checking the emergency suctioning equipment in your department each day to be certain that it is in good working order and that all necessary items for suctioning are available. The items necessary for suctioning the oropharynx or nasopharynx are as follows:

1. A wall outlet or a working portable suction machine

2. Adapters for wall outlets

3. Clean and sterile gloves

4. Tubing

5. Sterile disposable suction sets that contain suction catheters of various sizes and either a Y- or thumb-control connector

6. Sterile containers for sterile solution

7. Sterile water or sterile normal saline solution

8. Tongue depressors padded with gauze

9. An oxygen source and oxygen-administering equipment

10. Packets of sterile, water-soluble lubricant

11. Gowns, masks, and goggles

Catheters for emergency suctioning may vary in size from a 10F to 18F lumen for adults (22 inches long) and 5F to 8F lumen for children (Fig. 11–9A). Pressure settings vary depending on the patient's age and are usually higher than those used for NG suctioning. Sterile technique is recommended for nasopharyngeal and oropharyngeal suctioning because the respiratory tract is easily infected. Introducing new microorganisms into the respiratory tract must be avoided. Maintenance of sterile technique is discussed in Chapter 5.

Before suctioning begins, wash your hands and assemble the necessary equipment for the physician or nurse. The patient should be placed in a semi-Fowler's position with head turned toward the side if he or she is alert and has a functioning gag reflex. An unconscious patient or a child should be placed in a lateral (side-lying) position with no pillow. Adequate lighting must be available. (A portable gooseneck lamp may be used). A towel is then placed over the patient's chest.

After the patient is prepared, the person who will perform the suctioning will put on a gown, mask, and goggles and will open the sterile packet containing the catheter and the connector. He or she will then put on sterile gloves, pick up the catheter, and connect it to the suction adapter. You must keep the hand that will touch the suction catheter sterile; the other hand becomes contaminated. You may pour a small amount of normal saline into the sterile container, turn on the suction machine, and adjust the pressure as directed by the physician or nurse. The suction pressure for adults is approximately 110 to 150 mm Hg on a wall-mounted outlet. Wall outlets are usually more powerful than portable machines. For infants, the requirements vary from 50 to 95 mm Hg for wall-mounted outlets. For older children, the setting for wall outlet suction varies from 100 to 120 mm Hg.

The person doing the suctioning may test the suction by placing the catheter tip into the sterile water and drawing a small amount through the tubing. This also moistens the catheter tip and thereby lubricates it.

The patient should be encouraged to breathe slowly as the catheter is positioned. The catheter tip is advanced into the patient's oropharynx or nasopharynx. Suctioning must not begin until the catheter is in place. The suction is activated by placing the thumb over the

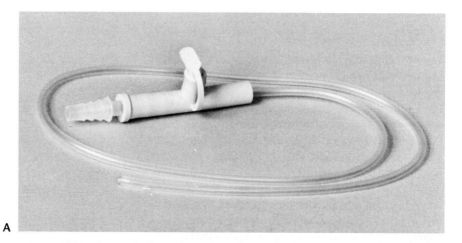

A

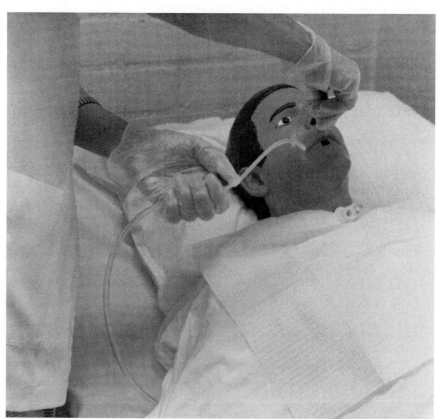

B

Figure 11–9. (**A**) A suction catheter. (**B**) Activating the suction.

opening on the connector (see Fig. 11–9*B*). The actual suctioning should not take more than 10 seconds. Suctioning for longer periods compromises the patient's oxygen supply. Suctioning may also damage the mucosa.

Care must be taken not to snag or irritate mucous membranes during the procedure. The catheter is withdrawn in a gentle rotating motion. The catheter tip is then placed into the sterile water or saline and the solution is passed through the catheter to cleanse it. A padded tongue blade may be used to keep the tongue depressed during oropharyngeal suctioning.

If further suctioning is needed, a period of 3 minutes is allowed for the patient to rest between catheter inser-

tions. This is particularly important for infants and children. The patient often receives oxygen between suctioning and should be suctioned no more than two times during one session. If the patient is able, he or she should be asked to cough and deep-breathe between suctionings.

If both oropharyngeal and nasopharyngeal passages are to be suctioned, a fresh catheter is used for each. Sterile, water-soluble lubricant is applied to the tip of a catheter to be inserted into the nasal passages. During this procedure, you should reassure the patient. If he or she fights the procedure, it may have to be discontinued.

After suctioning is completed, place the used disposable equipment into a plastic bag, which should be sealed and disposed of in the proper waste receptacle. Clean and replace the drainage tubing and collecting bottle from the portable suction machine. You must wear clean, disposable gloves while cleaning and disposing of this equipment because you may come into direct contact with the patient's secretions during the process. Sterile supplies should be replenished immediately. If the patient's condition permits, the radiographic imaging procedure may continue.

The Patient with a Tracheostomy

A tracheostomy is an opening into the trachea created surgically either to relieve respiratory distress caused by an obstruction of the upper airway or to improve respiratory function by permitting better access of air to the lower respiratory tract. This may be done as either a temporary or a permanent measure. Patients who require this procedure may have suffered traumatic injury or may be paralyzed, unconscious, or suffering from a disease that interferes with respiration.

After the surgical incision is made and the opening exists, a tracheostomy tube is inserted into the opening. Tracheostomy tubes are equipped with an obturator to ensure safe insertion; the obturator is removed as soon as the tube is in place (Fig. 11–10A).

There are several types of tracheostomy tubes. They are usually made of plastic but may be metal. They have a cuff that helps seal the tracheostomy to prevent air leaks and aspiration of gastric contents (see Fig. 11–10B). Most tracheostomy tubes have an inner cannula that is locked into place (see Fig. 11–10C). The tracheostomy tube is held in place at the back of the neck with ties or tapes. The tubes used for infants and small children do not usually have the cuff because they fit tightly enough without one.

Patients with newly inserted tracheostomy tubes are very fearful. They are unable to speak because the opening in the windpipe prevents air from being forced from the lungs past the vocal cords and into the larynx. They are afraid of choking because they are unable to remove secretions that accumulate in the tracheostomy tube. These secretions must be suctioned out by a registered nurse (see Fig. 11–10D). If a patient with a new tracheostomy is brought to the diagnostic imaging department, a nurse qualified to care for this patient should accompany him or her. Sterile suction catheters, suctioning equipment, and oxygen-administration equipment must be prepared before the patient arrives in the department. The semi-Fowler's position is usually most comfortable for these patients, and you should provide bolsters or pillows so that the best position for the patient may be maintained.

While caring for the patient with a tracheostomy, you must plan the care with the patient's nurse and the patient before any diagnostic imaging procedure is begun. The tracheostomy tube must not be removed, and the tapes holding it in place must not be untied for any reason, because the tracheostomy tube may be dislodged and may not be able to be replaced immediately. You must explain all procedures that the patient will receive to alleviate anxiety. You may provide a pencil and writing pad for the patient on which to write any comments or responses that he or she wants to make. If the patient appears to be breathing noisily or with difficulty, immediately stop working and allow the nurse to suction the patient or otherwise relieve the discomfort.

The Patient on a Mechanical Ventilator

You will be frequently called to the intensive care unit of the acute care hospital to take radiographs of patients who are being ventilated mechanically. Patients who continue to need mechanical ventilation may be transferred to extended care facilities or to their homes, and you may be sent there to radiograph a ventilator patient. Because mechanical ventilators support life, it is of great importance that you understand the precautions you must take in caring for a patient whose breathing is supported by mechanical means.

A patient who cannot breathe spontaneously or whose respiration is inadequate to oxygenate the blood is a candidate for mechanical ventilation. The need for this may be the result of a pathological condition that alters gas exchange, oxygen perfusion, or both. These are called gas exchange disorders. Examples of these might be pulmonary emboli or severe respiratory disease.

The need for mechanical ventilation may be the result of a disease process that affects the mechanics of breathing by interfering with the neurologic or neuromuscular functions related to breathing. These are called extrapulmonary disorders. Examples of extrapulmonary disorders that may require mechanical ventilation to support respiration are cerebral vascular accidents and Guillain-Barré syndrome.

There are two general classifications of mechanical ventilators: positive-pressure and negative-pressure ventilators. Negative-pressure ventilators are most likely to be seen in the home. They exert a negative pressure on the chest wall. When this occurs, air rushes into the negatively pressurized space to refill it, and it is again removed. While negative-pressure ventilators are cumbersome, they have the advantage of not requiring an artificial airway for use.

Positive-pressure ventilators are the more commonly used type. There are three general categories of positive-pressure ventilators: pressure-cycled, time-cycled, and volume-cycled. They inflate the lungs by

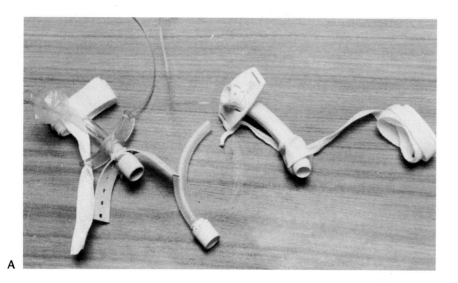

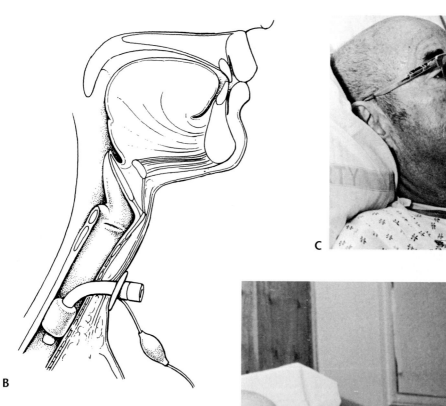

Figure 11–10. (**A**) Two types of tracheostomy tubes. Tube on right with obturator removed. Inner cannula is beside tube. (**B**) Tracheostomy tube placement. (Brunner LS and Suddarth DM: *Lippincott Manual of Nursing Practice.* Philadelphia: JB Lippincott, 1986.) (**C**) Removing the inner cannula from a tracheostomy tube. (**D**) Nurse suctioning a tracheostomy tube.

exerting positive pressure on the lungs, stopping inspiration when a preset pressure is attained. The lungs are then allowed to expire passively. All positive-pressure ventilators require an artificial airway, either an endotracheal tube or a tracheostomy. The volume-cycled ventilator is the most often used. The machine stops inspiration when it has delivered a predetermined volume of gas in spite of the amount of pressure needed to deliver it. Expiration is passive (Fig. 11–11).

When you are assigned to radiograph a patient who is on a positive-pressure ventilator, you must consult with the nurse assigned to care of the patient before beginning your work. You must identify with the nurse any special problems that you might have and plan the procedure carefully. Take the following precautions for a patient who is being ventilated by positive pressure:

1. Obtain as much assistance as necessary to move the patient safely.

2. Do not place tension on any intravenous tubing or on the tube to the ventilator.

3. Do not displace the endotracheal tube or tracheostomy tube.

4. Do not disconnect the power to the ventilator.

5. Do not disconnect the spirometer.

6. Have the patient's nurse stand by. Provide the nurse with a radiation protection garment.

7. If the patient becomes suddenly restless or confused or seems to be fighting the respirator, notify the nurse immediately.

8. Use meticulous medical aseptic technique when working with the patient to prevent infection. Put on gloves if you may possibly be in contact with blood or body fluids.

If displacement or malfunction of any part of the equipment occurs, an alarm will sound on the machine. This may indicate a life-threatening problem that must be attended to immediately. You must know where the nurse is and seek assistance immediately.

The potential complications due to a positive-pressure ventilator equipment displacement or malfunction include cardiovascular compromise related to inadequate oxygenation; pneumothorax resulting from excessive ventilator pressure; or infection resulting from exposure to microorganisms introduced into the pulmonary system.

The patient who is on a positive-pressure ventilator is unable to communicate because of the endotracheal

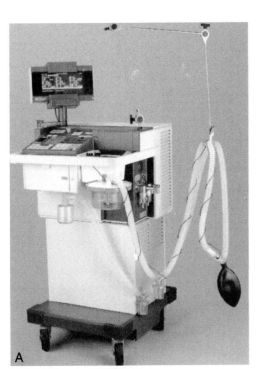
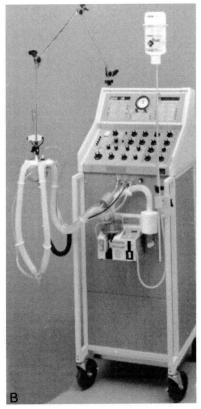

Figure 11–11. Two commonly used brands of volume-controlled ventilators. (A) Puritan-Bennett 7200A (courtesy of Puritan Bennett Corp). (B) Bear 2 Adult (courtesy of Bear Medical Systems, Inc).

tube or a newly acquired tracheostomy. This is extremely frustrating for the patient. Your explanation of what you intend to do for the patient goes a long way toward relieving this frustration, as does providing the patient with a means to give written feedback if he or she is able to write.

Endotracheal Tubes

Tubes are often inserted through the mouth into the trachea as a means of establishing or opening an airway on patients. After being placed in the trachea, a cuff is inflated, which keeps the airway open. At the same time, the tube prevents aspiration of foreign objects into the bronchus.

Correct placement of the tube is approximately 5 to 7 cm above the tracheal bifurcation (carina). A chest radiographic should always be obtained after intubations to ascertain proper placement of the tube. Up to 20% of all endotracheal tubes require repositioning after initial insertion. Because of the anatomical position of the right main bronchus, tubes that are inserted too far usually enter the right bronchus. This will cause collapse of the left lung. A tube positioned too high in the trachea may cause air to enter the stomach, causing the patient to regurgitate any gastric contents. This regurgitation may lead to aspiration pneumonia.

Radiographs should be taken on a daily basis to ensure that the tube has not accidentally shifted. The tube can be moved by the patient's coughing, the weight of the ventilator tubing, or the movement of the patient by a health care worker. Because you will have frequent interaction with patients who have an endotracheal tube, it is vitally important that you understand the consequences of any careless handling of the patient.

The Patient with a Chest Tube and Water-Sealed Drainage

The pressure in the pleural cavity is normally lower than atmospheric pressure, but disease or injury can alter this. Air in the pleural cavity known as a pneumothorax causes a collapse of the lung. A condition created by a collection of blood or fluid in the pleural cavity that prevents the lungs from expanding normally is called a *hemothorax*.

A thoracotomy, the surgical creation of an opening into the chest cavity, is performed to diagnose or treat diseases or injury to the lungs or pleura.

Conditions such as these require the placement of one or more chest tubes inserted into the pleural cavity. The chest tube is attached to a water-sealed drainage unit to remove any air or fluid from the pleural cavity (Fig.

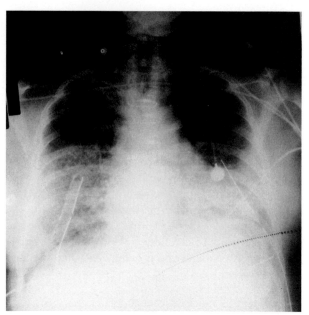

Figure 11–12. Chest tube inserted into the right pleural cavity of a patient with a pneumothorax.

11–12). This is done to reestablish the correct intrapleural pressure and to allow the lungs to expand normally.

A water-sealed drainage system is established by connecting the chest tube that originates in the pleural cavity to a clear tube that ends in a chamber containing sterile water or sterile normal saline solution. The tube leading from the chest tube remains below water level at all times to maintain the seal. When the patient inspires, air and fluid from the intrapleural spaces are drawn into the drainage tube and emptied into a chamber prepared to receive it. Since the fluid in the drainage chamber is heavier than air, it cannot be drawn back into the tube on inspiration, nor can air from the atmosphere enter because of the water seal.

There are several variations of the water-sealed system. There may be one, two, or three chambers. Additional chambers, also with water seals, are needed for drainage from the patient's pleural cavity and for suction regulation if suction is also attached to the chest tube. If two chest tubes are coming from the pleural cavity, a Y connector joins the two tubes near the patient's body and continues to the water-sealed drainage apparatus. Several commercial water-sealed drainage systems are on the market; most are disposable (Fig. 11–13).

When you are caring for a patient with a chest tube with water-sealed drainage, you must remember the following:

1. Keep the tubing from the pleural cavity to the drainage chamber as straight as possible. If it is long, loosely coil it on the patient's bed, and do not allow it to fall below the level of the patient's chest.

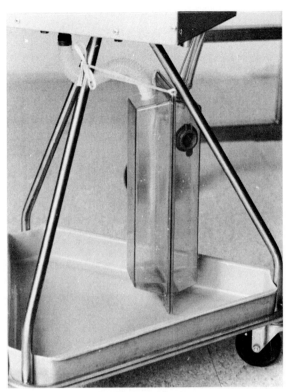

Figure 11–13. A disposable water-sealed pleural drainage set.

2. All connections must be tightly taped to the tubing, and stoppers must fit tightly into receptacles.

3. A heavy sterile dressing and tape are kept at the patient's bedside so that if the tubing is accidentally dislodged from the pleural cavity, the dressing can be taped to the open area immediately.

4. Do not empty water-sealed chambers or raise them. The water seal must remain below the patient's chest at all times.

5. Do not clamp chest tubes.

6. If a water-seal chamber is continuously bubbling, notify the patients' nurse immediately, since this may indicate a leak in the system. There should be a steady rise and fall of the water as the patient breathes.

7. Immediately report to the patient's nurse rapid, shallow breathing, cyanosis, or a complaint from the patient of a feeling of pressure on his chest.

8. The drainage tube from the chest should be long enough to allow free patient movement. If the patient must be moved for radiographic exposure, do not allow tension to be placed on the chest tube or the patient to be positioned in a way that causes the tubing to be kinked or sealed off.

CALL OUT!

You must ascertain whether the patient has a chest tube before moving him or her and placing the image receptor, since these tubes are often hidden under the blankets.

Tissue Drains

Tissue drains are placed at or near wound sites or operative sites when large amounts of drainage are expected. This drainage interferes with the healing process because the body reabsorbs it too slowly. In some circumstances, it may produce infection or result in formation of a fistula.

The Hemovac, Jackson-Pratt, and Penrose drains are three of the most common postoperative tissue drains. They are often placed in areas in which the surgical procedure calls for large amounts of tissue dissection or in areas with an increased blood supply, such as the breast, the neck, and the kidney. They are also placed in the abdominal area. One end of the tube or drain is placed in or near the operative site, and the other end exits through the body wall. The surgeon removes them when the drainage diminishes.

The Penrose drain is a soft rubber tube, which is kept from slipping into the surgical wound or beneath the body wall by a sterile safety pin (Fig. 11–14). It is allowed to drain into the surgical dressing.

The Jackson-Pratt and Hemovac drains are plastic drainage tubes that maintain constant, low, negative pressure by means of a small bulb, which is squeezed together and slowly expands to create low-pressure suction (see Fig. 11–14B and C). The drainage goes from the tubing into the bulb. You are most likely to encounter the Hemovac drain in the recovery room while radiographing a patient just out of hip surgery. Great care must be taken not to dislodge or pull on this drain while placing the image receptor.

Other types of drains are placed into the hollow organs of the body and may be sutured in place and attached to a collection bag. Some of these are the T tube, which may be placed into the common bile duct; the cecostomy tube, which is placed in the cecum; and the cystostomy tube, which is placed in the kidney.

All these drains must be identified during your assessment of the patient; you must plan care to prevent any tension on these drains, which might dislodge them partially or completely. You must also consider infection control. The presence of a tissue drain indicates that the patient has an opening directly into the body where infection may be easily introduced. If the care that you must give to your patient includes touching an area in which a drain is inserted,

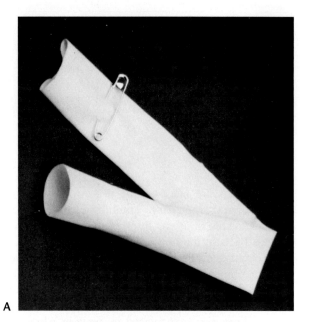

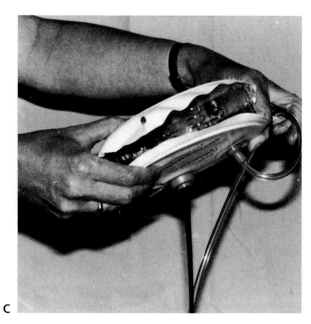

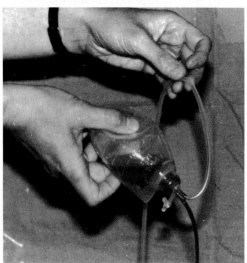

Figure 11–14. (**A**) Penrose drain. (**B**) Jackson-Pratt drain. (**C**) Hemovac drain. (Patrick ML, Woods SL, Craven RF, et al: *Medical-Surgical Nursing*. Philadelphia: JB Lippincott, 1986.)

you must use surgical aseptic technique to prevent introduction of new microorganisms into the wound. This requires hand-washing and donning of sterile gloves (see Chapter 5). If you come into contact with drainage from these areas, wear gloves and wash your hands correctly after their removal.

Summary

Nasogastric (NG) and nasoenteric (NE) tubes are inserted into the stomach and small intestine for varying medical purposes. They are used for gastric decompression, for diagnosis of diseases of the GI tract, for treatment of diseases of the GI tract, and for feeding persons who are unable to swallow food in the normal manner. Mechanical suction often accompanies NG and NE intubation. You must be prepared to assist with passage

of an NG tube and to transfer patients who have NG or NE tubes in place, including those who need suction.

Before transferring a patient who has a gastric tube in place and is receiving continuous gastric suction, you must learn whether it is permissible to discontinue the suction and, if so, for how long. The patient should be moved carefully. If the suction is continuous, it must be restarted at the same pressure as in the hospital room as soon as the patient reaches the radiographic imaging department.

The sump gastric tube is a double-lumen tube designed to maintain a continuous flow of atmospheric air into the stomach. This tube must never be clamped with a regular clamp or hemostat, since such clamping may destroy the double-lumen effect of the tube.

The gastric tubes most often used in the diagnostic imaging department are the Levin tube and the Cantor tube. The Levin tube enters the stomach, and the Cantor enters the small intestine. You must learn to assist with their passage and care.

You may remove Levin tubes if you receive a physician's order to do so. Gently withdraw the tube and wrap it in several thicknesses of paper toweling, place it in an impermeable bag, and dispose of it with the contaminated waste. If you cannot easily removed the tube, call the physician to remove it. The radiographer does not remove NE tubes. Either a registered nurse or the physician removes them, or they are allowed to pass through the intestinal tract and to be removed rectally.

Gastrostomy tubes are surgically inserted directly into the stomach for the purpose of providing a means of nourishing a person unable to take food or fluids by mouth for an indefinite period of time. When caring for a patient with a gastrostomy tube in place, you must take precautions not to dislodge the tube or to introduce infection at the insertion site. You must also understand that a person with a recently inserted gastrostomy tube may be grieving over the alteration in his or her body image and must therefore be treated with sensitivity.

Patients who are unable to receive nutrients through the GI tract may need to be nourished by partial or total parenteral nutrition (TPN). Partial parenteral nutrition is delivered by the peripheral intravenous route. TPN is delivered by the central venous route. This is because the nutrients in the TPN formula may injure the intima of small blood vessels. There are many others reasons for the use of central venous catheters; therefore, you must be able to recognize their presence and take the necessary precautions if they are in place.

You will not perform nasopharyngeal or oropharyngeal suctioning procedures, but you must be able to assess the patient's need for suctioning. You are responsible for having the equipment prepared and for assisting with the procedure. When it is required, it is usually an emergency procedure done to prevent aspiration of secretions into the lungs or respiratory arrest.

The patient with a tracheostomy may require radiographic imaging. You must understand that these patients may be extremely apprehensive. They are unable to speak and unable to clear their tracheostomy tube of secretions that accumulate. A nurse who is able to suction a tracheostomy should accompany the patient who has a new tracheostomy to the diagnostic imaging department. It is your responsibility as the radiographer to stop whatever you are doing for the patient at any time that the patient needs to be suctioned.

Mechanical ventilators are used to support respiratory function when a disease process or an obstruction prevents normal respiration. Mechanical ventilators support life when no other means is available; therefore, you must understand the precautions necessary when caring for a patient who is ventilator dependent. Most patients are on positive-pressure ventilators, which require an artificial airway for their use. This may be either a tracheostomy or an endotracheal tube. You must use caution to prevent dislodging or displacing the artificial airway when caring for the patient. Never disconnect the ventilator from its power source and obtain adequate assistance when radiographing a ventilator patient to prevent other life-threatening problems.

You must be able to care for patients who have chest tubes connected to water-sealed drainage. Remember to keep the tubing coiled at the patient's chest level, to keep all connections tightly sealed, to maintain the water seal at all times, not to lift the water-sealed bottle higher than the patient's chest level, not to clamp or kink the drainage tube, and to notify the patient's nurse immediately if the patient is in respiratory distress or if there is a continuous bubbling in the water-sealed chamber.

There are various tissue drains used for the purpose of removing excessive fluid from an operative site to hasten the healing process and prevent infection. You must be aware of the presence of a tissue drain in any patient for whom you are caring. If a tissue drain is present, do not allow tension to be placed on the drain that might dislodge it. You must also take appropriate infection-control precautions when caring for the patient who has a drain in place.

Chapter 11 Test

_____ 1. When you are caring for a patient who has an NG tube in place in your department, you need to
1. Find out if the tube is to be reconnected to suction; if so, the amount of pressure needed
2. Take care not to dislodge the tube
3. Remove the tube before the patient leaves the department
a. 1 and 2
b. 1, 2, and 3
c. 2 and 3
d. None of the above

_____ **2.** The items that must be on hand for patients who may need suctioning in the diagnostic imaging department are

1. A wall outlet or portable suction machine   a. Items 1, 2, 3, 4, and 8
2. A rectal tube   b. Items 2, 3, 5, 7, and 8
3. Sterile gloves of all sizes   c. Items 2, 4, 5, 6, and 8
4. An oil-based lubricant   d. Items 1, 3, 6, 7, and 8
5. A hemostat
6. Sterile, disposable suction sets (or sterile basins and suction catheters)
7. Sterile normal saline solution
8. An oxygen source

_____ **3.** You should place an alert patient whose swallowing reflex is intact into which position in preparation for nasopharyngeal or oropharyngeal suctioning?
   a. Prone
   b. Sims'
   c. Semi-Fowler's
   d. Lateral

_____ **4.** The following are two points to remember when caring for a patient with a new tracheostomy in place:
   a. He or she may need to be suctioned and will be talkative.
   b. He or she will be anxious and unable to speak.
   c. He or she will be in the stage of denial and will express his anger.
   d. He or she will be unconscious and will be accompanied by a nurse.

5. List the precautions you must take when caring for a patient who has a central venous catheter in place.

6. List the precautions you must take if you are sent to the intensive care unit to radiograph a patient who is receiving positive-pressure ventilation.

_____ **7.** When caring for a patient who has a chest tube with water-sealed drainage, what must you remember?
   a. The water seal must be maintained at all times.
   b. Continuous bubbling into the water-sealed chamber is an indication that all is well.
   c. The tubing may be clamped if necessary.
   d. Most patients with chest tubes complain of respiratory distress.

_____ **8.** Signs and symptoms that indicate a patient's need for oropharyngeal suctioning are

1. Audible rattling and gurgling sounds from the patient's throat   a. 1 and 2
     b. 1, 2, and 3
2. Gagging   c. 2 and 3
3. Breathing with difficulty   d. None of the above

_____ **9.** If you are caring for a patient who has a tissue drain in place, you must
   a. Disregard these drains, because they are not your concern
   b. Prevent tension on the drain and use surgical aseptic technique if in direct contact with the drain
   c. Measure intake and output from the drain
   d. Remove the drain because it will impede the success of the radiograph

10. List three reasons why a patient might have NG or NE intubation, and explain your responsibilities if such a tube is in place in a patient to whom you are assigned.

11. Explain your patient care responsibilities if your patient has a recently placed gastrostomy tube.

_____ **12.** When disconnecting a sump gastric tube (a tube with a double lumen), you must
   a. Clamp the tube with a regular clamp and then place sterile gauze over each end
   b. Clamp the tube closed with a hemostat
   c. Increase the amount of suction pressure
   d. Place a piston syringe in the open end of the gastric tube or place the "pig tail" over it
   e. Decrease the amount of suction pressure

_____ **13.** Examples of NG tubes include
   1. Levin tube   a. 1 and 2
   2. S-B tube   b. 2 and 3
   3. Gastrostomy tube   c. 1 and 3
                             d. 1, 2, and 3

14. Name the three types of tissue drains discussed, and identify which type you are likely to see most often.

_____ **15.** Which statement regarding chest tubes is not true?
   a. The patient may have difficulty breathing.
   b. Gurgling sounds coming from the patient is an indication for the need to suction.
   c. The tube must have one end open to the air for decompression of a pneumothorax.
   d. The water sealed drainage system must not be raised higher than the level of the chest tube insertion site.

16. Name two types of mechanical ventilators, and state which type is most commonly used.

12

Pharmacology for Radiographers

Objectives

After studying this chapter, you will be able to:

1. List the precautions and restrictions all health care professionals must take when administering drugs.
2. Explain the legal accountability of all health care professionals who administer drugs.
3. Discuss drug standards and methods of controlling drugs with a potential for abuse.
4. Explain how drugs are named and the sources of drugs.
5. Define "over-the-counter" drugs and explain alternative medications.
6. Define pharmacokenetics and pharmacodynamics.
7. Differentiate between side effects and adverse drug reactions.
8. Describe the processes involved in drug absorption, distribution, metabolism, and excretion.

9. Define and discuss the routes of drug administration.
10. Explain the manner in which drugs exert their action on the body.
11. Differentiate between drug action and drug effect; between drug agonists and drug antagonists.
12. Identify common drugs in each category that you as the radiographer may work with in diagnostic imaging, and identify the body systems affected by these drugs.
13. Explain the properties of iodinated contrast agents and the adverse reactions that may result from their administration.
14. List the items to be included in the patient assessment before the administration of a contrast agent.

Glossary

Agonists: A drug capable of combining with receptors to initiate drug action; passes affinity and intrinsic activity

Antagonists: Something opposing or resisting the action of another

Antipyretic: An agent that reduces fever

Arrhythmia: An irregularity in or loss of rhythm of the heartbeat

Baroceptor: Any sensor of pressure change

Biotransformation: The conversion of molecules from one form to another within an organism; often associated with change in pharmacologic activity

Enteric coated: A covering added to oral medication that is designed to be absorbed in the intestinal tract

Enterohepatic: Inflammation of both intestines and liver

Sclerosed: To become hardened

Viscosity: Thickness, resistant to flow

Pharmacology is the study of drug actions on and drug interactions with living organisms. Drugs are chemical substances that are not required for normal sustenance and that produce a biological effect in an organism. The word *pharmacology* comes from the Greek word *pharmacon*, meaning drug or poison. All drugs are—or can be, if misused—poisons (Agins, 1995).

The regulations regarding the licensed radiographer's ability to administer drugs and perform venipuncture vary from state to state and in each institution where he or she might work. However, the position of the American Society of Radiologic Technologists is that "venipuncture falls within the profession's Scope of Practice and Practice Standards and that it shall be included in the didactic and clinical curriculum with demonstrated competencies of all appropriate disciplines regardless of the state or institution where such curriculum is taught." The clinical component if drug administration is discussed Chapter 13.

As a professional radiographer who administers drugs (medications), you are expected to know the safe dosage, safe route of administration, limitations of the drug, side effects, potential adverse and toxic reactions, and the indications and contraindications for its use. You must also understand the potential hazards of any drug that is incorrectly or unsafely administered. If drug administration errors occur because of lack of knowledge, the person who administers the drug is legally liable. Radiologic technology students who are permitted to administer drugs either parenterally or orally must adhere to the specific ethical and legal guidelines established for drug administration for patient safety. The student must be supervised by a licensed professional; professional liability coverage must be adequate; and the student must follow appropriately established laboratory objectives. The student must also demonstrate competency before performing drug administration without supervision.

Pharmacology and its clinical application is a scientific discipline unto itself and cannot be covered adequately without combining theoretical knowledge with clinical coursework. Chapters 12 and 13 in this text introduce you to pharmacology and give you the information necessary to practice the skills of medication administration in a formal classroom setting with a licensed instructor.

Drug therapy is a highly complex and ever-changing aspect of patient care. Health care professionals who prescribe medications must spend years becoming proficient in this aspect of patient care. As a radiographer, you are not licensed to dispense drugs. You cannot enter a hospital pharmacy and select a drug. You are legally liable if any drug you take from a dispensary results in adverse effects. If you make a drug error, you must document the incident completely and fill out an institutional incident report according to the policy of the facility in which you are employed.

CALL OUT!

Radiographers are not licensed to dispense drugs.

Drug Standards

Drugs vary in strength and activity. This variation depends on the source of the drug, the technique by which the strength and purity of the drug are measured (called assay) or, in cases in which there is no available method of analyzing their strength, a method called *bioassay* is performed. Bioassay determines the amount of a preparation required to produce a predefined effect in the laboratory on an animal under standardized conditions.

The federal government of the United States has strict standards for control of drug safety, which are strictly enforced. The Food and Drug Administration (FDA) is charge with enforcing the federal Food, Drug and Cosmetic Act, which began the legislation of drug control when it was passed in 1906. The FDA also has an adverse reactions reporting program. Before a new drug may be marketed, it must go through a long series of animal and human testing. The properties that are regulated are as follows:

1. *Purity:* the type and acceptable amount of extraneous material that may safely be added to the active ingredient of a drug

2. *Bioavailability:* the amount of a drug that becomes available for activity in the targeted tissue

3. *Potency:* the strength or power of the drug needed to achieve the desired effect

4. *Efficacy:* the effectiveness of each drug used in treatment

5. *Safety and toxicity:* determined by the number and severity of adverse effects reported after use of the drug; these standards are monitored and refined constantly

Since 1980, the only official books or publications of drug standards in the United States are the *United States Pharmacopeia* (USP) and the *National Formulary* (NF). The drugs listed in these books meet the high standards of quality, purity, and strength. There are several other good references for drugs that you may consult in the clinical area; however, drugs that meet the criteria of the US Pharmacopeia can be identified by the letters USP after the drug's official name.

Great Britain and Canada also have strict drug legislation programs. The United Nations through the World Health Organization provides technical assistance with drug research and use. Drug enforcement agencies throughout the world cooperate to control the use and problems associated with habit-forming drugs internationally.

Drug Control

All drugs that must be administered parenterally; drugs that are hypnotic, narcotic, or habit-forming or contain derivatives of habit-forming substances; drugs that may be toxic if not administered under the supervision of a physician, dentist, or nurse-practitioner; or new drugs limited to investigational use that are not safe if indiscriminately used must bear the legend, "Caution: federal law prohibits dispensing without prescription." Drugs that are considered safe for self-administration are called over-the-counter drugs (OTC drugs). Some drugs that must be prescribed may also be purchased as OTC drugs because they are marketed in a lesser potency when sold in this manner. OTC drugs must also be reviewed by a panel of reviewers appointed by the FDA and deemed safe for self-administration. When you take a patient's drug history as part of an initial interview, note that the patient's use of any OTC drug is important information because these agents may affect treatment.

Alternative Medications

In the recent past, patients' use of unconventional medical practitioners and self-administration of herbal remedies have increased tremendously. However, the scientific efficacy and safety of these therapies is lacking. The terminology of these practices bears explaining. *Alternative medicine* generally refers to practices that have no scientific foundation or research into their effectiveness or safety. *Complementary medicine* indicates that there is some scientific foundation and research into the effectiveness and safety of the practice. Some examples of complementary medicine are diet therapy, exercise programs, counseling, biofeedback, and massage therapy.

Herbal products are marketed as dietary supplements in the United States. As such, they do not demand proven safety or effectiveness. The FDA was unable to adapt standards for these products, so the Dietary Supplement and Health Education Act of 1994 was created to separate supplements from food and drug (Salerno, 1999). This act deemed these products independent of FDA rules. Herbs, vitamins, minerals, and many other dietary supplements are in this

category. You must also incorporate the use of dietary supplements into your patient history, since some of these herbal remedies affect the use of recognized drugs and may be toxic if used in conjunction with other drugs.

Controlled Substances

Drugs that have a potential for abuse are dealt with in a special manner in the United States. In 1971, the Controlled Substances Act was enacted. It was intended to increase research into and prevent drug abuse. The act was also meant to assist persons dependent on these drugs with rehabilitation and to improve regulation of drugs in these categories. In 1973, the Drug Enforcement Administration (DEA) in the Department of Justice became the nation's only legal drug enforcement agency.

Drugs labeled as controlled substances have been categorized by the Controlled Substances Act into schedules according to numbers related to their potential for abuse. The drug schedules are listed in the Table 12-1.

Drug Sources, Names, and Actions

Drugs come from many natural and synthetic sources. They are produced from animal sources, such as hormones and heparin. Many come from plant sources, such as digitalis and atropine. Some are produced from microorganisms, such as some antibiotics. Minerals are the source of calcium, iron, and other dietary supplements. Most drugs are made from synthetic materials in laboratories. In recent years, drugs have begun to be genetically engineered; Epogen (epoetin alfa), a drug used to treat some anemias, is an example of such a drug.

The same drug may be sold under many different proprietary or trade names. The *trade name* is assigned to a drug by a particular manufacturer. This name is copyrighted and cannot be used by another manufacturer. The same drug may be manufactured by another company and be given a different trade name.

The *chemical name* of a drug presents its exact chemical formula and always remains the same. A drug's *generic name* is the name given to the drug before its official approval for use; like the chemical name, it remains unchanged. Generic names of drugs begin with lower-case letters. Trade names begin with capital letters. Drugs are also given *official names*; frequently the official name is used in an official publication such as the *United States Pharmacopeia*. For instance, a drug frequently used as a preprocedure drug in radiologic imaging is parenteral diazepam.

TABLE 12-1
Drug Schedules

SCHEDULE	CHARACTERISTICS	DISPENSING RESTRICTIONS	EXAMPLES
I	High abuse potential; not recognized for medical use; may lead to severe dependence	Approved protocol necessary	Heroin, opioids, hashish, PCP (Phencyclidine; angel dust), marijuana derivatives, LSD (lysergic acid diethylamide), others
II	High abuse potential; accepted for medical use; may lead to severe dependence	Written prescription by a licensed person; verbal orders must be signed within 72 hours; no prescription refills; container must have warning label	Opioids, codeine, fentanyl, morphine, barbiturates, amphetamine, cocaine, others
III	Less abuse potential; accepted medical use; may lead to dependence	Written or oral prescription required that expires in 6 months; container must have warning label	Codeine of less than 1.8 grains per dL; opioid combined with one or more noncontrolled active ingredients; steroids, benzphetamine
IV	Less abuse potential than schedule III; may lead to limited dependence	Written or oral prescription required that expires in 6 months; no more than 5 refills	Benzodiazepines, chloral hydrate, meprobamate, phentermine, and so on
V	Less abuse potential than Schedule IV; may lead to limited dependence	May or may not require a prescription, depending on state law	Antitussives, antidiarrheals, codeine expectorants

Diazepam is the generic name for Valium, and the chemical formula is 7-chloro-1,3-dihydro-1-methyl-5-phenyl-2H-1,4-benzodiazepin-2-one. You must be able to identify drugs by their trade name and their generic name. It is not essential to learn the chemical formula of each drug.

A drug does not have the capacity to change cellular structure, but acts to either increase or decrease the rate and range of a normal or abnormal physiologic process going on within the cells of the body. Drugs are administered for a number of reasons—to relieve undesired symptoms, to prevent disease, to cure disease, or to diagnose disease. You will be involved in administering drugs primarily for diagnosis of disease or pathological conditions. Occasionally, you may administer a drug to relieve anxiety or pain before or during a diagnostic procedure.

Drugs are absorbed, distributed, metabolized, and then excreted from the body. As this process takes place, the drug reaches a point at which it has its intended effect. This is called the *onset* of action. As it continues to be absorbed, it reaches a peak concentration level. This is the time during which the drug attains its maximum therapeutic response. The time during which the drug is in the body in an amount large enough to be therapeutic is called its *duration of action*. As the drug is excreted, the concentration level subsides to a point at which there is little or no intended effect.

It is not possible to keep up with all new drugs marketed and used; however, any health care practitioner who administers drugs must be able to obtain information from reliable sources before administering a drug with which he or she is not familiar. Some of these reliable references are as follows: *The American Hospital Formulary Service Drug Information; Drug Facts and Comparisons; Handbook of Nonprescription Drugs; Physicians' Desk Reference; United States Pharmacopeia.* All these references are updated yearly. You must know where a reliable drug reference is available in your workplace to consult as necessary. A current pharmacology textbook should be a part of the library of any person who administers drugs.

Pharmacokinetics

As a radiographer, you must understand how drugs interact with body tissues. The processes that control absorption, distribution, metabolism, and excretion of drugs by the body are called *pharmacokinetics*. Individuals process drugs differently depending on their age, nutritional status, ethnicity, existing pathological condition, immune status, state of mind or psychological factors, sex, weight, environmental factors, and the time of day.

Drug Absorption

A drug must advance from its dosage form into a form that makes it biologically available for passage into the systemic circulation. Tablets or dry powders must be reduced to liquid form before they can be absorbed and begin their journey. Drugs taken by mouth in liquid form are processed more quickly than tablets and capsules. In other words, a drug must be absorbed and taken through the bloodstream to its intended site in order to act. The amount of drug that actually reaches the systemic circulation becomes *bioavailable* or reaches a state of bioavailability.

The amount of time needed to absorb a drug and the extent to which it becomes bioavailable depend on the route of administration, gastrointestinal (GI) motility, dosage form, interaction with food, and interaction with other drugs. Food in the stomach generally delays gastric emptying time and the time it takes a drug to become bioavailable. Combining a drug with another drug may reduce or increase the amount available for absorption.

Drug absorption varies from person to person and depends on the absorptive surface available. A damaged or absent intended drug surface alters the length of time it takes a drug to reach its intended site. Drugs may be absorbed by either passive or active transport or by *pinocytosis*, a form of active transport.

A drug must be made up of the same components as those at its intended absorption site. A fat-soluble (lipid-soluble) drug is unable to penetrate a water-soluble site and a water-soluble drug cannot penetrate a lipid site. Lipoid (lipid) tissues are highly impenetrable. The central nervous system, which includes the brain and the spinal cord, is composed of these highly impenetrable lipoid tissues. The capillaries of the brain have tight junctions, and the intercellular spaces are without the pores present in other cells of the body. This construction, the *blood-brain barrier*, makes the brain less easily penetrable by chemicals that might damage it. Only lipid-soluble drugs may pass this barrier. The placenta is also composed of lipoid tissue; however, it is believed that the fetus is exposed to and can be damaged by all drugs and toxins ingested by the mother.

Drugs move to their site of absorption and then must penetrate the cell membrane at that site. This is accomplished by varying methods. One method is passive diffusion, which requires no cellular energy. The drug simply moves across a cell membrane from an area of lower concentration to one of higher concentration. When the concentration equalizes on both sides of the cell membrane, the transport is complete. Lipid solubility is the most important determinant in deciding whether a drug will cross cell membranes, although water solubility is also of importance. Most drugs cross cell membranes by passive diffusion.

Active transport is another method of drug absorption. This method requires energy from the cell and a carrier that forms complexes with drug molecules on the membrane surface to carry them through the membrane and then leave them by disassociation. Active transport is necessary to move some drugs and electrolytes such as sodium and potassium from outside to inside a cell.

Pinocytosis is a type of active transport in which a cell engulfs a drug particle, forms a protective coat around it, and transports it across the cell membrane. Fat-soluble vitamins are transported in this manner.

Drugs taken orally are usually absorbed in the small intestine, which has a large surface for absorption. If a portion of the small intestine has been removed or is scarred, the ability to absorb a drug is reduced.

The quantity of blood flow to absorption surfaces affects the rate at which a drug is absorbed. For instance, a drug is absorbed much more rapidly when it is administered intramuscularly in the deltoid muscle than in the gluteal muscle because the blood flow is greater in the deltoid.

A person who is in severe pain or in a state of acute stress may have decreased ability to absorb a drug. The cause is not certain; however, it is theorized that it is because there is a change in blood flow, decreased GI motility, and gastric retention due to autonomic nervous system activity resulting in pyloric sphincter contraction.

First-Pass Effect

It is important for you to recognize what is called the *first-pass effect* of drugs taken by mouth (orally). When a drug is taken by mouth and swallowed into the stomach, it goes from the small intestine to the mesenteric vascular system, and then to the portal vein, and from there into the liver before it is transported into the systemic circulation. Because of this travel throughout the gastric and hepatic circulation, a portion of the drug is metabolized en route and becomes inactive.

The partial metabolism of a drug before it reaches the systemic circulation is called *a first-pass effect*. The effect requires, in the case of many drugs taken orally, that they be given in larger doses so that a portion of the drug will remain to perform its intended effect. Drugs that can be administered by a sublingual, vaginal, or parenteral route avoid the first-pass effect by going directly into the systemic circulation; however, these methods of administration may be contraindicated for other reasons.

> ### /// WARNING \\\
> The dosages of most drugs given by the oral route are generally much larger than those given by parenteral routes because they are susceptible to the first-pass effect!

Some drugs, after they are absorbed, are moved from the bloodstream into the liver and then through the biliary tract, where they are excreted in bile to return to the small intestine and then back into the bloodstream. This action, called *enterohepatic recycling*, allows the drug to persist in the body for long periods of time.

Drug Distribution

After absorption of a drug into the body, it must be distributed to its intended site of action by way of the circulatory system. The rate and extent of distribution depend on adequate blood circulation, protein binding, and the drug's affinity for lipoid or aqueous tissues. Drugs move quickly to body organs that have a rich blood supply such as the heart, liver, and kidneys. They reach muscles and fatty tissues more slowly.

As a drug travels through the circulatory system, it may come into contact with plasma proteins and bind to them or remain free. A drug that is bound to a plasma protein becomes inactive. Only the free drug is able to act on the cells; however, as the free drug acts, there is a decrease in plasma drug levels, which allows a portion of the bound drug to be released and become active. This slow release allows blood levels of the drug to remain somewhat constant. This differs for each drug and for each patient, depending on health status and other characteristics. Drugs do not always distribute well throughout the body. Pathological conditions such as abscesses and other infective material impair or impede drug distribution.

When two or more drugs are present and competing for a limited number of plasma-binding sites, the drug with the strongest affinity for the site acquires it. This leaves a greater amount of one drug free to act.

This may result in a toxic level of that drug or result in a drug-drug interaction.

Lipid-soluble drugs are stored in lipoid tissues. Fat is not soluble; therefore, lipid-soluble drugs are not present in the blood as such. Highly lipid-soluble drugs remain stored in fatty tissues, where they are released very slowly, with sometimes less than the intended therapeutic effect. Drugs that are intended to penetrate the blood-brain barrier must be highly lipid soluble and bind minimally with plasma proteins to achieve their intended effect.

Because of the nonselective nature of the placenta, most drugs are able to pass that barrier and affect the developing fetus. The toxicity of drugs to the fetus during the first trimester of pregnancy makes it mandatory that the pregnant mother receive no medications without the explicit orders of her physician. Only drugs that are absolutely necessary to maintain the optimum health of the mother should be given. This is important for you to remember as you care for female patients of childbearing age.

> ### /// WARNING \\\
> All female patients of childbearing age must be screened before receiving any drug to ascertain whether they are pregnant.

Biotransformation

The process by which the body alters the chemical structure of a drug or other foreign substance is called *biotransformation* or *metabolism* (interchangeable terms). Generally, this process reduces lipid solubility to render the drug ready for excretion. Most drug metabolites are less biologically active than the initial drug; however, in some instances the metabolite may be more active, more toxic, or similar to the initial drug in its activity. Some drugs remain inactive until they are biotransformed into an active metabolite.

Most drugs are metabolized in the liver by the hepatic microsomal enzyme system. A key element in the enzyme system is the cytochrome P450 system. These enzymes act on a wide variety of compounds. In certain drugs, tissues from plasma, kidneys, lungs, and the intestinal mucosa may be involved. Biotransformation occurs through four major pathways. They are oxidation; reduction or the addition of hydrogen; hydrolysis in the case of esters and amides; and conjugation, which involves the addition of other groups. These reactions may occur at the same time or in a sequence.

Age, overall health, time of day, emotional status, the presence of other drugs in the body, genetic variations, and disease states may alter the rate of drug metabolism. For instance, an infant has a reduced rate of metabolism because of the immaturity of the hepatic enzyme system. A person with liver or heart disease also has a reduced rate of metabolism. The elderly person has a decreased blood supply and a decreased number of liver enzymes, which decreases the ability to metabolize drugs. An altered metabolic state may allow a drug to accumulate in the body and produce an adverse reaction. Conversely, rapid metabolism of a drug may interfere with the intended effect. Drugs administered orally are significantly metabolized by the first-pass effect through the liver, which also affects their metabolism.

Drug Excretion

Excretion of drugs from the body takes place chiefly in the kidneys. The kidneys can excrete only water-soluble substances; therefore, an important aspect of drug metabolism is the transformation of lipid-soluble substances into water-soluble metabolites. Some drugs are excreted virtually unchanged through the kidneys, whereas others are extensively metabolized with only a small amount of the original drug remaining. Urine pH affects the excretion of drugs. Weak acids are excreted more quickly in alkaline urine and more slowly in acidic urine. Weak bases are affected in the opposite manner.

Other sites of drug excretion are through the biliary tract and into the feces or through the enterohepatic cycle and later into the kidneys. Gases and volatile liquids used for anesthesia are excreted by the pulmonary route. Sweat and saliva are of minimal importance in drug excretion.

Some drugs or drug metabolites may cross the epithelium of the mammary glands and be excreted in breast milk. This is important if the mother is breast-feeding an infant, and a drug, particularly a narcotic drug, is transferred in high concentrations to the infant.

CALL OUT!

You must take a detailed drug history from female patients of childbearing age. A nursing mother must only have drugs as ordered by her physician. Inform the physician if the patient is a nursing mother!

Half-life

The time it takes for a 50% decrease in a drug's presence in the body is called its half-life. This is determined by the time it takes a drug to transform into water-soluble

metabolites and to be eliminated from the body. For a drug to have its intended effect, it must reach a steady-state concentration in the body. Four or five drug half-lives are required for this to occur. Drugs have variable half-lives. For a steady-state concentration to be maintained, the same amount of a drug must be taken in as is eliminated in each 24-hour period. A prescribing physician treating a particular illness must determine the amount of drug needed to maintain a steady state in the body to obtain the drug's intended effect. A larger dose may be given initially to obtain a therapeutic effect more quickly than it would otherwise take to reach a steady state. When the intended therapeutic level is reached, the dosage is reduced to maintain a steady state.

A drug's removal from the body is called its *clearance rate*. If a drug has a rapid clearance rate, it must be administered more frequently to maintain the therapeutic level. If the drug is slow to clear, it will need to be administered less frequently. This is an important consideration, because a drug with a slow clearance rate that is given too often may accumulate and reach a toxic level.

Pharmacodynamics

Pharmacodynamics is the study of the method or mechanism of drug action on living tissues or the response of tissues to chemical agents at various sites in the body. Drugs may alter the physiologic effects of blood pressure, heart rate, urinary output, and response to the central nervous system as well as cause changes in all other body systems. However, drugs do not produce new functions on tissues or organs of the body. Usually, a primary site of drug action is targeted by a drug administered systemically; nevertheless, all body tissues are affected in some way by every drug. The intent of drug therapy is to produce a therapeutic effect that may be to control pain, cure a particular disease, alleviate symptoms of a disease, or diagnose a disease. The particular area for which a drug is intended and that receives the maximum effect of a drug is called the *drug receptor*. A drug receptor is a macromolecular component of body tissue.

Drug receptors have an *affinity* for a particular drug. This means that there is an attraction between the drug and the receptor. Affinity is the determining factor in the concentration of the drug necessary to initiate the intended physiologic effect. If there is a strong affinity at the receptor site, the concentration of drug necessary to accomplish an effect is low. This may also be referred to as the *efficacy* of the drug. A drug that attaches to a receptor and possesses both an affinity for the site and the ability to produce *intrinsic activity* at that site is said to be an *agonist*. Intrinsic activity is the ability of a drug to initiate a chain of events. If a drug attaches to a receptor site and prevents the agonist from responding in its intended manner, it is said to be an *antagonist.*

There are also believed to be partial agonists, competitive antagonists and noncompetitive antagonists. The *partial agonist* is an agonist with affinity and some efficacy at a receptor site, which can antagonize a drug action that has more efficacy. A *competitive antagonist* has an affinity for the same receptor as another drug and may inhibit the action of the agonist. A *noncompetitive antagonist* combines with receptors in the same tissues and inactivates the response of the agonist no matter how high its concentration.

The molecular structure of each drug determines the affinity for a receptor. Very small changes in a drug molecule can leave the drug's affinity to a receptor unchanged but drastically change the pharmacological action of the drug.

Many drugs exert more than one effect on the body. For instance, a drug given at the recommended dosage will have the intended effect; however, if given in a larger dose, it may have an undesirable effect. The relation between the dosage at which the intended effect of a drug is obtained and the amount that produces an unwanted effect is called the *therapeutic index.* The greater the therapeutic index, the safer the drug is, since more can be tolerated without adverse effects.

Nonspecific Drug Interaction

There are drugs that seem to have no specificity and act more generally on cell membranes and cell processes. They seem to accumulate on cell membranes and interfere physically or chemically with cell function or metabolism. Some of these are systemic drugs such as general anesthetics. Others are topical agents such as ointments and emollients. More destructive nonspecific drugs are phenol derivatives that destroy the functional integrity of living cells.

Adverse Drug Reactions

Any person who participates in drug administration must be aware of the potential harm that may result from drugs. They can produce many adverse or unintended effects. Some adverse effects occur almost immediately after drug administration, and some take weeks or months of administration before an untoward reaction is produced. When an unintended effect is expected to occur and is essentially not harmful, it may be termed a *side effect.* An effect that is harmful is called an *adverse reaction.*

A *toxic reaction* is an unwanted effect that is an extension of the therapeutic effect, such as an overdose of a drug that, when given in the prescribed amount, is therapeutic. A toxic reaction does not include an allergic reaction or anaphylactic shock, which is classified as an adverse reaction.

Immediate adverse reactions to drugs can include drowsiness, gastric distress, and allergic or hypertensive reactions that may range from mild urticaria to severe anaphylactic shock. Some drugs are disease-producing themselves and may produce blood dyscrasias, hepatic disease, GI ulcerations, bleeding, or thrombosis. Since drugs are tested extensively before they are permitted to be marketed, most adverse reactions have been documented, and it is known that these reactions may occur. The therapeutic or diagnostic purpose of a drug is weighed against the risk factors before administration. If the need outweighs the risk, it is prescribed by the physician with caution.

The patient is educated regarding the potential adverse effects of the drug before its administration and instructed to notify the physician if adverse reactions occur. Particular care must be given to pregnant women and nursing mothers. All health care workers who administer drugs have the responsibility to understand and educate their patients about any drugs that they administer.

CALL OUT!

It is the responsibility of all health care workers who administer drugs to understand and educate their patients about any drug that they administer.

An unexpected or exacerbated effect from a drug the first time a patient receives it is called a *metareaction.* This type of reaction is often genetic or familial in nature. If the metareaction manifests as an allergic reaction, it may be called an *idiosyncratic reaction.*

Drugs that have a mind-altering effect may produce a *dependency reaction.* This dependence may be physiological or psychological in nature. A drug that creates a physiological dependence has an unpleasant effect called a *withdrawal effect* if it is not received or if it is discontinued. A drug to which psychological dependence is developed may lead to drug abuse patterns.

Tolerance to a drug that is received continually for a length of time creates a change in the response to that drug. Usually, the drug is needed in increasingly larger doses to attain the desired effect. The drugs to which one develops a dependent or tolerant reaction are the narcotic, analgesic, sedative-hypnotic and anti-anxiety drugs, and the amphetamines. *Tachyphylaxis* is a rapid

TABLE 12-2

Special Considerations for Receiving Drugs

AGE GROUP	PHYSIOLOGIC CHANGES	PRECAUTIONS
Pregnant women	Many drugs cross the placental barrier. Drug effects depend on fetal age and can result in harm to the fetus.	Drug use during pregnancy must be avoided or administered only to women who absolutely require treatment. If in doubt, inform patient's physician of possible pregnancy before administering the drug.
Infants	Infants lack the protective mechanisms of older children and adults. Skin is thin and permeable; stomachs lack acid; lungs lack mucous barrier; temperature control is poor; they become dehydrated easily and have immature dehydrated easily and have immature liver and kidneys that cannot manage foreign chemicals.	Only persons educated in drug administration to infants must administer medications to them.
Breastfed infants	May have all drugs in maternal circulation transferred to colostrum and breast milk.	Mothers who are breastfeeding must cease to breastfeed for a prescribed time if they are to receive radioisotopes or radiation. All other drug therapies must be considered, since they may harm the infant. Take a detailed history and report breastfeeding to physician. Do not administer any drug without establishing that it will not harm the infant.
Pediatric patients	At 1 year of age, liver metabolizes more rapidly than that of adults; renal function may be more rapid than adults after 1 year of age. Standard dosage for children is nonexistent and depends on child's weight or body surface area. Their skin surface is large and more permeable. Topical drugs are more absorbable through skin.	Children are not small adults! Physiologic differences vary and only those experienced in medicating children must administer drugs to them! Topical drugs and solutions, including antiseptics, can cause poisoning in children. Cleanse only with mild soap and water.
Elderly patients	Blood-brain barrier is more easily penetrated, with increasing rate of dizziness and confusion. Reduced baroreceptor response increases hypotensive effects of some drugs. Liver size, blood flow, and enzyme production decrease, increasing the half-life of some drugs and leading to possible toxic reaction. Increased adipose tissue in abdominal area may lead to toxicity from fat-soluble drugs. Decreased renal blood flow and filtration decrease elimination of drugs from body. Slower gastric emptying time and increase in pH of gastric juices increase risk of gastric irritation.	Drugs affecting the CNS and cardiovascular system must be given with extreme caution. Patients must be monitored closely and assisted with ambulation to prevent falls. Do not allow elderly patients who have been given drugs to leave department unattended.

development of tolerance to a drug. *Cross-tolerance* is tolerance to a particular drug that results from administration of a different drug with the same action.

A drug that adversely affects the fetus, causing abnormal development, is said to have a *teratogenic effect*. Some drugs may be cancer producing. These are called *carcinogens*. Drugs that adversely affect the kidneys are called *nephrotoxic*.

> ### WARNING
> Drugs must be stored according to manufacturer's directions. If a drug has a sediment or is discolored, it must not be used.

Drug Incompatibility

Drugs must never be mixed in the same syringe without being certain of their compatibility. Many drugs, when combined with another drug, can either become inactivated or form a toxic compound. Some drugs must always be given individually.

> ### WARNING
> Before mixing two drugs for administration, a drug compatibility chart or a pharmacist must be consulted if any uncertainty exists about the drugs' compatibility. Never assume that related drugs can be combined, because this may not be the case.

Medical personnel who use drugs and equipment from an emergency cart in departments where medical care is rendered must have special education in emergency drug use. These drugs, if used incorrectly, can have lethal effects. Although emergency drugs are listed in this text, the explanations given here are not adequate to qualify you as a radiographer to administer them. Health care institutions must have on their staff persons specifically trained in emergency drug procedures and equipment use.

You have an obligation to know the location of the emergency cart, how to gain access to it when it is needed, and how to summon the emergency team in a timely manner. In a department with limited staff, you may be responsible for maintaining the completeness and currency of the drugs and equipment on the emergency cart. If this is the case, you must be educated to do this, and the maintenance must be done on a daily basis and after each use.

> ### WARNING
> During an emergency is not the time to update emergency drugs and equipment, since every minute lost in this pursuit is life threatening for the patient!

Age-Related Changes in Drug Administration

Pregnant women, nursing mothers and infants, and pediatric and elderly patients must have special consideration when they are receiving drugs. Each group has special needs if they are to receive any type of drug therapy. It is not possible in this text to list all of the drugs that may result in adverse effects; however, you must be aware of the special problems each group represents. These are listed in Table 12-2.

Routes of Drug Administration

Enteral Routes

The enteral routes are broken down into oral, sublingual, buccal, and rectal subroutes. Drugs taken by mouth can be immediately absorbed by the oral mucosa if they are placed under the tongue (the sublingual route) or on the buccal area at the inside of the cheek (the buccal route). Medications given at these sites are absorbed into the bloodstream immediately and are exempt from the first-pass effect of drugs that go into the stomach. Only very small amounts of non-irritating drugs that demand rapid action can be administered in this manner, because the area for absorption is small.

Drugs taken by mouth and swallowed into the stomach are said to be given orally or by the oral route (PO). This is often the most efficient and the most cost-effective method of drug administration. The oral route is used if the drug will not be destroyed by secretions in the gastrointestinal tract and when slower absorption and longer duration of drug activity are desired.

The drug taken by mouth disintegrates and dissolves in the stomach, then travels to the small intestine, where most absorption takes place. The large intestine plays a small role in absorption by absorbing water and electrolytes. If a person cannot swallow oral drugs, he or she may take them enterally by having them administered through a nasogastric or gastrostomy tube.

> ## CALL OUT!
>
> Do not break or crush enteric-coated tablets because they may act as gastric irritants or become less effective!

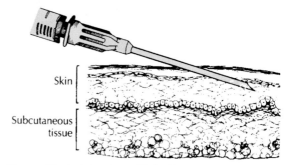

Figure 12–1. Intradermal injection.

There are several valid reasons for not giving drugs orally. The drug may have an unpleasant taste, it may cause nausea and vomiting, it may be destroyed by digestive juices, there may be a danger of aspiration, the patient may be uncooperative, or a more rapid absorption may be desired. Drugs that are irritating to the gastric mucosa are sometimes given in an enteric-coated form so that they can be taken orally.

If a drug is to be administered in an enteric-coated form, the patient must be instructed not to chew the tablet before swallowing it, since it can irritate the stomach or be rendered less effective. If the medication is in tablet form and is not scored, it should not be broken. You must request the correct dose from the pharmacy. Capsules should not be tampered with, because this may result in incorrect dosage.

Drugs may be administered by rectum if a patient is nauseated and unable to retain oral drugs. This method of administration has the advantage of avoiding the first-pass effect; however, it has disadvantages. Correct dosage is difficult to determine because absorption may be erratic. Lack of fluid in the rectum also makes absorbability questionable.

Parenteral Routes

Parenteral routes of drug administration include subcutaneous (SC) (into the subcutaneous tissues), intramuscular (IM) (into the muscle), intravenous (IV) (into the vein), intrathecal (into the spinal subarachnoid space), epidural (into the spinal canal on or outside the dura mater surrounding the spinal column), intra-articular (within the joint), intra-arterial (into an artery), pulmonary (into the lungs), and intradermal (beneath the skin surface). Physicians and specifically educated personnel administer medications by way of the intrathecal, epidural, and intra-articular routes.

Administration of drugs by any of the parenteral routes requires surgical aseptic technique, since each is an invasive procedure. Techniques of administration are discussed in Chapter 13.

Intradermal administration of a drug is usually used for testing sensitivity to a drug or an antigen or for local anesthesia. It is administered between the layers of the skin just below the surface (Fig. 12–1). Very small doses of a drug are used at this site. If the drug is given to test for a sensitivity reaction, the patient must be monitored carefully for signs of an anaphylactic reaction.

Subcutaneous drugs are administered below the epidermis (Fig. 12–2). Absorption is through the capillaries at a fairly rapid rate. The dosage administered at subcutaneous sites should be not more than 1 to 2 mL.

Intramuscular absorption of drugs is variable, depending on how the drug is formulated and also on the muscle into which the drug is injected (Fig. 12–3). The deltoid, gluteal, and vastus lateralis muscles are most frequently used for intramuscular injections. Blood flow is more rapid through the deltoid than the gluteal muscles; however, the amount of drug that may be safely administered into the gluteal muscles is larger. The composition of the drug also affects the rate of absorption from the intramuscular site. A solution absorbs most rapidly; suspensions and oil-based emulsions absorb more slowly.

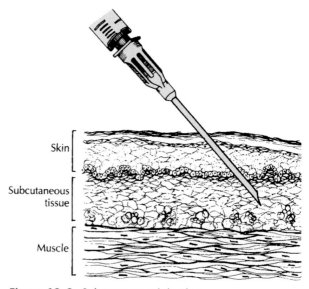

Figure 12–2. Subcutaneous injection.

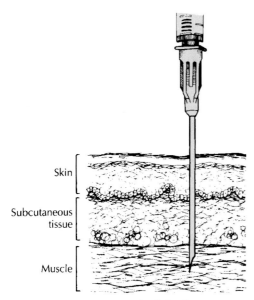

Figure 12–3. Intramuscular injection.

**/ / / WARNING \ \ **

Oil-based drugs and micro-fine crystalline solutions must never be injected intravenously or intra-arterially because they may cause emboli. Cloudy or thick solutions are not for intravenous or intra-arterial administration!

Since there are no barriers to absorption, the intravenous route achieves the most rapid systemic response. This method is selected if rapid effect is desired or if a drug cannot be injected into body tissues without damaging them. This can be one of the most hazardous routes of drug administration because once a drug is injected directly into the circulatory system, the reaction is immediate. Intravenous administration of drugs is discussed in Chapter 13.

Intrathecal, epidural, intra-articular, and intra-arterial sites for drug administration are used to achieve a high local concentration of a drug for pain relief, analgesia, or treatment of neoplasms or to inject contrast media for diagnosis, or, in some instances, to administer anti-infective drugs. Drugs administered by intrathecal route bypass the blood-brain barrier. You will not administer drugs by these methods, but you may assist when they are used to administer contract agents.

The pulmonary route is used to administer drugs in the form of fine mists called *aerosols* or gases. These drugs are used to assist with normal oxygen-carbon dioxide exchange in the lungs. The lungs have a large surface area for drug absorption and a rich capillary network to absorb drugs. This route is used to treat patients in respiratory distress. You will not usually administer drugs by this route; however, many patients with chronic pulmonary disease may bring their own aerosol medications with them to the diagnostic imaging department and use them as necessary. Respiratory therapists are often seen at a patient's bedside administering these drugs as treatment for respiratory diseased and infections.

Topical Routes

Topical drug administration is used for local treatment of skin ailments, as well as systemic treatment. The skin, when unbroken, is slow to absorb drugs into the systemic circulation. The rate of topical absorption is accelerated if there is an open lesion or if the drug is applied to mucous membranes or to the area behind the ear (the postauricular area).

Drugs are considered to be administered by topical route if they are administered to the eyes, nose, throat, respiratory mucosa, or vagina and, in some cases, to the rectum. Drugs administered to the eyes or by inhalation to the respiratory mucosa are also absorbed systemically to some degree.

Some drugs are applied to the skin for intended systemic effect. When this is the case, the route is called *transdermal*. It is believed that drugs administered transdermally are absorbed slowly, and a constant blood level of the drug is achieved. You may care for patients with transdermal patches applied at various areas of the body, generally the upper thoracic area.

Drug Classification

Drugs may be classified in several ways. They can be grouped according to their physiologic effects on receptors, their physiologic effects on specific body systems, or their overall physiologic effects. This chapter provides a brief overview of the physiologic effects of drugs on body systems and drugs used to treat specific conditions. Contrast agents are discussed, as are some drugs used in radiographic imaging, particularly those found on the emergency drug cart. *The drug descriptions that follow do not adequately explain the nature of these drugs to anyone who plans to participate in drug administration.*

Drugs used in radiographic imaging and elsewhere in the practice of medicine are constantly changing. New and better preparations are appearing on the market monthly, and the personnel administering them must be educated in their use before working with them. This is true of contrast agents as well as other drugs.

Drugs chosen in each classification for this text are chosen at random or as prototypical in each category and do not in any way mean to influence drugs selected for use or preference for any drug.

CALL OUT!

The drug descriptions herein do not adequately explain the nature of these drugs to anyone who plans to participate in drug administration. More knowledge is mandatory!

Drugs That Act on the Nervous System

The nervous system is the most complex of the body systems. It takes in and processes all information and communication from the outside environment. It stores information and coordinates all body functions and behaviors. It is beyond the scope of this text to describe the nervous system in any detail, but we will give a very simple and cursory description of the workings of that system necessary to understand the work of various drugs that affect it.

The nervous system is divided into the central and peripheral system. The neuron is the basic functional

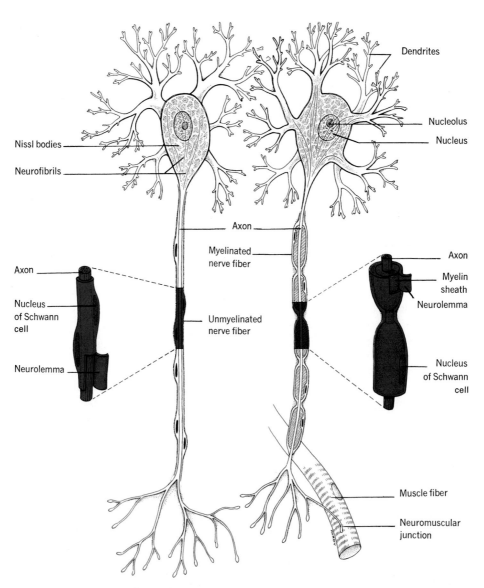

Figure 12–4. Structure of typical unmyelinated and myelinated neurons. (Rosdahl CB: *Textbook of Basic Nursing,* 7th ed. Philadelphia: JB Lippincott, 1999.)

unit of the nervous system. Neurons affect memory, influence thinking processes, and regulate the function of organs and glandular activity in the body. Neurons do not undergo cellular reproduction and cannot be replaced if destroyed. The anatomical structure of the neuron is briefly described in the following text:

- *Neuron*: has only one cell body that contains a nucleus; sensory neurons receive messages (afferent); motor neurons transmit messages (efferent); interneurons connect.

- *An axon*: an extension that carries impulses away from the neuron's cell body.

- *Myelin sheath*: a fatty covering surrounding an axon that electrically insulates one nerve cell from another (Fig. 12–4).

- *Dendrites*: short, branched extensions of the cell body that receive impulses from the axons of neurons and transmit impulses toward the cell body.

- *Synapse*: the junction between the axon of one neuron and the dendrites of another.

- *Neurotransmitter*: a chemical that an axon releases that allows a nerve impulse to cross the synapse and reach a dendrite; synaptic transmission is in one direction, from the presynaptic to the postsynaptic neuron. The cell that receives the impulse rapidly inactivates the neurotransmitter with an opposing chemical to prevent repeated or continuous impulses.

The central nervous system (CNS) is more complex than the peripheral nervous system, and there are major differences between the neurons in the peripheral nervous system and those in the CNS. The CNS contains a network of inhibitory neurons that work to modulate the rate of neuron transmission. The CNS also uses from 10 to 50 different neurotransmitters, whereas the peripheral nervous system uses primarily two: acetylcholine and norepinephrine.

Drugs That Act on the Central Nervous System

The CNS consists of the brain and the spinal cord. The basic functional unit of the CNS is the neuron (nerve cell), which responds to stimulation by conveying electrical impulses. Neurons are arranged in chains separated by spaces called synapses (Fig. 12-5). As an electrical impulse reaches the end of a neuron, a synaptic vesicle releases a chemical called a *neurotransmitter*. Molecules of a neurotransmitter are able to cross the synapse to receptors on the postsynaptic fiber and activate a new wave of electric current. In this way the impulse travels to its intended destination in the brain.

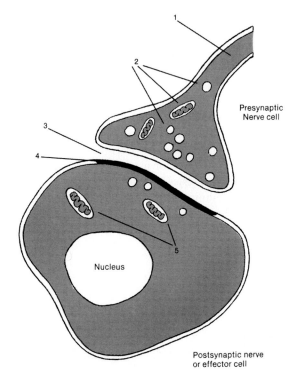

Figure 12–5. Steps in the synaptic transmission process. (*1*) Transport of substrate down the presynaptic axon. (*2*) Organelles and enzymes in the nerve terminal that synthesize, store, release, and actively reuptake the transmitter chemical. (*3*) Synaptic contact zone, where extracellular enzymes catabolize the transmitter chemical. (*4*) Postsynaptic receptor that triggers postsynaptic response to the transmitter chemical. (*5*) Organelles within the postsynaptic cells that respond to receptor trigger. (Spencer et al: *Clinical Pharmacology in Nursing Management,* 4th ed. Philadelphia: JB Lippincott, 1993.)

The spinal cord functions as a pathway for carrying impulses to and from the brain. It is also the center for reflex actions of the body. Neurotransmitters are composed of acetylcholine, dopamine, norepinephrine, histamine, serotonin, endorphins, and enkephalins. They have inhibitory or excitatory potential. The inhibitory neurotransmitters increase negative responses; excitatory neurotransmitters decrease negative responses between the synaptic clefts.

Drugs that act on the CNS are broadly categorized as depressants and stimulants. CNS depression may range from mild to severe. The most severe CNS depression results in respiratory failure, coma, and death. Some CNS depressants are able to produce a selective depression if used in the prescribed range. There are CNS antagonists that are used to counteract severe depression resulting from drug overdose. There are also CNS stimulants that produce hyperactivity and insomnia. The effects of CNS stimulants that are used less frequently for treatment are difficult to control.

Opioid Analgesics and Antagonists

Opioid analgesics are used to control intense pain and the anxiety that results. These are natural and synthetic agents that have an effect like morphine. Unfortunately, these drugs are often abused because of the feelings of well-being and euphoria that often accompany their administration. Because of this, they are controlled substances that must be kept in locked cabinets and signed out for use by authorized persons only. If opioid analgesics are administered to children, they must be administered by a person educated in pediatric medicine or nursing. Several drugs in this category and the methods of administration follow.

STRONG AGONISTS

Morphine sulfate: PO

Morphine tartrate: injection, IM, SC, epidural, intrathecal, rectal

Methadone hydrochloride (Dolophine, Methadose): PO, IM, SC

Fentanyl: IV, IM, transdermal, transmucosal.

Meperidine hydrochloride (Demerol): IM, IV, SC; slow IV in individualized dilution dosage

MODERATE AGONISTS

Oxycodone with acetaminophen (Percocet): PO

Propoxyphene hydrochloride (Darvon, Dolene): PO

Codeine sulfate: PO, IM

Adverse Reactions: All opiates may result in tolerance and dependence. They may cause nausea, restlessness, hyperactivity, respiratory depression, hypotension, constipation, urticaria, hypersensitivity, depressed renal function, shock, and death.

ANTAGONISTS

Drugs in this category have a high affinity for opioid receptor sites but reverse the effects of opioids and synthetic opioids in persons addicted to them. They have little effect on normal persons and are used to counteract severe depressive symptoms resulting from an intake of excessive amounts of opioid drugs. The following are examples of those widely used for this purpose.

Naloxone hydrochloride (Narcan): IM, IV, SC; *found on emergency drug carts*

Naltrexone (Nalorex), (Trexan): PO

Adverse Reactions: Few adverse effects reported from naloxone; if given before detoxification, acute withdrawal symptoms may occur from naltrexone.

Anxiolytic (Anti-anxiety) and Hypnotic Drugs

The benzodiazepines are the most commonly used drugs for the treatment of debilitating anxiety and have greatly decreased the use of barbiturates as hypnotics because they do not interfere with the REM (rapid eye movement) sleep cycle. They are also used in some instances to treat psychosis and other behavior disorders. The benzodiazepine receptors are found only in the CNS. Their action is to reduce anxiety. At higher doses, they produce hypnosis, relax muscles, and several reduce seizure activity. They are controlled substances, since they may cause physical and psychological dependence. They are also used for preoperative and pre-procedure sedation. The benzodiazepines used as anti-anxiety drugs are as follows.

Alprazolam (Xanax): PO

Lorazepam (Ativan): PO, IM, IV

Chlordiazepoxide (Librium): PO, IM, IV

Diazepam (Valium): PO, IM, IV; *found on emergency drug carts*

Adverse Reactions: All benzodiazepines have a potential for addiction and may have severe withdrawal reaction after prolonged use. Possible adverse reactions are excessive drowsiness, restlessness, skin rash, nausea, bradycardia, tachycardia, urinary symptoms, extrapyramidal symptoms, and cardiovascular collapse. Patients who have taken this drug must not operate motor vehicles.

/// **WARNING** \\\

When administering diazepam intravenously, administer into large veins; monitor for extravasation. Do not administer intra-arterially because this may cause gangrene or arteriospasm. Do not mix in a syringe with other medications or solutions!

BENZODIAZEPINE ANTAGONIST

Flumazenil (Romazicon): IV

Adverse Reactions: Seizures; possible withdrawal in dependent patients; dizziness, nausea, agitation, and vomiting.

HYPNOTIC DRUGS

Midazolam (Versed): IM, IV; short half-life

Estazolam (ProSom): PO

Temazepam (Restoril): PO

OTHER ANXIOLYTIC AND HYPNOTIC DRUGS

Buspirone (BuSpar): PO; used for anxiety relief

Zolpidem (Ambien): PO; hypnotic, a controlled substance

Zaleplon (Sonata): PO; hypnotic, a controlled substance

Adverse Reactions: All for short-term use only; all have potential for dependence, headache, peripheral edema, abnormal vision, pruritus, fever, anxiety, hallucinations, tremor, and malaise.

BARBITURATES

Barbiturates are hypnotic drugs that were widely used in the past; however, they are seldom used today because they have several unfavorable side effects. They alter normal sleep patterns, decrease REM sleep, and have a high rate of abuse. Barbiturates continue to be used as adjuncts to anesthesia and for control of convulsive seizures in acute care settings. Barbiturate drugs must be used with extreme caution in treatment of the elderly and must not be administered to children under the age of 12 years unless a person educated in pediatrics is present to administer the drug and remains with the patient. All barbiturate drugs have the potential for dependency and are for short-term use only. Drugs in the category are as follows.

Pentobarbital (Nembutal): PO, rectal, IM, IV, short-acting

Secobarbital (Seconal) PO, rectal, IV, IM, short-acting

Amobarbital (Amytal): PO, IM, IV; long-acting

Phenobarbital (Luminal): PO, IM, IV; long-acting

Adverse Reactions: Short- and intermediate-acting barbiturates have a high rate of dependence and abuse. They may produce agitation, confusion, somnolence, apnea, respiratory and circulatory collapse, bradycardia, syncope, nausea, vomiting, epigastric distress, tissue necrosis, physical and psychological dependence, tissue necrosis, hypersensitivity reactions, and death. Barbiturates must not be mixed with other medications for parenteral administration! Administer intravenously only if no other route is feasible. Do not give more than 5 ml in one intramuscular injection site, and give deep intramuscular injections into a large muscle.

Psychotherapeutic Drugs

ANTIDEPRESSANT DRUGS

Antidepressant drugs are used to treat clinical depressive disorders, panic disorder, obsessive-compulsive disorder, and the depressive state of bipolar disorders. Antidepressants have also been used with some success in treating older children with enuresis. When symptoms of depression are prolonged for more than a 2-week duration and prevent the afflicted person from performing activities of daily living as well as obtaining pleasure from any life experiences, a physician must be consulted. Antidepressant drugs are often helpful; however, persons in states of severe depression must be monitored carefully, since they may be a danger to themselves or others. Persons suffering from panic disorders or obsessive-compulsive disorders also suffer debilitating symptoms that may result in harm to themselves or others. Antidepressant drugs are frequently very helpful for these conditions also.

Persons taking antidepressant medications must be monitored with caution. This is especially true for persons with renal, hepatic, and cardiovascular disease, and these persons must be under the care of a physician. There are four categories of antidepressant drugs on the market. They are the tricyclic antidepressants (TCAs), selective serotonin reuptake inhibitors (SSRIs), monoamine oxidase inhibitors (MAOIs), and atypical antidepressants. The intended therapeutic effect of all of the drugs is to increase affect, energy, motivation, and self-image and to correct dietary, sleep, and sexual abnormalities.

> ### /// WARNING \\\
> Persons taking MAOI drugs must not take another antidepressant drug or sympathomimetic drug until the MAOI drug has been discontinued for at least 2 weeks. Concurrent use of these drugs may lead to an adverse reaction!

TCAs and MAOIs are the older antidepressant drugs. They have side effects that make them somewhat unpleasant to take, such as dry mouth, orthostatic hypotension, sedation, and weight gain. MAOIs are used less frequently because they interact adversely with foods containing tyramine (aged foods, such as cheese) and a large number of other drugs. SSRIs and the atypical antidepressant drugs have fewer side effects and are quite effective. All antidepressant drugs must be taken for 2 to 4 weeks before symptoms are noticeably improved. There is a high potential for suicide in the early stages of treatment with antidepressants. Patient education and monitoring are vital! Some widely used drugs in each group are as follows.

TRICYCLICS

Amitriptyline (Elavil): PO

Imipramine (Tofranil): PO

Doxepin (Adapin, Sinequan): PO

Adverse Reactions: Cardiac toxicity, seizures, and urine retention.

MAOIs

Phenelzine (Nardil): PO

Tranylcypromine (Parmate): PO

Adverse Reactions: CNS stimulation; orthostatic hypotension; seizures; if taken with sympathomimetic drugs or foods containing tyramine, hypertensive crisis may result.

SSRIs

Fluoxetine (Prozac): PO

Sertraline (Zoloft): PO

Paroxetine (Paxil): PO

Adverse Reactions: Skin rash, diarrhea, fever, chills, respiratory infections, palpitations, seizures, impaired renal function, impaired hepatic function, and anorexia.

ATYPICAL ANTIDEPRESSANTS

Trazodone (Desyrel): PO

Bupropion (Wellbutrin): PO

Venlafaxome (Effexor): PO

Nefazodone (Serzone): PO

Adverse Reactions: Sedation, CNS stimulation, seizures, headache, anxiety, and tremor.

> ### ⫻⫻⫻ WARNING ⫻⫻⫻
> Do not use tricyclic agents, SSRIs, or atypical antidepressants with MAOIs or sympathomimetic drugs.

Antipsychotic Drugs

Antipsychotic drugs are also referred to as *neuroleptics* or major tranquilizers. They are used primarily to treat persons with schizophrenia and other psychotic illnesses and bipolar disorder in the manic phase. They are occasionally used to treat combativeness and severe agitation in persons with organic illnesses; however, they are considered to be chemical immobilizers (restraints) and must be used within the constraints of other immobilization techniques, as discussed in Chapter 4.

Antipsychotic drugs block dopamine receptors in the CNS. The newer drugs are believed to block serotonin receptors as well. They are classified as low-potency, medium-potency, high-potency, and atypical drugs. All antipsychotic drugs may have side effects and adverse reactions, and patients taking these drugs must be carefully monitored by qualified personnel. Patient and caregiver education is also important for compliance with these drug regimens. Several of the widely used antipsychotic drugs follow.

LOW POTENCY

Chlorpromazine (Thorazine): PO, IM

Thioridazine (Mellaril): PO

MEDIUM POTENCY

Loxapine (Loxitane): PO

Molindone (Mobane): PO

HIGH POTENCY

Halperidol (Haldol): PO, IM

Trifluoroperazine (Stelazine): PO, IM

ATYPICAL

Clozapine (Clozaril): PO

Risperidone (Risperdal): PO

Olanzapine (Zyprexa): PO

Quetiapine fumarate (Seroquel): PO

Adverse Reactions: The drugs listed have the potential for causing acute dystonia, parkinsonian symptoms, akathisia, and tardive dyskinesia. If these symptoms occur, they are often controlled by use of an antiparkinsonian drug or an anticonvulsant drug. Other potential adverse reactions are anticholinergic effects, orthostatic hypotension, seizures, sedation, blood dyscrasias, and neuroleptic malignant syndrome, which is potentially fatal.

Clozapine has less tendency to cause parkinsonian symptoms than tardive dyskinesia; however, blood dyscrasias may result, and persons taking this drug must be carefully monitored for this adverse reaction.

DRUG USED TO TREAT BIPOLAR DISORDER

Lithium (Eskalith, Lithicarb): PO

(There are several anticonvulsant drugs currently used to treat this disease that will be discussed as anticonvulsants).

Adverse Reactions: Nausea, vomiting, tremors, confusion, ataxia, seizures, tinnitus, oliguria, renal failure, and death. Persons on lithium therapy must have regular blood tests to maintain a therapeutic level while avoiding toxicity.

Anticonvulsant Drugs

Seizure disorders are described in Chapter 7. There are five groups of drugs used to control seizures, but none is able to cure the problem. Generalized tonic-clonic seizures are usually treated for long periods of time. The goal of therapy is to stabilize cell membrane excitability in the brain and reduce the spread of discharge that results in the seizure without sedating the patient. The same drugs are often used to treat partial seizures and grand mal seizures. Partial seizures are treated only for short periods of time, usually until the underlying condition is treated. There are five classes of anticonvulsants: hydantoins, barbiturates, succinimides, benzodiazepines, and a miscellaneous group. Barbiturates and benzodiazepines were discussed earlier in this chapter and are often used alone or in conjunction with other drugs to control seizures. Major drugs in each group are listed below.

HYDANTOINS

Phenytoin (Dilantin): PO, IM, IV; *found on emergency drug carts*

SUCCINIMIDES

Ethosuximide (Zarontin): PO

MISCELLANEOUS (ALSO PRESCRIBED TO TREAT BIPOLAR MANIA)

Carbamazepine (Tegretol): PO

Valproic acid (Depakene): PO

Adverse Reactions: Gastric upset, drowsiness, CNS depressions, skin rash, hypotension, and blood dyscrasias. All anticonvulsant drugs must be monitored carefully because they may become toxic. No anticonvulsant therapy should be stopped abruptly.

Specific Drug Reactions

Phenytoin: gingival hyperplasia, ataxia, hirsutism

Carbamazepine: blood dyscrasias

Valproic acid: seizures and disturbances of liver function. *Do not use this drug in conjunction with clonazepam. It may cause seizures!*

Antiparkinsonian Drugs

Parkinson's disease is a neurologic disorder that manifests with symptoms of tremor, rigidity, bradykinesia, disturbed posture, and disturbances in balance. As the disease progresses, dementia, depressions, and other psychological disturbances become evident. Unfortunately, this disease is relatively common among the elderly, so you will encounter patients in your practice with parkinsonian symptoms. It is a degenerative disease that decreases dopamine in the brain and increases availability of acetylcholine, thereby producing the symptoms listed above. Treatment is aimed at increasing dopamine availability in the brain and inhibiting acetylcholine by use of anticholinergic agents. The drugs used to treat this disease control symptoms but do not stop disease progression.

A secondary parkinsonism occasionally follows viral encephalitis or other diseases that result in multiple small vascular lesions in the brain. The older generation of antipsychotic drugs may also result in parkinsonian symptoms. The following are drugs widely used to treat Parkinson's disease and pseudoparkinson's disease.

DOPAMINERGIC AGENTS

Levodopa (Larodopa, Dopar): PO

Carbidopa (Lodosyn): PO

Amantadine (Symmetrel): PO

Carbidopa-levodopa (Sinemet): PO

Adverse Reactions: Nausea, vomiting, increased abnormal movements, psychiatric symptoms, and cardiac arrhythmias.

ANTICHOLINERGICS

Benztropine (Cogentin): PO

Trihexyphenidyl (Artane): PO

Adverse Reactions: Mental confusion, agitation, and hallucinations.

Anesthetic Drugs

There are essentially three types of anesthetic agents: local, short-acting IV, and general inhalation anesthetics. Also several adjunct medications are used to achieve a successful general anesthesia. These are preanesthetic medications to calm anxiety, lower body metabolism, and relieve pain. Muscle relaxants are used to suppress undesirable reflexes and ease in the intubation of the patient. Anticholinergic drugs are used to decrease secretions and reduce reflux irritability. Administering anesthesia requires years of specialized academic and clinical education. Persons without this education must not administer anesthetic drugs. If administered incorrectly, they are life threatening. A very brief list of some of the more widely used anesthetic drugs follows.

GENERAL INHALATION ANESTHETICS

Halothane (Fluothane): nonexplosive, nonflammable liquid, used in conjunction with nitrous oxide and muscle relaxants

Enflurane (Ethrane): nonexplosive, nonflammable liquid, rapid acting

INTRAVENOUS AGENTS

Thiopental sodium (Pentothal): ultra-short-acting barbiturate usually administered via bolus

Methohexital sodium (Brevital): short-acting barbiturate usually administered via bolus

Alfentanil (Alfenta): used alone for short-duration procedures

LOCAL ANESTHETICS

Procaine hydrochloride (Novocain): used for topical anesthesia

Lidocaine (Xylocaine): used for topical or regional anesthesia and as an antiarrhythmic drug; *found on emergency drug carts*

Tetracaine (Pontocaine): used for topical or spinal anesthesia

Adverse Reactions: All anesthetic agents may produce hypotension, cardiac arrhythmias, respiratory distress, aspiration pneumonitis, malignant hyperthermia syndrome, interactions with other drugs, shock, and circulatory failure. Local anesthetics may result in anaphylactic reactions.

MUSCLE RELAXANTS

Skeletal muscle relaxants are used before general anesthesia to suppress muscle tone and facilitate intubation of the patient. Following are some frequently used muscle-relaxing drugs.

Succinylcholine chloride (Anectine): injection

Tubocurarine chloride (Tubarine): injection

Vecuronium (Norcuron): injection; *found on emergency drug carts*

Adverse Reactions: Hypotension, arrhythmias, cardiac arrest, bradycardia, respiratory depression, apnea, and bronchospasm.

Drugs Used to Treat Alzheimer's Disease

This is a degenerative disease of the CNS that leads to progressive dementia and ultimately to death. It is an increasingly common disease of the elderly population, and a successful treatment has not been discovered. It is attributed to loss of neurons on the hippocampus area of the brain, which is the area for memory. Since acetylcholine is an important neurotransmitter in memory, it is believed that if acetylcholine levels are increased, the progress of this disease may be retarded. The drugs currently used to treat this disease are as follows.

Tacrine (Cognex): PO

Donepezil (Aricept): PO

Adverse Reactions: Seizures, abnormal crying, headache, nausea and vomiting, syncope, depression, diarrhea, depression, and insomnia.

Central Nervous System Stimulants

There are two groups of drugs that stimulate the CNS. The psychomotor stimulants decrease feelings of fatigue and increase motor activity and feelings of euphoria, and hallucinogens alter thought patterns and mood with little effect on the brain stem or spinal cord. Most CNS stimulant drugs are not used clinically but are frequently abused and must be recognized. Some of the most commonly used follow.

PSYCHOMOTOR STIMULANTS

The following group of drugs are controlled substances, Schedule II. They are common drugs of abuse.

Amphetamine: PO; used to treat attention deficit disorder

Dextroamphetamine (Dexadrine): PO; used to treat narcolepsy

Methylphenidate hydrochloride (Ritalin): PO; used to treat attention deficit disorder

Cocaine: PO, IV; intranasal; occasionally used as topical anesthesia for eye, ear, nose, and throat surgery

Adverse Reactions: Anxiety, hypertension, tachycardia, sweating and paranoia, cardiac arrhythmias, restlessness, impotence, insomnia, and death with excessive dose.

Nicotine: no clinical use; however, it is a highly addictive drug that is used in smoking cessations therapy as a chewing gum and a transdermal patch

Adverse Reactions: Peripheral vascular disease, emphysema, tremors, diarrhea, increased heart rate in high doses, death.

Caffeine: CNS stimulant; contained in many over-the-counter drugs for stimulation

Adverse Reactions: Insomnia, restlessness, headache, agitation, tachycardia, and diuresis.

Hallucinogens

Lysergic acid diethylamide (LSD): PO

Tetrahydrocannabinol (THC): Smoked

Phencyclidine (PCP, "angel dust"): PO

Adverse Reactions: Tolerance and physical dependence may occur with these drugs. All decrease motor skills, impair mental activity, visual hallucinations, stupor, hostile, bizarre behavior, and coma.

Miscellaneous Drugs Acting on the Central Nervous System

These drugs are presumed to act as agonists at serotonin receptors on the extracerebral intracranial blood vessels to treat acute migraine headaches.

Rizatriptan benzoate (Maxalt):PO

Sumatriptan succinate (Imitrex, Imigran): PO, SC, intranasal

Adverse Reactions: Dizziness, vertigo, drowsiness, malaise, tingling, atrial fibrillation, and ventricular fibrillation.

Sibutramine hydrochloride monohydrate (Meridia): PO (a controlled substance, Schedule IV); used for management of obesity

Adverse Reactions: Headache, insomnia, anxiety, tachycardia, hypertension, and elevated liver function tests.

Drugs Used to Treat Muscle Spasms

Drugs used to treat muscle spasms and spasticity of muscles may be classified as central-peripheral because they may act on the CNS as well as on the peripheral nervous system to reduce muscle spasms and spasticity. Several drugs in this category follow.

Dantrolene (Dantrium): PO, IV; for use during surgical procedures for treatment of malignant hyperthermia; acts peripherally on the muscle itself

Baclofen (Lioresal): PO; not to be used if patient has impaired renal function or is under 12 years of age

Methocarbamol (Robaxin): PO, IM, IV

Cyclobenzaprine (Flexeril): PO; should not be used for longer than 3 weeks

Adverse Reactions: CNS depression, sedation, dizziness. If used for long periods, drug must be withdrawn slowly, since user may have severe withdrawal reaction. Some of the drugs in this group, if used for a long period of time, create a physical dependence.

Drugs That Act on the Peripheral Nervous System

The peripheral nervous system has two branches, the voluntary, or somatic, nervous system and the involuntary, or autonomic, nervous system (ANS). The voluntary branch conveys information from the external environment to the CNS, which controls the responses of the musculoskeletal system. The person in good health has control of these responses. The ANS controls the enervation of the smooth muscles and body organs, such as the heart and the glands. The ANS is divided into the sympathetic and parasympathetic divisions. The sympathetic nerves originate in the thoracic and upper lumbar regions of the spinal cord. The parasympathetic nerves originate in the brain stem and sacral region of the spinal cord.

The two principal neurotransmitters responsible for transmission of nerve impulses through the ANS are acetylcholine and norepinephrine. The nerve fibers that secrete acetylcholine are called *cholinergic fibers*. The nerve fibers that secrete norepinephrine are called *adrenergic fibers*. Both acetylcholine and norepinephrine act on the organs and tissues of the body to produce either excitatory or inhibitory effects, depending on the organ involved. Most organs of the body are controlled by either the sympathetic or parasympathetic system. Often when the sympathetic nervous system excites a particular organ, the parasympathetic system inhibits it.

When the sympathetic nerves are stimulated, an adrenergic response occurs. This response may produce the following reactions:

Dilation of blood vessels

Increase in heart rate

Decrease in gastric motility and sensation

Contraction of the gastric sphincters

Contraction of the urinary bladder sphincter

Constriction of the blood vessels of the skin

Secretion of adrenalin

When the parasympathetic nerves are stimulated, a cholinergic response occurs causing the following reactions (Fig. 12–6)

Constriction of the pupils

Bronchial constriction

Decrease in heart rate

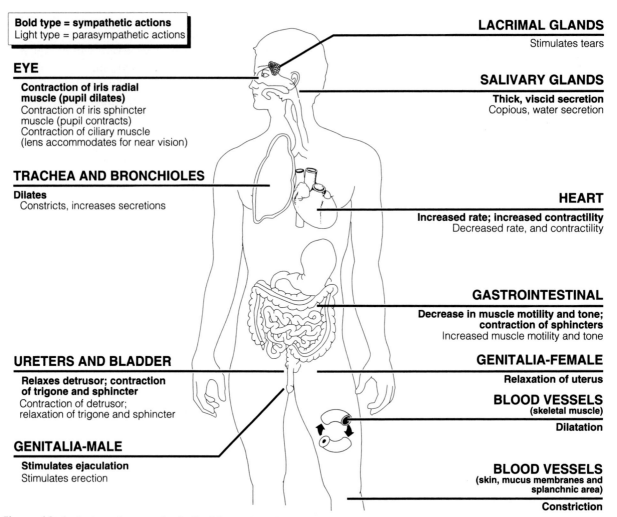

Bold type = sympathetic actions
Light type = parasympathetic actions

EYE

Contraction of iris radial muscle (pupil dilates)
Contraction of iris sphincter muscle (pupil contracts)
Contraction of ciliary muscle (lens accommodates for near vision)

TRACHEA AND BRONCHIOLES

Dilates
Constricts, increases secretions

URETERS AND BLADDER

Relaxes detrusor; contraction of trigone and sphincter
Contraction of detrusor; relaxation of trigone and sphincter

GENITALIA-MALE

Stimulates ejaculation
Stimulates erection

LACRIMAL GLANDS
Stimulates tears

SALIVARY GLANDS

Thick, viscid secretion
Copious, water secretion

HEART

Increased rate; increased contractility
Decreased rate, and contractility

GASTROINTESTINAL

Decrease in muscle motility and tone; contraction of sphincters
Increased muscle motility and tone

GENITALIA-FEMALE

Relaxation of uterus

BLOOD VESSELS
(skeletal muscle)

Dilatation

BLOOD VESSELS
(skin, mucus membranes and splanchnic area)

Constriction

Figure 12–6. Action of sympathetic **(bold type)** and parasympathetic (light type) nervous systems of effector organs. Mycek, MJ, Harvey, RA, Champe, PC: *Lippincott's Illustrated Reviews: Pharmacology*, 2nd ed. Philadilhia: Lippincott Williams & Wilkins, 2000.

Increase in gastric motility and secretion

Relaxation of the urinary sphincter

Increased secretion from the salivary and lacrimal glands

Drugs may affect the autonomic nervous system by increasing release of a neurotransmitter, decreasing release of a neurotransmitter, mimicking a neurotransmitter, blocking receptors, or inhibiting breakdown of a neurotransmitter. Symptoms of diseases controlled by use of drugs acting on the ANS include ulcers, urinary retention, glaucoma, asthma, angina pectoris, congestive heart failure, bradycardia and tachycardia, nasal congestion, hypertension, constipation, and diarrhea. Examples of drugs that are used for the purpose of affecting the autonomic nervous system follow.

Adrenergic Drugs

Adrenergic drugs produce effects that are in many ways the same as the stimulating effects of some drugs

that act on the sympathetic nervous system. The most notable action of these drugs is to constrict blood vessels and to stimulate the heart. Many of the drugs in this category are used in cardiovascular, respiratory, and allergic emergencies.

Dopamine (Intropin): IV, used to treat hypotension and shock; *found on emergency drug carts*

Adverse Reactions: Cardiac arrhythmia, extreme hypertension; tissue necrosis if extravasation occurs, dyspnea; and nausea and vomiting.

Epinephrine (Adrenalin): IV, SC, inhalers; used as a bronchodilator and vasoconstrictor in acute asthma, anaphylactic shock, and hypersensitivity reactions; *found on emergency drug carts*

Adverse Reactions: Hypertensive headache, intracranial hemorrhage, cardiac arrhythmias, pallor, palpitations, anxiety, dizziness, dyspnea, and pulmonary edema.

Ephedrine: IM, SC, IV, topical; used as a bronchodilator, for cardiac stimulation, hypotension, nasal decongestant

Adverse Reactions: Extreme hypertension; intracranial hemorrhage; tachycardia; cardiac arrhythmias; anxiety, pallor, and circulatory collapse.

Norepinephrine bitartrate (Levophed): IV; used to treat hypotension and shock; *found on emergency drug carts*

Adverse Reactions: Bradycardia; headache; extreme hypertension; skin irritation and tissue necrosis, if extravasation occurs.

Albuterol (Proventil, Ventolin): PO, inhalation; used as a bronchodilator

Adverse Reactions: Anxiety, CNS stimulation, insomnia, tremor, vertigo, cardiac arrhythmias, tachycardia, pulmonary edema, bronchospasm, sweating and pallor, nausea, and heartburn.

Dobutamine (Dobutrex): IV; *found on emergency drug carts*

Adverse Reactions: Increased heart rate; hypertension; angina; anaphylaxis.

Isoproterenol (Isuprel): sublingual, IV; potent bronchodilator used to treat shock and acute renal failure; for hypotension to promote perfusion to vital organs; *found on emergency drug carts*

Adverse Reactions: May be harmful in cardiogenic shock, tachycardia, palpitations, angina-type pain, flushing, tremors, headache, nausea, and bronchial edema.

Antiadrenergic Drugs

Drugs are used to block the effects of nerve impulses transmitted by adrenergic fibers of the sympathetic nervous system. They cause increased peripheral circulation and decreased blood pressure. Alpha-1 receptor-blocking agents dilate blood vessels and decrease peripheral vascular resistance. Alpha-2 blocking agents block sympathetic nervous system impulses in the brain. Beta-adrenergic blocking agents decrease heart rate, force of myocardial contraction, cardiac output, and renin release from the kidneys. Alpha- and beta-blocking agents are widely used and must be recognized by the radiographer.

ALPHA-1-ADRENERGIC BLOCKING DRUGS

Prazosin (Minipress): PO; used to treat hypertension and Raynaud's vasospasm

Terazosin (Hytrin): PO; used to treat hypertension

Adverse Reactions: Dizziness, headaches, vertigo, depression, tachycardia, orthostatic hypotension, dyspnea, nausea, urinary symptoms, blurred vision, epistaxis, and syncope after first dose of prazosin.

ALPHA-2-ADRENERGIC BLOCKING DRUGS

Clonidine (Catapres): PO; used to treat hypertension, Tourette's syndrome, migraine

Adverse Reactions: Vomiting, parotitis, sedation, nightmares, hallucinations, depressions, orthostatic hypotension, tachycardia, bradycardia, impotence, rash, and hyperpigmentation.

Methyldopa (Aldomet): PO; used to treat hypertension

Adverse Reactions: Sedation, weakness, bradycardia, aggravation of angina, nausea, blood dyscrasias, rash, and gynecomastia.

Beta-adrenergic Blocking Agents

Atenolol (Tenormin): PO; used to treat hypertension, angina, myocardial infarction, and migraine

Metoprolol (Lopressor): PO; used to treat hypertension and myocardial infarction

Propanolol (Inderal): PO, IV; used to treat hypertension, angina, cardiac arrhythmias; *found on emergency drug carts*

Nadolol (Corgard): PO; used to treat angina and hypertension

Adverse Reactions: Bradycardia, congestive heart failure, arrhythmias, vertigo, fatigue, bronchospasm, dyspnea, gastric pain, nausea, impotence, joint pain, rash, and eye irritation.

Antimuscarinic Drugs

Antimuscarinic drugs belong to a category known as classic anticholinergic drugs, which block activity at postganglionic parasympathetic receptor sites found in cardiac and other smooth muscle. Widely used drugs in this group are the following.

Atropine: PO, IV, IM, topical; used to treat gastric diseases as an antispasmodic and to treat bradycardia by increasing heart rate; also used preoperatively to prevent salivary and bronchial secretions and in ophthalmology to relax pupil of eye; *found on emergency drug carts*

Adverse Reactions: Dry mouth, nausea, vomiting, blurred vision, urine retention, impotence, bradycardia, tachycardia, and suppression of lactation.

Scopalamine: PO, SC, IM, IV diluted with water for injection; used to treat motion sickness and GI disorders and as a preliminary to anesthesia

Adverse Reactions: Tachycardia, dry mouth, blurred vision, CNS toxicity, delirium; not for use in patients with side-angle glaucoma.

Calcium Channel Blockers

Calcium channel blockers are drugs that inhibit the flow of calcium ions across the membranes of smooth muscle cells. Calcium is important in cardiac and smooth muscle contraction and in the generation and conduction of electrical impulses in the heart. By reducing calcium flow, the smooth muscle tone is relaxed, thereby reducing muscle spasm. These drugs have been used extensively to treat heart diseases caused by arterial spasms. Recently, there has been some question concerning the effectiveness of these drugs. Some of those widely used follow:

Verapamil (Calan, Isoptin): PO; comes in sustained-release form; used to treat angina, cardiac arrhythmias, and hypertension; *found on emergency drug carts*

Nifedipine (Procardia, Adalat): PO; comes in sustained-release form; used to treat angina, and hypertension

Diltiazem (Cardizem): comes in sustained-release form; used to treat angina and hypertension; *found on emergency drug carts*

Adverse Reactions: Peripheral edema, hypotension, arrhythmias, bradycardia, dizziness, nausea, flushing, rash; may cause heart block if patient is taking digitalis preparation.

Vasodilators

Vasodilators are used for severe hypertension. Tachycardia, renin release, and fluid retention are common adverse effects from these drugs. Therefore, when they are prescribed, a diuretic or a beta-blocking agent is prescribed with them.

Hydralazine (Apresoline): PO, IM, IV; used for hypertensive crisis and severe hypertension

Minoxidil (Loniten): PO; used for severe hypertension

Adverse Reactions: Same as for calcium channel blockers.

Hydralazine: lupus-like syndrome

Loniten: pericardial effusion, hirsutism

Cardiac Glycosides

These drugs are all derived from the foxglove plant (*Digitalis purpurea*). There are several forms of the drug; however, they all basically perform the same function. That is, they all increase the force of cardiac contractility and slow the heart rate. Drugs in this group are the following:

Digoxin (Lanoxin): PO, IV; used to treat congestive heart failure and some cardiac arrhythmias

Digitoxin (Crystodigin): PO; used to treat congestive heart failure and some cardiac arrhythmias

Adverse Reactions: Fatigue, muscle weakness, dizziness, vertigo, stupor; cardiac toxicity, anorexia, nausea, vomiting, abdominal pain, diarrhea, gynecomastia, and cardiac arrest.

Organic Nitrates

Organic nitrates are used to relax smooth muscles of both arteries and veins; their ability to relax (dilate) veins makes them useful in treating anginal pain. Venous capacity is increased, thereby reducing, temporarily, the amount of blood entering the heart. This has the effect of reducing the heart's workload. Organic nitrates may be very short-acting or long-acting drugs. Several of the most widely used are as follows:

SHORT ACTING

Nitroglycerin (Nitrostat, Tridil, Nitrostat IV, Nitrolingual): sublingual, IV; used to treat sudden onset of anginal pain

Isosorbide dinitrate (Isordil, Sorbitrate): sublingual

LONG ACTING

Nitroglycerin (Nitrogard, Nitro-Dur, Transderm Nitro): PO, buccal, topical ointment, transdermal patch; used to prevent anginal pain; by buccal route, used to treat sudden-onset cardiac pain

Isosorbide dinitrate (Sorbitrate, Isordil): PO; used to prevent anginal pain

Adverse Reactions: Headache, vertigo, faintness, hypotension, syncope, flushing, dermatitis, and burning sensation at contact point.

Antidysrhythmics

All cardiac arrhythmias are the result of abnormalities or errors in electrical impulse formation or conduction. The arrhythmia that is generated creates a change, either in the heart's rate of contractility or in its rhythm. These changes may be life threatening. Several of the widely used antiarrhythmic drugs are:

Quinidine: PO, IM, IV; used to maintain normal cardiac rhythm and, in emergencies, to restore normal cardiac rhythm; *found on emergency drug carts*

Adverse Reactions: Cardiac arrhythmias, heart block, hypotension, nausea, diarrhea, liver toxicity, vision changes, rash, ringing in ears, and tremor.

Procainamide (Pronestyl, Procan): PO, IV; controls cardiac arrhythmias; *found on emergency drug carts*

Adverse Reactions: Lupus-like syndrome; hypotension, cardiac disturbances, nausea, depression, convulsions, psychosis.

Lidocaine (Xylocaine): IV, IM; used as a local anesthetic and as the drug of choice for treating serious ventricular arrhythmias after myocardial infarction, cardiac surgeries, and diagnostic examinations; *found on emergency drug carts*

Adverse Reactions: Cardiac arrhythmias, heart block, cardiac arrest, respiratory depression, hypotension, and septic meningitis.

Adenosine (Adenocard): IV; *found on emergency drug carts*

Adverse Reactions: Shortness of breath, dizziness, tingling, headache, dyspnea

Amiodarone hydrochloride (Cordarone): PO, IV; *found on emergency drug carts*

Adverse Reactions: asthenia, headache, weakness, sleep problems, bradycardia, arrhythmias, and heart failure.

Sotalol hydrochloride: PO

Adverse Reactions: Asthenia, headache, fatigue, sleep problems, bradycardia, heart failure, ventricular fibrillation, and chest pain.

Diuretics

Diuretics are drugs used to treat hypertension, congestive heart failure, pulmonary edema, and other medical conditions that create an edematous state in the body. When diuretic therapy is begun, cardiac output decreases as blood volume decreases. Diuretics are often used in combination with other cardiac and antihypertensive drugs. Some of the commonly used diuretics are:

Furosemide (Lasix): PO, IV; used to treat hypertension, congestive heart failure, and pulmonary edema; *found on emergency drug carts*

Thiazides (Esidrix, HydroDIURIL, Hygroton): used to treat hypertension and other medical conditions that cause fluid retention

Acetazolamide (Diamox): PO; used to treat open-angle glaucoma

Hydrochlorothiazide (Dyazide, Maxzide): PO; used to treat hypertension

Mannitol (Osmitrol): IV; used to treat the oliguric phase of renal failure, used in radiographic imaging to prevent nephropathy or acute renal failure; *may be found on emergency drug carts*

Adverse Reactions: Hypokalemia, hyperkalemia, alkalosis, hyponatremia, and vascular collapse.

Spironolactone (Aldactone): PO: a potassium-sparing diuretic

Adverse Reactions: headache, diarrhea, ataxia, increased BUN (blood urea nitrogen) levels, agranulocytosis.

Analgesics, Antipyretics, and Anti-inflammatory Drugs

This group of drugs is called NSAIDs, for *nonsteroidal anti-inflammatory analgesic drugs.* Every drug in this category has the same effect; that is, they are all analgesic (reduce pain), antipyretic (reduce fever), and anti-inflammatory (reduce inflammation in tissues) agents. They are highly effective and widely used to relieve moderate pain, especially pain related to myalgia (muscle pain), neuralgia (pain of nerve origin), and cephalalgia (headache that may be of histamine origin). They are also used to reduce fever and to reduce inflammation in osteoarthritis, rheumatoid arthritis, bursitis, and rheumatic fever. Because they reduce platelet aggregation and decrease prothrombin formation, they are used to prevent venous emboli and cerebral ischemia associated with heart disease.

NSAIDs affect both the central and peripheral nervous systems. All inhibit cyclooxygenase (an enzyme: prostaglandin endoperoxide synthase). This action reduces the sensitivity of peripheral pain receptors and may interfere with pain impulses at subcortical brain centers. Some of the most widely used NSAIDs are as follows:

Salicylates and aspirin: PO; used for all disease states mentioned above; most widely used of the NSAIDs (at low doses) for preventing platelet aggregation and prevention of thrombi

Indomethacin (Indocin): PO, most potent NSAID; not used as an analgesic; used to treat osteoarthritis, rheumatoid arthritis, patent ductus arteriosus in infants, and gout

Ibuprofen (Advil, Motrin, Nuprin): PO; used to relieve symptoms of dysmenorrhea and other mild to moderate pain

Naproxen (Naprosyn): PO; approved for use in juvenile arthritis; also used for gout and arthritic conditions

Piroxicam (Feldene): PO; long-acting drug used to treat arthritic diseases; may cause severe GI bleeding

Sulindac (Clinoril): PO; used for chronic pain; *must not be used for children!*

Ketorolac (Toradol): PO, IM; used as a more potent analgesic; *may cause severe GI problems*

Relafen and Daypro: PO; newest of NSAIDs; used as long-acting drug for pain relief

Adverse Reactions: GI pain, nausea, dyspepsia, dysuria, renal impairment including renal failure, headaches, somnolence, tinnitus, dyspnea, bleeding, platelet inhibition, blood dyscrasias, peripheral edema, and fatal anaphylaxis.

/ / / **WARNING** \ \ \

Use NSAIDs with extreme caution in elderly persons. Use in children only with physician in attendance.

Other Nonnarcotic Analgesics

Acetaminophen (Tylenol): PO; used to treat moderate pain without anti-inflammatory effects; the antipyretic of choice for small children

Adverse Reactions: The most severe adverse reaction is liver toxicity associated with large doses. It may cause dizziness, excitement, disorientation, and renal tubular necrosis.

Drugs Affecting The Blood

Anticoagulants

Frequently, drugs are used prophylactically to prevent thrombus formations before surgical procedures. These same drugs are used to prevent extension of thrombi after myocardial infarction, pulmonary embolism, venous thrombosis, and strokes. These drugs are called *anticoagulants. You will see some of these drugs used in special procedures and in the operating room.*

There are drugs that facilitate the dissolution of blood clots by converting plasminogen to plasmin, the body's natural anticoagulant. These drugs are called *thrombolytics.* Some are relatively new and are quite

effective. These drugs are used to facilitate the dissolution of blood clots in acute thromboembolic disorders, as in myocardial infarction and acute pulmonary thromboembolism. Thrombolytics are to be used only by persons who have been educated to treat acute care situations because when bleeding occurs, it is very difficult to control.

Agents used to prevent thrombus formation in persons who have the potential for developing myocardial infarction or cerebral emboli are called *antithrombotics.* The most effective and widely used of these is aspirin, as discussed in the previous section.

Some of the commonly used anticoagulant and thrombolytic drugs follow.

Heparin: IV, SC; must not be given to persons with preexisting bleeding disorders, active ulcer, hemophilia, before or after brain, spinal cord, or eye surgery; contraindicated in pregnancy and for persons taking NSAIDs; *antidote*: protamine sulfate.

Warfarin (Coumadin): PO; used to prevent and treat emboli, used prophylactically for persons who have prosthetic heart valves; *antidote:* phytonadione (vitamin K, Mephyton), PO, SC, IM; increases blood clotting ability

Adverse Reactions: Bleeding, hemorrhage, urinary tract bleeding, urticaria, alopecia, nausea, blood dyscrasias, osteoporosis, and suppression of renal function.

Alteplase (tissue plasminogen activator, recombinant: t-PA): IV; used for lysis of thrombi obstructing coronary arteries in acute myocardial infarction; to manage acute massive pulmonary embolism; and ischemic strokes

Adverse Reactions: Cerebral hemorrhage, hypotension, arrhythmias, nausea, and anaphylaxis.

Streptokinase (Streptase): IV

Adverse Reactions: bleeding, pulmonary edema, headache, nausea, and anaphylaxis.

Clopidogrel bisulfate (Plavix): PO

Adverse Reactions: Hemorrhage, abdominal pain, edema, hypertension, and arthralgia.

Vitamin K (Mephyton): PO, SC, IM, IV: used to stop bleeding

Drugs Used to Treat Anemia

Anemia, which may be either a disease or a symptom of disease, manifests as a decrease in the number of red blood cells (RBCs, erythrocytes), a decrease in the hemoglobin content of the RBC, or a change in the size of the RBCs. The causes are varied: blood loss, hemolysis (breakdown of RBCs); bone marrow dysfunction; a deficiency in iron, vitamin B$_{12}$, or folic acid—the essential cofactors in maintaining a normal RBC count. The symptoms vary, depending on the severity of the disease, and may range from mild fatigue to severe hypoxia, tachycardia, angina, cardiac arrhythmias, and heart failure.

Treatment depends on the severity of symptoms and the cause. Iron deficiency, a common cause of anemia, is treated by replacement of iron if the condition is not severe. Drugs used to treat anemia include the following.

Ferrous sulfate: PO; used to treat mild iron-deficiency anemia

Adverse Reactions: Nausea, heartburn, constipation, diarrhea; may aggravate gastric ulcers; to be taken with food.

Erythropoietin (Epogen): IV, SC; used to treat anemias

Adverse Reactions: Headache, seizures, hypertension, edema, gastric symptoms, increased BUN, hyperkalemia, arthralgia, and pyrexia.

Iron dextran: IM; used when unable to ingest oral product

Adverse Reaction: Anaphylaxis.

> ### ⫽⫽⫽ WARNING ⫻⫻⫻
> Iron can be extremely toxic in children and some adults. It may result in gastric necrosis and pulmonary and hepatic failure. Antidote: desferoxamine.

Vitamin B$_{12}$: IM; used for treatment of pernicious anemia; treatment is lifelong; no significant adverse reactions; patient must report for therapy, since this is a life-threatening illness

Folic acid: PO; used to treat folic acid deficiency

Antihyperlipedemic Drugs

A common cause of stroke and myocardial infarction is atherosclerosis. This is caused by deposits of fatty plaques that eventually cut off circulation to the heart of the brain, resulting in a life-threatening illness. In recent years, drugs have been developed that have been relatively successful in preventing formation of atherosclerotic plaques. They are called *antilipemics* and *vasodilators*.

Antilipemic drugs decrease hyperlipoproteinemia by altering production, metabolism, and removal of lipoproteins from the bloodstream. Following are some of the widely used antilipemic drugs.

Atorvastatin calcium (Lipitor): PO

Lovastatin (Mevacor): PO; decreases hepatic synthesis of cholesterol

Gemfibrozil (Lopid): PO; decreases hepatic production of triglycerides

Cholestyramine (Questran): PO; increases oxidation of cholesterol and decreases blood cholesterol

Simvastatin (Zocor): PO; reduces total cholesterol

Adverse Effects: GI upset, headache, rash, hepatotoxicity, and blood dyscrasias.

Nicotinic acid: hyperglycemia

Peripheral Vasodilators

Peripheral vasodilating drugs are of questionable use in dilating atherosclerotic vessels; however, a newer type of drug that affects the cellular components of the blood improves blood flow by decreasing blood viscosity. Following are some of the commonly used peripheral vasodilators.

Nylidrin hydrochloride (Adrin, Arlidin): PO; used to treat Raynaud's disease and diabetic vascular disease

Isoxsuprine hydrochloride (Vasodilan): PO; used to treat arteriosclerosis obliterans

Adverse Reactions: Hypotension, tachycardia, chest pain, nausea, dizziness, and rash.

Drugs Affecting the Respiratory System

Respiratory disorders range from acute, life-threatening diseases to brief, minor ailments. The range between these extremes is great. It is not within the scope of this text to discuss all illnesses and medications available for these disorders; however, a brief overview is relevant for you as the radiographer, since you will be caring for many persons with these disorders.

The acute, life-threatening diseases most commonly seen in the acute care hospital setting are asthma and chronic obstructive pulmonary disease (COPD). The following are medications widely used to treat these diseases.

Epinephrine and ephedrine: used to treat asthma, as discussed earlier under adrenergic drugs

Xanthine derivatives: theophylline: PO, IV; used for relief or prevention of symptoms of bronchial asthma, bronchospasm, and COPD

Theo-Dur: PO; a long-acting theophylline preparation used as a bronchodilator

Aminophylline: PO, IV; dilates bronchial smooth muscles; same use as for theophylline preparations

Adverse Reactions: Loss of appetite, epigastric pain, tachypnea, respiratory arrest; if blood levels high, may produce seizures, brain damage, and death.

Isoproterenol (Isuprel): IV, sublingual, inhalation; relaxes bronchial smooth muscles; used to treat acute respiratory distress; *found on emergency drug carts*

Ipratropium (Atrovent): inhalation; used to treat bronchospasm

Adverse Reactions: Seizures, blurred vision, weakness, dizziness, tremors, and nervousness.

Nasal Decongestants

There are many drugs used to relieve allergic rhinitis, sinusitis, colds, and flu. Some of the most widely used of these drugs are the following.

Phenylephrine (Neo-Synephrine): PO, topical; used as nasal decongestant, ophthalmic vasoconstrictor, and to treat shock

Phenylpropanolamine (Propagest): PO; used as a nasal decongestant

Pseudoephedrine (Sudafed): PO; used as a nasal decongestant

Adverse Reactions: Fear, anxiety, drowsiness, tremors, hypertension, arrhythmias, cardiovascular collapse, tachycardia; with prolonged abuse, symptoms of paranoia, nausea, vomiting, necrosis, and slouching when given IV.

Antitussives, Expectorants

These drugs may be used as expectorants to render a cough more productive by increasing respiratory secretions. Expectorants do not contain opiates when they are used to suppress cough. They may or may not contain opiates such as codeine or hydrocodone when they are used to affect the cough center in the CNS.

EXPECTORANT

Guaifenesin (Robitussin): PO

NARCOTIC ANTITUSSIVE

Hydrocodone bitartrate, codeine: PO

Adverse Reactions: May create dependency with prolonged use.

NONNARCOTIC ANTITUSSIVES

Benzonatate (Tessalon): PO

Dextromethorphan (Pertussin, Benalyn DM, St. Joseph Cough): PO

Adverse Reactions: Respiratory depression with overdose.

Antihistamines

Histamine is a compound discharged from the mast cells of the body into the bloodstream when particular stimuli influence it to be released. Stimuli such as an antigen-antibody response, tissue injury, extreme cold, and some drugs produce histamine release. Once released into the bloodstream, histamine acts on the body to contract smooth muscles; increase capillary permeability to fluids resulting in an outflow of fluid into the body tissues; dilate cerebral blood vessels producing severe headache; stimulate secretion of gastric fluid in large amounts of high acidity; and stimulate sensory nerve endings causing pain and itching. These are the events of an anaphylactic reaction. When this type of event occurs, an antihistamine drug is administered.

There are many antihistamines on the market. Some are strong CNS depressants and produce a sedative effect. The newer drugs are not as sedating. Antihistamines are used to treat anaphylactic shock; upper respiratory disorders; acute urticaria; edema; hypersensitivity reactions; motion sickness; and nausea. They are also used as over-the counter sleep medications. Some of the more widely used antihistamines are:

Diphenhydramine hydrochloride (Benadryl): PO, IM, IV, topical; used for anaphylactic reactions and many other uses; *found on emergency drug carts*

Chlorpheniramine maleate (Chlor-Trimeton): PO SC, IM, IV; used to treat symptoms of colds and allergies

Promethazine hydrochloride (Phenergan): IM, IV, PO; very potent antihistamine with pronounced sedative effects; used as sedative and in motion sickness

Adverse Reactions: Must be used with caution in patients with hypersensitivity to these drugs, narrow-angle glaucoma, prostatic hypertrophy, peptic ulcer, and bladder neck obstruction and in pregnant women. *Not for use in patients with asthma!* Reactions are drowsiness, dizziness, dry mouth, hypotension, paradoxical excitement, hyperirritability, blurred vision, urinary retention. Patients must be warned not to operate motor vehicles after administration of antihistamines.

Antiemetic Drugs

The blood-brain barrier is poorly developed in the chemo-emetic trigger zone (CTZ); therefore, many drugs and environmental conditions may result in nausea and vomiting. The neuroreceptors, dopamine and possibly serotonin, are important in inhibiting gastric motility occurring during nausea and vomiting. A dopamine antagonist is of some help in preventing nausea. Anticholinergic agents and H_1 antihistamines also help to reduce motion sickness, nausea, and vomiting. Several of the commonly used drugs in this area follow.

ANTIDOPAMINERGIC AGENTS

Metoclopramide hydrochloride (Reglan): PO, IV, IM

Adverse Reactions: Seizures, suicide ideation, blood dyscrasias, anxiety, depressions, akathisia, tardive dyskinesia, extrapyramidal symptoms.

Prochlorperazine maleate (Compazine): PO, IM, IV, rectal

Adverse Reactions: Pseudoparkinsonian symptoms, extrapyramidal symptoms, dizziness, and orthostatic hypotension.

ANTICHOLINERGIC AGENTS

Scopolamine (Hyoscine, transderm-Scop): IV, PO, SC, transdermal

H_1 ANTIHISTAMINES

Dimenhydrinate (Dramamine): PO, IV, IM

Hydroxyzine (Atarax, Vistaril): PO, IM

Adverse Reactions: Drowsiness, dizziness, headache, hallucinations, tachycardia, bradycardia, dry mouth, and epigastric distress.

Drugs That Act on the Gastrointestinal System

The drugs in this category are used to treat gastric ulcers, gastroesophageal reflux, constipation, and diarrhea. The causes of gastrointestinal diseases are multiple and range from moderate to severe; some are even life threatening. Gastric ulcers may be caused by the *Helicobacter pylori* bacteria. If this is the causative organism, the ulcers are treated with a combination of antimicrobial drugs for 14 days. The drug descriptions listed in this text are very brief and do not include drugs used to treat neoplasms and other serious illnesses.

Drugs Used to Treat Peptic Ulcer Disease

Cimetidine (Tagamet): PO; used to modify the acidity of the gastric secretions

Ranitidine (Zantac): PO, IV, IM; used to modify acidity of gastric secretions

Famotidine (Pepcid) and nizatidine (Exid): PO; used to modify gastric secretions

Adverse Reactions: Interferes with action of several commonly used drugs such as lidocaine and quinidine among others, to cause toxicity; must be used with caution in persons with renal and hepatic disease; not for use in pregnant women or children.

Sucralfate (Carafate): PO; protects lining of stomach with coating to prevent further damage

Omeprazole (Prilosec): PO; inhibits activity of acid pump; blocks formation of gastric acid

Adverse Reactions: Headache, diarrhea, nausea, constipation, and flatulence.

Antacids

These drugs may be purchased over the counter to treat symptoms of heartburn and indigestion. Several of the widely used preparations are listed below:

Amphogel: PO; contains aluminum hydroxide

Di-Gel: PO; contains magnesium hydroxide and aluminum hydroxide

Gelusil: PO; contains magnesium hydroxide and aluminum hydroxide

Gelusil-M: PO; contains magnesium hydroxide and aluminum hydroxide

Maalox suspension: PO; contains magnesium hydroxide and aluminum hydroxide

Mylanta: PO; contains magnesium hydroxide and aluminum hydroxide

Sodium bicarbonate: PO, IV; used to relieve gastric hyperacidity; used in cardiac arrest to reduce acidosis; *found on emergency drug carts*

Adverse Reactions: Diarrhea.

Aluminum derivatives: intestinal impaction, anorexia, weakness, impaired reflexes, depression, tremors, bone pain

Magnesium derivatives: profound diarrhea, dehydration, nausea, vomiting, impaired reflexes, hypotension, respiratory depression, bradycardia, renal stones

Sodium bicarbonate: systemic alkalosis, sodium overload, rebound hypersecretion

Drugs Used to Treat Constipation

Four types of drugs are used to relieve or prevent constipation. They are classified as either *cathartics* or *laxatives*. Cathartics cause evacuation of the bowel by increasing peristalsis, usually by irritating the intestinal mucosa. Laxatives promote bowel evacuation by increasing the bulk of the feces, by softening the stool, or by lubricating the intestinal wall. Laxatives are generally less harsh than cathartics. There are saline and irritant, or stimulant, cathartics and bulk-forming and surfactant laxatives. Examples of those widely used follow.

SALINE CATHARTICS

Magnesium citrate solution: PO

Magnesium hydroxide (Milk of Magnesia): PO

IRRITANT CATHARTICS

Castor Oil: PO

Cascara sagrada: PO

BULK-FORMING LAXATIVES

Methylcellulose: PO

Psyllium preparations (Metamucil, Serutan): PO

SURFACTANT LAXATIVES (STOOL SOFTENERS)

Docusate sodium (Colace, Doxinate): PO

Docusate potassium (Dialose): PO

Adverse Reactions: All cathartics may create dependence and electrolyte imbalance; should not be used in undiagnosed abdominal pain.

Drugs Used to Treat Diarrhea

Bismuth subsalicylate (Pepto-Bismol): PO; may darken tongue and stools

Diphenoxylate hydrochloride and atropine sulfate (Lomotil): PO

Adverse Reactions: Sedation, dizziness, confusion, tachycardia, and paralytic ileus.

Loperamide (Imodium): PO

Adverse Reactions: Drowsiness, fatigue, abdominal pain.

Opium tincture (Paregoric): PO; controlled substance, may cause dependency after long-term use

Drugs Used to Treat Endocrine Disorders

Endocrinology is a medical specialty area for treatment of a wide range of diseases that include diabetes mellitus, thyroid dysfunction, sexual dysfunction, and the autoimmune diseases. The endocrine system is composed of the hypothalamus, pituitary, thyroid, parathyroid, pancreas, adrenals, ovaries, and testes. All of these glands produce hormones that work with the nervous system to regulate body functions.

It is highly complex and beyond the scope of this text to consider this aspect of medicine; however, as the radiographer you will frequently work with persons who have thyroid diseases and diabetes mellitus and those who are taking corticosteroid preparations. Several of the widely used preparations are presented briefly.

Drugs That Affect the Thyroid and Parathyroid Glands

The thyroid and parathyroid glands function to regulate growth and development, metabolic rate, energy level, and reproductive organs. Parathyroid dysfunction affects serum calcium and vitamin D levels and results in bone demineralization. Diseases of these glands are not infrequent and are often managed by drug therapy. Some of those frequently prescribed follow.

DRUGS USED TO TREAT OSTEOPOROSIS AND HYPERPARATHYROIDISM

Calcitonin-salmon (Calcimar): IM, SC; may cause anaphylaxis–skin test required before use!

Pamidronate (Aredia): IV

Etidronate (Didronel): IV

Alendronate (Fosamax): PO

Adverse Reactions: All may cause muscle pain, GI symptoms, taste perversions, and headache. Etidronate may cause bone fractures and osteomalacia and must not be used in persons with hypercalcemia, heart failure, bone fractures, enterocolitis and impaired kidney function. *All of these drugs must be managed carefully and by persons knowledgeable about adverse effects of each of these drugs!*

DRUGS USED TO TREAT DISEASES OF THE THYROID GLAND

The thyroid gland produces two iodine-containing hormones, thyroxine and tri-iodothyronine. These hormones are essential for normal growth and development and for normal metabolic function. Thyroid dysfunction may result in the under- or overproduction of thyroid hormones. Both produce adverse effects on the body and must be treated. Treatment of hypothyroid commonly includes some of the following drugs.

Levothyroxine (Synthroid): PO, IV

Thyroid: PO

Adverse Reactions: Nervousness, insomnia, tremor, arrhythmias, weight loss, and cardiac arrest.

Drugs used to treat hyperthyroidism include the following:

Sodium iodide (Iodopen): PO; a radioactive isotope of iodine that selectively damages or destroys thyroid tissue

Adverse Reactions: Sore throat, neck swelling, pain, loss of taste, nausea, vomiting, and bleeding episodes.

Adrenocorticosteroids

Adrenocorticosteroids are essential for life and are produced in the adrenal cortex. They influence all nutrient metabolism in the body and affect the function of the cardiovascular system, kidneys, skeletal muscles, and nervous system. They also affect hepatic deposition of glycogen and sodium retention and have anti-inflammatory effects. The two most important adrenocorticosteroids are cortisol and aldosterone. Adrenocorticosteroids are used as replacement therapy in diseases of the adrenal glands; for relief of inflammatory symptoms; for severe allergic reactions; and for relief of the stress caused by trauma or other stress reactions resulting in physical insults to the body. Some of the most frequently used steroid drugs are listed here.

Hydrocortisone sodium succinate (Solu-Cortef): injection; *found on emergency drug carts*

Cortisone (Cortone): PO, IM; used to treat inflammatory and allergic disorders and as replacement therapy for adrenal insufficiency

Dexamethasone (Decadron): PO; used to treat inflammatory and allergic disorders; *may be found on emergency drug carts in IV form*

Dexamethasone sodium phosphate (AK-Dex, Decadron Phosphate): intra-articular, topical, inhalant, ophthalmic preparations; used for many inflammatory and allergic disorders, dermatologic diseases, and cerebral edema

Methylprednisolone (Medrol): PO

Methylprednisolone (Solumedrol): IM, IV; anti-inflammatory; used in radiography as premedication for high-risk patients who have had previous allergic reactions or a history of allergies

Hydrocortisone (Hydrocortone, Cortef): PO, topical, parenteral (route depends on purpose and type of preparation)

Adverse Reactions: Hyperglycemia, exacerbation of diabetes, fat redistribution, moon face, peptic ulcers, weakness, behavioral disturbances, psychosis, edema, cardiac arrhythmias, heart failure, metabolic toxicity, and infections.

CALL OUT!

Do not stop adrenocorticosteroids abruptly after long-term therapy. To do so may be fatal! They must be administered by a person who is knowledgeable. Great caution must be exercised if given intravenously or intramuscularly, and these drugs may not be given intrathecally!

Drugs Used to Treat Osteoporosis

Osteoporosis is a disease that results in the deterioration of the substance of bones. It is associated with pain, loss of stature, and deformities. Fractures of the fragile bones occur very easily, sometimes as the result of very little or no direct trauma. It is a problem of postmenopausal women, sedentary or immobilized persons, and persons on long-term steroid therapy. Drug therapy is not totally effective but may slow the process of body deterioration. At present, the most widely used drugs to treat this condition are:

Estrogen replacement therapy: PO, IM, vaginal, transdermal patch; currently the most effective method of prevention for menopausal women

Adverse Reactions: Nausea, headaches, hypertension, endometrial cancer (without added progesterone), fluid retention, gallstones, and jaundice.

Calcium preparations (Os-Cal, Kalginate, calcium chloride): PO

Calcium chloride: given by slow injection to treat tetany and in CPR to increase cardiac contractibility; *found on emergency drug carts*

Adverse Reactions: Anorexia, nausea, vomiting, constipation, severe tissue necrosis when extravasation occurs, bradycardia, peripheral vasodilatation, and drop in blood pressure (IV).

Vitamin D: PO; used with calcium preparations for treatment of osteoporosis, rickets, and osteomalacia; increases effects of calcium

Adverse Reactions: Hypercalcemia, the symptoms of which are anorexia, nausea, abdominal pain, apathy, poor memory, depression, disorientation, and coma.

Insulin and Oral Hypoglycemic Drugs

Diabetes mellitus is not a single disease but a group of syndromes with the central characteristic of hyperglycemia. The disease is characterized by either a relative or absolute insulin deficiency. The major forms of the disease are type I or insulin-dependent diabetes mellitus (IDDM) and type II or non–insulin-dependent diabetes mellitus (NIDDM). Patients with IDDM are treated with insulin, and those with NIDDM are treated with oral hypoglycemic agents. Most insulin presently used is of the human form and is classified according to its duration of action. Insulin continues to be administered by subcutaneous injection, although there are a number of pumps that provide for continuous or as needed dosage.

Adverse Effects of Insulin: Hypoglycemia as demonstrated by sweating, tremor, blurred vision, slurred speech, weakness, hunger, confusion, loss of consciousness, coma, and death.

Glucagon: by injection; used to elevate glucose level when hypoglycemia occurs; *found on emergency drug carts*

Diazoxide (Proglycem): PO; elevates glucose levels

Adverse Reactions: Nausea, vomiting. Diazoxide may cause congestive heart failure, cardiac arrhythmias, hypotension. *Do not give glucagon or diazoxide during pregnancy or lactation.*

Oral Hypoglycemic Drugs

All are used to treat mild, stable NIDDM. The older agents require larger doses and have more drug interactions. The newer drugs are more potent and have fewer side effects.

Tolbutamide (Orinase): PO

Glipizide (Glucotrol): PO

Glyburide (Micronase): PO

Metformin (Glucophage): PO

Adverse Reactions: Older drugs (Orinase, Micronase): must be administered with care to the elderly, since they are at risk for renal and hepatic impairment. With newer drugs (Glipizide, Metformin), weight loss, diarrhea, abdominal discomfort, hypoglycemia, and GI upset can occur in patients of any age.

> /// **WARNING** \\\
> Oral hypoglycemic drugs must not be administered to insulin-dependent diabetics, persons in severe stress, or those with fevers or infections.

Drugs Used to Treat Infections

The drugs listed in each category are randomly chosen and do not indicate author preference or recommendation.

Antimicrobial Drugs

Antimicrobial drugs do not all react in the same way, nor do they all destroy the same types of microorganisms. They are chosen selectively for use by the physician according to their ability to inhibit or destroy particular bacteria, fungi, protozoa, viruses, or other parasites.

Although it is widely believed that anti-infective drugs can cure any infection without ill effects, this is not entirely true. There are continuing problems with administration of anti-infective drugs that remain unsolved. They are as follows:

1. *Tissue damage:* The GI mucosa becomes irritated when these drugs are taken by mouth, resulting in nausea, vomiting, and diarrhea. Local reactions at parenteral sites of injection may also occur. The most serious effects to body tissues are kidney damage and neurotoxicity. Neurotoxic symptoms can range from vertigo and deafness to convulsive seizures.

2. *Allergic reactions:* These may range from mild hypersensitivity to severe, life-threatening anaphylactic shock.

3. *Superinfections:* Use of anti-infective drugs destroys the pathogenic organisms but also inhibits the growth of natural flora of the body.

Without these natural inhabitants of the body, stronger microbes, or those that are not susceptible to these antimicrobial medications, grow uncontrollable and produce life-threatening infections.

4. *Misuse of anti-infective drugs*: Many people who have common upper respiratory infections (such as the common cold), which are caused by viruses unresponsive to these agents, request treatment with anti-infective drugs. This may result in a sensitivity to the drug prescribed, and when the drug is needed for treatment of a serious infection, an allergy to the drug requires that it be discontinued. Development of a resistance to the drug can also result, which renders it ineffective at a time when it is needed.

Antimicrobial drugs are sometimes used to prevent infection in susceptible patients. This is called *prophylactic use*. Some conditions that may require prophylactic use of antimicrobial drugs are bacterial endocarditis, neutropenia, HIV, and tuberculosis. These drugs may also be prescribed before major surgery.

Antimicrobial drugs should be used in a concentration and dosage high enough to destroy or inactivate the infectious microorganisms. They should also be used over a long enough period of time for this action to result. If this is not done, resistant strains develop and treatment is not successful. There are many antibacterial agents that are used when other drugs are not effective; these will not be mentioned in this brief synopsis. At times, antimicrobial drugs are used in combinations to increase effectiveness.

Anti-infective drugs vary in their effectiveness against microbes. This means that they have differing *spectrums* of activity or may be destructive to only a particular class of microbes. Some anti-infective drugs have a broad spectrum of effectiveness, meaning that they are useful for destroying many different types of microbe. Others have a narrow spectrum, meaning that they are of use for a limited number of microorganisms. There are also extended-spectrum anti-infective drugs, which are effective against gram-positive and some gram-negative bacteria. Antimicrobial families of drugs include the following:

Penicillins, cephalosporins, monobactams, vancomycin, carbapenems (antibacterials): these bactericidal (bacteria-destroying) drugs are administered at dosages that vary depending on the patient's age, type of infections, and weight.

Aminoglycosides, tetracyclines, macrolides, sulfonamides, trimethoprim: these drugs are bacteriostatic (growth-stopping) and/or bactericidal.

Isoniazid, rifampin, fluoroquinolones: general bacteriostatic agents.

PENICILLINS

The penicillins are widely used in various forms to treat gram-negative, gram-positive, and anaerobic bacteria. Some forms of penicillin are used as broad-spectrum antimicrobials (effective against a wide range of microorganisms). An enzyme produced by many bacteria, called penicillinase, is able to inactivate many forms of penicillin and promotes resistance to it. Many strains of staphylococci are able to produce penicillinase. The newest agents in the penicillin group of drugs are combined with penicillinase inhibitors. They perform the same as the previously listed penicillins; however, they also are able to work against penicillinase-producing bacteria. The following are some of these:

Ampicillin + sulbactam (Unasyn)

Amoxicillin + clavulanic acid (Augmentin)

Piperacillin + tazobactam (Zosyn)

Many drugs in the penicillin group of antimicrobials are given parenterally. Some are given by mouth.

Adverse Reactions: Allergic reactions ranging from skin rashes to anaphylaxis; fever, pain, phlebitis, nausea, diarrhea, and superinfection.

CEPHALOSPORINS

Cephalosporins are divided into four different groups, called *generations*, which are based on their activity against particular bacteria. Several of the widely used drugs in each generation are as follows:

- *First generation*: act against gram-positive bacteria (*Staphylococcus*, group A and B hemolytic streptococci) and gram-negative bacteria (*Escherichia coli*, *Klebsiella*, *Proteus mirabilis, and Haemophilus influenzae*). These drugs are not able to penetrate cerebrospinal fluid. Widely used drugs in this category are:
  Cephalexin (Keflex, Keflet, Keftab): PO
  Cefazolin (Ancef, Kefzol): IM, IV
  Cephalothin (Keflin): administered parenterally
- *Second generation*: act against gram-negative bacteria and some gram-positive bacteria. They are not able to penetrate the CNS. Widely used drugs in this category are:
  Cefaclor (Ceclor): PO
  Cefprozil (Cefzil): PO
  Cefoxitin (Mefoxin): administered parenterally
- *Third generation*: have reduced gram-positive action; act against gram-negative bacteria such as *Salmonella, Enterobacter, Pseudomonas aeruginosa, Serratia*. These drugs are able to enter the cerebrospinal fluid. Drugs in this category are:
  Cefixime (Suprax): PO
  Ceftriaxone (Rocephin): administered parenterally

Adverse Reactions: Hypersensitivity, bone marrow suppression, nephrotoxicity, bleeding disorders, nausea, and vomiting.

Cefepime (Maxipime): IV, IM

Adverse Reactions: Headache, phlebitis, GI disturbances, urticaria, pain, inflammation, and fever. Pseudomembranous Colitis. Use with Caution.

MONOBACTAMS

This new class of antimicrobial drug has a narrow spectrum of activity. Monobactams act against gram-negative bacteria only. The drug representing this class is aztreonam (administered parenterally).

Adverse Reactions: Diarrhea, abdominal cramps, nausea, and vomiting.

Vancomycin: IV, PO; only as prophylaxis against bacterial endocarditis; highly toxic and used when other drugs are no longer effective

Adverse Reactions: Hearing loss, renal failure, superinfections, and "red man syndrome." This reaction manifests with severe hypotension, fever, chills, paresthesias, and redness of neck and back.

AMINOGLYCOSIDES

Aminoglycoside drugs are both bacteriostatic and bactericidal and act against gram-negative and gram-positive microorganisms. Drugs in this category are toxic and are used when other antimicrobial drugs are not effective. Drugs in this class include the following:

Gentamicin (Garamycin): IM, IV

Streptomycin: IM

Adverse Reactions: Ototoxicity and nephrotoxicity. These drugs are not to be administered with other antibacterial drugs.

TETRACYCLINES

Tetracyclines are bacteriostatic and are true broad-spectrum antibacterial drugs. They are used to treat rickettsial infections, chlamydia, cholera, mycoplasma pneumonia, and Lyme disease. Widely used drugs in this category are:

Doxycycline: PO

Minocycline: PO

Adverse Reactions: GI irritation; discoloration of teeth in children and depression of bone growth; renal and liver toxicity, suprainfections.

MACROLIDES

Macrolides are bacteriostatic in low doses and bactericidal in high doses. They are broad-spectrum antibacterial drugs used to treat diseases caused by gram-positive microbes such as Legionnaire's disease. Widely used drugs in this category are:

Erythromycin: administered PO and IV

Azithromycin: PO, IV

Clarithromycin: PO, IV

Adverse Reactions: GI distress, nausea and vomiting, thrombophlebitis when administered intravenously, anaphylactic reactions, cholestatic hepatitis. These drugs must not be mixed with other drugs.

SULFONAMIDES AND TRIMETHOPRIM

Sulfonamides are most commonly used to treat urinary tract infections and chlamydia. Trimethoprim is frequently used in combination with sulfamethoxazole (TMP-SMX) to treat *Shigella*, systemic salmonellosis, and prostatitis. These drugs are administered orally.

Adverse Reactions: Nausea and vomiting, rash, crystalluria, toxic nephrosis, and hypersensitivity reactions; adverse effects increased in combination with SMZ.

FLUOROQUINOLONES

These drugs are bactericidal and are effective against gram-negative microbes and some gram-positive microbes. They are used to treat urinary tract infections, gonorrhea, resistant respiratory infections and acute diarrheal illnesses. Widely used drugs in this category are:

Ciprofloxacin (Cipro): PO

Norfloxacin (Noroxin): PO

Lomefloxacin (Maxaquin): PO

Adverse Reactions: Nausea and vomiting, diarrhea, headache, drowsiness, seizures, and visual disturbances.

/ / / **WARNING** \ \ \

Fluoroquinolones must not be used for pregnant women, nursing mothers, or children under 18 years of age, because these drugs produce articular cartilage erosion in immature laboratory animals.

Antifungal Agents

Major fungal infections may be treated systemically or by topical route. Widely used drugs in this category are:

Amphotericin B: IV or intrathecally

Nystatin: PO or topically to mucous membranes

Adverse Reactions

Amphotericin B: fever, chills, nephrotoxicity, anemia, pain, anaphylaxis, intra-alveolar hemorrhage; highly toxic

Nystatin: highly toxic systemically; topical administration can result in skin irritation, hypersensitivity when given PO

Antimycobacterial Drugs

The drugs in this category are used to treat mycobacterial diseases, primarily tuberculosis and leprosy. The drugs frequently used to treat tuberculosis are:

Isoniazid: PO

Adverse Reactions: Hypersensitivity.

Rifampin: PO

Adverse Reactions: Nausea, vomiting, rash, and fever.

The drugs used to treat leprosy are as follows and are recommended to be used as a triple drug regimen by the world Health Organization:

Dapsone: PO

Adverse Reactions: Hemolysis, peripheral neuropathy, erythema nodosum leprosum, and blood dyscrasias.

Clofazimine: PO

Adverse Reaction: red-brown discoloration of the skin.

Rifampin is the third drug recommended for treatment of leprosy.

Antiviral Drugs

Antiviral drugs are used to prevent or treat viral infections including genital herpes simplex virus, AIDS-related infections, hepatitis, leukemia, and Kaposi's sarcoma. Drugs frequently used in this class are:

Amantadine: PO to treat respiratory viral infections

Adverse Reactions: Nausea and vomiting, insomnia, nervousness, and urine retention. Use with caution in patients with glaucoma, in pregnant women, and in nursing mothers.

Acyclovir (Zovirax): PO, IV, and as a topical ointment; used to treat herpes and cytomegalovirus infections

Adverse Reactions: Irritation and local reactions at injection site, phlebitis, renal impairment, and blood dyscrasias. Orally may cause vertigo, depression, diarrhea, and fever.

Famciclovir (Famvir): PO; used only to treat acute herpes zoster

Adverse Reactions: Headache, fever, nausea, and arthralgia.

Stavudine (Zerit): PO; used to treat persons with advanced HIV

Adverse Reactions: Blood dyscrasias, chest pain, peripheral neuropathy, abdominal symptoms, and liver toxicity.

Zidovudine (AZT and Retrovir): used to treat HIV infections

Adverse Reactions: Blood dyscrasias, bone marrow suppression, headache, nausea and vomiting, mouth ulcers, nosebleeds, acne, and pruritus. Must be used with caution in pregnant and breast-feeding women.

Interferon alfa-2b recombinant (Intron-A): IV, IM, SC; other preparations used to treat hepatitis, leukemia, and Kaposi's sarcoma; this preparation used to treat hairy cell leukemia

Adverse Reactions: Dizziness, confusion, depression, anxiety, GI symptoms, blood dyscrasias, and others.

Antiprotozoal and anthelmintic drugs are not included in this text but are available.

Fluids, Electrolytes, and Nutrients

Intravenous replacement of fluid, electrolytes, and nutrients is part of the medical care of most patients treated in acute care hospitals. It is also part of many home care medical treatments. Intravenous fluids are frequently used in radiographic imaging departments as part of the diagnostic plan of care. Often, the hospitalized patient comes to the radiographic imaging department with intravenous fluids being administered. It is not within the radiographer's scope of practice to select the intravenous solution to be used; however, you must recognize the reasons for their use and the potential hazards of these preparations.

Intravenous fluids are administered to patients to replace fluids, reestablish electrolyte balance, or provide vitamins or calories. They are also used as diluents for medication administration. Fluid must be replaced when a person becomes dehydrated. Dehydration occurs when more fluid is lost from the body than is taken in, usually because of a pathological disturbance of body function. Some electrolytes are lost with the fluid, and some become more concentrated within the body, thus creating an electrolyte imbalance. Electrolytes are elements or compounds that, when dissolved in a solvent (water in the human body), separate into ions capable of conducting electrical activity. Electrolytes in the body vary in concentration, depending on whether they are in blood plasma, interstitial fluid, or cellular fluid. This variability affects movement of substances between compartments within the body depending on concentration gradients.

Depletion of or an excess of one electrolyte affects the concentration of all others. For the body to function in a state of good health, the correct balance of fluids, electrolytes, and nutrients must be maintained. When a person is acutely ill, this balance is maintained by IV therapy.

There are many prepared combinations of fluid and electrolyte solutions for IV use. Vitamins, minerals, and medications may be added to these solutions or given separately as prescribed. Parenteral solutions for IV nutrition are also available.

There are hydrating solutions composed of water, carbohydrate, and varying amounts of sodium chloride. These solutions do not usually contain potassium, which is essential to body function but may be harmful if present in excess amounts.

There are solutions designed to help the body meet its energy requirements. The fluid in these solutions may be either normal saline or water. The dextrose content may be either 5% or 10%. Intravenous replacement solutions usually are packaged in containers of 250 mL, 500 mL, and 1000 mL. Some of the widely used parenteral fluids and their uses are listed in Table 12-3.

More simple solutions are also available, which contain dextrose in various concentrations and normal saline solutions. You will work with this type of solution when the patient needs an IV line available but does not require electrolytes or nutrients.

Electrolyte replacement therapy is not necessarily prescribed by IV route. Oral and intramuscular preparations are also available. Some of those widely used are:

Potassium chloride (e.g., K-Lor, Slow-K, K-Lyte): PO and in parenteral solutions; potassium is necessary to maintain cellular osmolarity, to transmit nerve impulses, and for muscle contraction

Adverse Reactions: Bradycardia, nausea, vomiting, diarrhea, cardiac arrest, dysphagic, respiratory distress, weakness, and muscle paralysis leading to death. By injection: tissue sloughing, necrosis, phlebitis, and venospasm.

Sodium chloride: IV, may take PO; needed to maintain osmotic pressure and serum osmolarity; sodium regulates fluid volume and controls muscle contraction

Adverse Reactions: With deficit, anorexia, nausea, mental confusion, giddiness, apprehension, convulsions, pallor, clammy skin, and low blood pressure. With excess, symptoms of fluid volume excess (edema, disorientation, twitching, hyperirritability, coma).

Magnesium: IV; used to treat convulsive states and cerebral edema, correction of nutritional deficiency and uterine tetany

Adverse Reactions: Absence of knee-jerk reflex, hypotension, respiratory depression, profuse perspiration, circulatory collapse, cardiac arrest.

Sodium bicarbonate: IV; used in emergencies to treat metabolic acidosis, ketoacidosis, and hyperkalemia; *found on emergency drug carts*

Vitamins and Minerals

The maintenance of good health requires an adequate daily intake of vitamins and minerals. These are usually acquired by eating animal and vegetable products that contain them. If vitamins or minerals are lacking in the diet for a period of time, diseases may result. Many people feel that a daily supplement of vitamins and minerals is needed to ensure that these nutritional needs are met.

Vitamins are either fat-soluble or water-soluble. The fat-soluble vitamins are vitamins A, D, E, and K.

TABLE 12-3 — **Parenteral Solutions**	
PARENTERAL FLUID	**USAGE**
Hydrating solutions	Dextrose in water—2.5%, 5%, 10% Dextrose in NaCl—2.5% in 0.45% NaCl Dextrose 5% in NaCl 0.45%
Maintenance solutions	PlasmaLyte 56 PlasmaLyte 148 (Isolyte s) Normal saline 0.9%
Isotonic solutions	Lactated Ringer's solutions Normal saline
Hypertonic solutions	Sodium chloride 3% for injection Sodium chloride 5% for injection

The water-soluble vitamins are vitamins B_1, B_2, B_5, B_{12}, C, folic acid, pantothenic acid, niacin, and biotin.

The minerals necessary to maintain health are iron, calcium, magnesium, sodium, potassium, phosphorus, copper, zinc, iodine, cobalt, chromium, manganese, and selenium. Most of these are necessary in only trace amounts.

It is not within the scope of this text to discuss each vitamin and mineral individually. Those that the radiographer may see in practice have been discussed in previous sections of this chapter.

Intravascular and Iodinated Contrast Media

Intravascular radiopaque contrast media (ROCM) are the drugs that you will work with most frequently in your professional practice as a radiographer. Contrast agents are categorized as drugs because they can be absorbed into the systemic circulation and may affect a physiologic response. When an anatomical area is filled or outlined by these agents, the image of the organ appears to be white or light (positive contrast), whereas negative agents make the organs appear dark. Negative contrast agents are discussed in Chapter 10.

Barium is the most common type of contrast used in the imaging of the GI system. Because barium is a metal, it does not dissolve; it is suspended in solution. Barium and Gastrografin as they are used in the GI system were discussed in Chapter 10 of this text.

The most frequently used intravascular contrast agents used in diagnostic imaging procedures contain iodine. Iodine has a high atomic density and can provide the contrast needed for visualization in areas of the body where there is no natural contrast, as in bones (Fig. 12-7). It is the iodine atoms in the contrast media molecules that are the primary attenuators of the new ionizing radiation.

Iodinated contrast agents are used in examinations of the GI tract, kidneys, gallbladder, pancreas, heart, brain, adrenal glands, arteries, veins, and joints. They are used to increase the visibility of body cavities, organs, and vascular system in diagnostic imaging, fluoroscopy, and other imaging modalities. Special imaging procedures are discussed in Chapter 16.

The most important variables that a physician considers when selecting a contrast agent are the ability of the agent to mix with body fluids, its viscosity, its ionic strength, its persistence in the body, its iodine content, its osmolality, and its potential for toxicity. Most contrast agents are water-based; however, a few imaging procedures require an oil-based contrast agent.

Iodinated contrast agents are administered by oral, vaginal, intravenous, and intra-arterial routes. They may also be directly instilled into joints (percutaneous

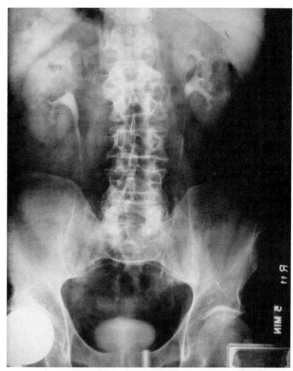

Figure 12–7. Intravenous pyelogram using an iodinated contrast agent. This image is reversed.

route) or into body cavities. They can be distributed easily to areas where visualization is needed for diagnosis and then excreted from the body in a relatively dependable manner.

Drugs used to treat most illnesses are administered in small dosages at selected intervals, whereas contrast agents are administered in a large dose at one time (by bolus). Another variation from other drugs used for treatment is that most other drugs administered intravascularly are isotonic. This means that they have the same concentration of solute as another solution; therefore, they exert the same amount of osmotic pressure as that solution (in this case, the fluids of the body). Contrast agents have osmolalities that are much higher than those of body fluids. They are also very viscous (thick and sticky). When they are administered intravascularly, the high osmolality and viscosity of iodinated contrast agents prompt a sudden shift in body fluid from the interstitial spaces and cells into the systemic circulation. This abrupt physiologic change is thought to cause the adverse effects that occur in some instances with administration of intravascular contrast agents.

There is a group of newer contrast agents that are nonionic and have a lower osmolarity (determined by the number of particles in solution). Use of these agents decreases the potential for adverse reactions. Whenever possible, these agents are chosen by the physician for use, because they have a wider margin of safety and comfort for the patient.

Ionic and Nonionic Contrast Agents

All positive (radiopaque) contrast agents contain iodine. The iodine in contrast agents provides the contrast (or density difference) between the organ and its surrounding tissues by attenuating the x-ray beam. The chemical makeup of ionic and nonionic contrast differs in the number of particles in solution, not in the number of iodine compounds. Ionic contrast agents are also known as high-osmolar contrast media (HOCM). Conversely, nonionic contrasts are considered low-osmolar contrast media (LOCM). Osmolarity can be thought of as the volume of the compound, whereas osmolality can be identified as the weight of the ion. A side chain of HOCM that creates the osmotic effect (known as the cation) is responsible for an increased risk of adverse reactions. When this cation is removed from the contrast compound and replaced with a group of lower osmolality, the risk of an adverse reaction is significantly reduced. The removal of this cation does not degrade the radiographic image.

A crucial factor to consider in the selection of a contrast agent is its osmolality. Conventional contrasts (ionic) are hyperosmotic to body fluids such as blood. Ionic contrast agents disassociate into separate ions in solution causing problems such as spasms of the veins, fluid retention and cardiac symptoms. Nonionic contrast agents have an osmolality that is much closer to that of human plasma and will result in fewer and less severe reactions. All contrast agents currently in use are considered safe; however, all may result in adverse reactions.

CALL OUT!

Ionic contrast agents (HOCM) differ from nonionic contrast agents (LOCM) only in the number of particles in solution.

Reactions to Contrast Agents and Treatment

Several reactions may occur when an iodinated contrast agent is administered. These reactions are most apt to occur when the agent is administered intravenously or intra-arterially. There are expected side effects that do no harm; but must be explained to the patient to alleviate anxiety while they are occurring. Expected side effects include a feeling of flushing and a metallic taste in the mouth. Adverse reactions are not predictable and may be a threat to the patient's life.

The ionic, high-osmolality iodinated contrast agents are most frequently associated with adverse reactions. These reactions range from mild to severe and life threatening. The rapidity and skill with which these reactions are observed and treated make a significant difference in the patient outcome. You will most often be the health care worker who is present to observe symptoms of a potential adverse reaction; therefore, it is your obligation to be skilled in assessment so that you may recognize problems quickly and initiate the emergency action necessary to resolve them.

The American College of Radiology has identified the following classifications of adverse reactions: mild (minor), intermediate, and major (severe), which can be life threatening. A fourth reaction has been identified as being a reaction to the procedure rather than to the contrast agent itself. This is a vasovagal response and occurs when the patient experiences high anxiety about the procedure and its result.

Invasive radiographic procedures are frequently stressful. The patient's mental state before and during a procedure that requires contrast media is of great importance. The professional radiographer must be able to identify the highly anxious patient during the initial assessment interview. You must use your critical thinking skills and your therapeutic communication techniques to alleviate the patient's anxiety. You must assess the patient's understanding of the procedure and inform him or her in detail about how it will proceed. Education about some expected side effects of iodinated contrast media that are not symptoms of an adverse reaction should also be explained to prevent feelings of anxiety. When the patient understands what to expect and what is occurring, his or her anxiety will be greatly reduced. The patient must also be allowed to express feelings of anxiety because this also reduces these feelings. Thoughtful care by you as the radiographer will establish a feeling of trust in the patient and adverse reactions may be avoided.

Clinical manifestations of a vasovagal reaction include pallor, cold sweats, and syncope. Symptoms of a vasovagal reaction may be tachycardia or bradycardia and hypotension.

The following are possible effects of iodinated contrast media.

CLINICAL MANIFESTATIONS

- A feeling of flushing or warmth: may result from a bolus injection of a high osmolarity contrast medium being injected rapidly

- Nausea and/or vomiting: feeling may pass quickly or may be a precursor to an anaphylactic reaction

- Headache: may pass without note or may also be a precursor to an anaphylactic reaction

- Pain at the injection site: a burning sensation that occurs as a result of leakage into the surrounding tissues or may simply be the result of the large-gauge needle needed for the contrast agent
- Altered taste, may be metallic: results from the iodine content of the contrast agent

RADIOGRAPHER'S RESPONSE

1. Notify the radiologist or the radiology nurse.
2. Stop or slow the rate of the contrast injection.
3. Observe the patient closely and reassure the patient.

MILD ADVERSE REACTIONS

- Complaints of itching of nose and eyes
- Anxiety
- Cough
- Hives or rash

RADIOGRAPHER'S RESPONSE

1. Stop the infusion, and notify the radiologist or radiology nurse.
2. Do not leave the patient unattended
3. Reassure the patient; however, understand that these symptoms may quickly escalate into a severe anaphylactic reaction.

INTERMEDIATE REACTION

- Coughing that results from laryngospasm or angioedema of the upper respiratory tract leading to a feeling of tickling in the throat
- Dyspnea and wheezing resulting from edema
- Initial symptoms of shock: anxiety, rapid pulse, rapid respirations, hypotension
- Complaints of chest pain

RADIOGRAPHER'S RESPONSE

1. Stop the infusion.
2. Notify the radiologist and the radiology nurse.
3. Call for the emergency team if symptoms progress rapidly from intermediate to severe.
4. Stay with the patient and offer reassurance.
5. Prepare to administer oxygen and intravenous medications such as Benadryl or epinephrine.

6. If the patient is in respiratory distress, place in a semi-Fowler's position.
7. Position patient who is vomiting so that aspiration does not occur.

MAJOR REACTION

You must understand that all clinical manifestations before this stage of adverse reactions may occur quickly and advance to a major reaction within 2 or 3 minutes. Never ignore early manifestations of an anaphylactic reaction.

- Shock
- Seizures
- Cardiac arrest

RADIOGRAPHER'S RESPONSE

1. Call a Code Blue.
2. Notify the radiologist.
3. Prepare to use AED (automated external defibrillator) equipment.
4. Prepare to administer oxygen and intravenous medications.

CALL OUT!

Patients who are receiving iodinated contrast media must not be left unattended. An anaphylactic reaction can occur quickly and without warning!

If symptoms are present and are allowed to progress, the patient may develop pulmonary edema, bronchospasm, cardiac arrhythmia, and cardiac arrest. For most diagnostic imaging procedures that require use of a contrast agent, a peripheral intravenous infusion is started to maintain hydration and to permit emergency administration of medications if the situation requires this. This ensures that there will be an intravenous access line established and saves valuable time in an emergency. Most reactions occur relatively soon after administration of the contrast agent is begun; therefore, you need to carefully observe the patient initially.

Although most reactions to contrast media occur within the first several minutes after administration, delayed reactions are possible. These reactions are infrequent, and you are usually not aware of them because the patient has left the department by the time they occur. You must instruct the patient to obtain medical care if they have symptoms such as fever, joint pain, malaise, skin rash, and swollen lymph nodes.

Precautions for Elderly and Pediatric Patients

Although the contrast agents used for the elderly patient and the pediatric patient are generally the same as those used for the average adult patient, the amount administered varies. The potential for fluid and electrolyte imbalance is far greater in this population; therefore, the dosage must be individualized with great care to prevent renal failure and other adverse reactions. Low-osmolar contrast media are often chosen for infants and children. If the child is to be sedated for a procedure, a person who is educated in pediatric care must be present to administer the drug.

Elderly patients have a greater potential for impaired renal or hepatic function, which makes them more prone to life-threatening fluid and electrolyte imbalance. They may also present for care in a dehydrated state. Careful consideration must be given to the care of persons in this age group.

Patient Assessment and Care

Before administering a contrast agent, you must perform an assessment. This is often preceded by requesting the patient to respond in writing to a printed assessment questionnaire that each department has formulated for an overview of the patient's health problems. You must read the patient's responses and make certain that the patient fully understands the questionnaire and that the responses are accurate. If there are positive responses that indicate a problem that may affect the procedure, you must notify the physician before beginning the procedure. For most invasive procedures, an informed consent must also be signed and in place. It is your obligation as the radiographer to confirm that consents are correctly signed and that the health assessment is complete and accurate. The assessment information that must be obtained is as follows:

1. Age of patient

2. History of impaired hepatic function (liver disease)

3. History of impaired renal function (kidney disease)

4. History of hypersensitivity reactions (allergic or anaphylactic reactions) (described in Chapter 7)

5. History of thyroid disease: hyperthyroidism or hypothyroidism

6. Possibility of pregnancy

7. Lactation (nursing mother)

8. Sensitivity to aspirin

9. Sensitivity to tartrazine (a coloring agent used in foods and beverages)

10. History of diabetes mellitus

11. History of multiple myeloma (a malignant tumor of the bone marrow)

12. History of sickle cell disease (a chronic, incurable anemic condition affecting red blood cells)

13. History of hypertension

14. History of heart disease including congestive heart failure

15. History of pheochromocytoma (a tumor of the adrenal gland resulting in excess secretion of epinephrine and norepinephrine)

16. History of homocystinuria (an inherited disease caused by enzyme deficiencies that may result in mental retardation and skeletal abnormalities)

17. Medication history (list all medications taken, including over-the-counter drugs taken occasionally)

18. History of previous reactions to medications or contrast agents

---

CALL OUT!

Patients who are highly anxious, have heart disease or renal insufficiency, or are generally debilitated or dehydrated are at risk for adverse reactions.

Other considerations when iodinated contrast agents are used are as follows:

1. Infants, children, and elderly patients are rapidly dehydrated by the osmotic diuretic action of iodinated contrast agents. Restriction of fluids in preparation for diagnostic examinations using these agents is not advised as it may produce life-threatening dehydration and renal failure.

2. Highly viscous contrast agents should not be directly injected into the carotid or vertebral arteries.

3. Extravasation (infiltration) of iodinated contrast agents may cause extensive tissue damage and must be prevented.

4. Overdosage of iodine may occur. Eighty to 90 g of iodine rapidly administered may produce symptoms of overdosage, which are tremors, irritability, and tachycardia (early symptoms). If such symptoms occur, stop administration of the contrast agent immediately and initiate emergency action.

5. All solutions of contrast agents should be administered at body temperature.

6. All solutions administered must be clear. If there are particles in the solution, it must be discarded.

7. Protect iodinated contrast media from exposure to light

8. Discard all unused agents that have been opened.

9. Do not mix contrast agents with other drugs.

10. Do not mix contrast agents with other contrast agents.

Nonionic, low-osmolar (determined by number of particles in the solution), iodinated contrast agents decrease the potential for adverse reactions. Use of such a contrast agent decreases the incidence of cardiovascular symptoms, nausea and vomiting, pain during injection, and adverse effects on the circulating blood volume. Whenever possible, low-osmolar nonionic agents are chosen for use for the safety and comfort of the patient.

Many iodinated contrast agents are quite viscid. This property contributes to discomfort during injection. Some agents are so viscid that they must be administered by power injector (Fig. 12-8). You must remember that all iodinated contrast agents, particularly the viscid agents, are most comfortable for the patient when administered at body temperature. Power injectors have heating mechanisms. If there is no power injector, raise the temperature of the contrast agents to body temperature by placing the solution to be injected into a basin of tepid water for 10 to 15 minutes before administration. This reduces the viscosity of the agent and thereby decreases the amount of physiologic basal constriction and pain produced by administration at room temperature. You must ensure that the temperature of contrast agent is not higher than body temperature when administered to prevent unnecessary pain and discomfort to the patient.

The patient must also be instructed to increase fluid intake after a procedure that involves a contrast agent and to seek medical care immediately if he or she is unable to urinate or has difficulty doing so. A list of contrast agents that are used for special procedures appears in Chapter 16.

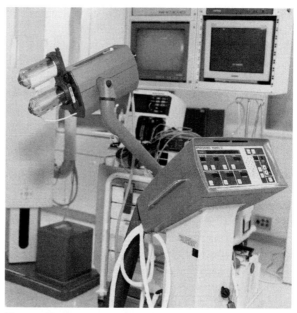

Figure 12–8. Injector pump.

Summary

Any health care worker who administers drugs must have both theoretical and clinical education in pharmacology. He or she must also understand the pharmacokinetics and pharmacodynamics of drugs, their intended physiologic actions, and the potential adverse reactions that each can cause.

Each drug that is marketed for medical use has several names: a chemical name derived from its chemical formula, a generic name given before official approval, and a trade name given and governed by a particular manufacturer. The chemical name and the generic name do not change, but the same drug may have more than one trade name. You must acquaint yourself with the generic name and the various trade names of the drugs used frequently in your department.

The federal government has established standards for control of drug safety. Drugs that create dependency are restricted and are categorized according to their margin of safety. These established categories are called drug schedules.

A drug is taken into the body and then must be made bioavailable for use at a particular receptor site. The route of administration determines the amount of time it takes for a drug to become bioavailable. The amount of blood flow; the size of the surface area available for absorption; and the patient's emotional state, age, and other factors determine how a drug is absorbed and utilized in the body. The routes of drug administration are enteral (oral or rectal), parenteral, and topical. The method of administration is determined by the chemical nature of the drug and the limitations of the particular individual.

Drugs are most commonly administered by the oral route. This is considered to be the most efficient and economical route and is used for drugs that will not be destroyed by gastric secretions or when the patient is not suffering from nausea and vomiting. This route is also used when a prolonged period of effectiveness is necessary.

The most common parenteral routes of drug administration are subcutaneous, intramuscular, intradermal, and intravenous. These routes of drug administration are used when rapid action and shorter duration of action are desired.

After a drug is administered, it is absorbed. The manner in which a drug enters the body determines the rate at which it is absorbed and the length of time it takes to achieve its desired effect. Once a drug has been absorbed, it is distributed to its intended site of action through the circulatory system. The rate and extent of distribution depend on the adequacy of circulating blood, protein binding, and the drug's affinity for lipoid or aqueous tissues.

After absorption and distribution, drugs are metabolized and excreted from the body. The liver is the center for drug metabolism, and most drugs are excreted through the kidneys after biotransformation. Age, overall health, time of day, emotional status, and the presence of other drugs in the body may alter the rate of drug metabolism. As the radiographer, you must proceed with caution when administering a drug to the very young and the very old patient, for these age groups have special problems with drug metabolism. A health care worker educated in administration of drugs to children should be called to give these drugs.

The potential for an adverse reaction to a drug must always be considered, since all drugs are potentially harmful and may be life threatening. As a radiographer administering any drug, you must be acquainted with its potential adverse reactions as well as its intended action. You must observe your patient for these reactions and educate the patient regarding the effects of the drugs that you administer. The right patient must receive the right drug in the right dose at the right time by the right route. A drug history must be taken for every patient before administering any drug.

Drugs may be categorized in various ways. In this chapter, they are categorized according to their intended purpose or the manner in which they affect a body system. You must become familiar with the drugs that will be found on the emergency drug cart and those frequently administered in your department. Contrast media are the drugs that you will see most frequently. You must be knowledgeable concerning their indications, contraindications, and adverse reactions.

Contrast media are categorized as positive or negative contrasts. Negative contrasts are also known as radiolucent and are in the form of a gas. Positive contrasts are also known as radiopaque and can be further categorized as ionic and nonionic contrast. The number of iodine particles found in solution of contrast agents influences the possibility and severity of an adverse reaction when administered to the patient. The osmolarity of the contrast agent is a factor in the severity of an adverse reaction; therefore, you must be aware of the chemical makeup of the contrast injected and be prepared to act in the event of such an incident.

You must also compile a patient history before administering a contrast agent. You must report any negative data gathered from the history to the physician caring for the patient. This must be done before the agent is administered. If the patient has an adverse reaction to a contrast agent, you must stop the administration of the agent and call for assistance. You must never leave unattended a patient who is receiving a contrast agent.

The patient's age, weight, sex, medication history, history of allergies, emotional status, occupation, and overall physical condition, as well as the reason for the drug administration and the route and time, are factors that must be taken into account in determining the strength and quantity of drug to be prescribed. You must be aware of these factors and be alert to any deviation from normal reactions to drugs by patients when in radiographic imaging.

Chapter 12 Test

_____ **1.** All drugs, if misused, are poisons.
   a. True
   b. False

2. Explain the legal accountability of any health care worker who administers drugs.

_____ **3.** The purpose of drug metabolism is to
   a. Initiate a physiologic response
   b. Break down the drug for absorption throughout the body
   c. Transform the drug for distribution throughout the body
   d. Break down the drug for distribution throughout the body

_____ **4.** Which of the following best describes drug efficacy?
   a. The maximal response produced by the drug
   b. The amount of drug required for an adverse reaction to occur
   c. The amount of drug needed to produce the desired response
   d. The amount of drug needed to reach the plateau response

_____ **5.** What change in an elderly person alters the absorption of an oral medication?
   a. Decreased gastric secretion
   b. Decreased total body mass
   c. Increased total body fat
   d. Decreased cardiac output

6. List the factors that will alter drug absorption in the body.

_____ **7.** Drugs given by mouth are generally given in larger doses. This is because
   a. They absorb more slowly
   b. They absorb more rapidly
   c. They are unreliable
   d. Larger doses ensure that some of the drug will remain to perform the intended effect

_____ **8.** For a drug to reach its therapeutic effect more quickly, a physician might order
   a. A larger initial dose and later smaller doses
   b. A smaller initial dose, then a larger dose
   c. A bolus
   d. A maximizing dose

9. Differentiate between an adverse reaction and a side effect of a drug.

_____ **10.** Marjorie Belweather takes oral morphine for chronic pain. After taking the prescribed dosage for 2 weeks, she notices that it no longer seems to be controlling the pain. This reaction is called
   a. Addiction
   b. Dependency
   c. Tolerance
   d. An adverse reaction

_____ **11.** Two drugs must never be mixed in the same syringe for administration before checking their
   a. Effectiveness
   b. Correct dosage
   c. Compatibility
   d. Expiration dates

12. List the problems with antimicrobial drugs other than adverse reactions.

13. List the composition of neurotransmitters.

_____ **14.** Identify the following symptoms as either (1) sympathetic response or (2) parasympathetic response.
   a. Heart rate increases.
   b. Epinephrine is secreted.
   c. Gastric motility and secretion increase.
   d. Salivation increases.
   e. Gastric motility decreases.

15. Differentiate between administration of an iodinated contrast agent and most other drugs administered.

16. List the side effects and the adverse reactions to iodinated contrast agents, and describe the radiographer's response to each.

17. Explain the problems with administering iodinated contrast agents to the elderly patient and the pediatric patient.

_____ **18.** The drug name given by a particular manufacturer is the
  a. Trade name
  b. Generic name
  c. Chemical name
  d. Proper name

_____ **19.** An analgesic is a drug used for
  a. Vasodilation
  b. Decongestion
  c. Relief of pain
  d. Enuresis

_____ **20.** Factors that may influence the effect of a drug are
  a. Age and weight
  b. Sex and time of day
  c. Medication history and the patient's temperament
  d. a and b
  e. a, b, and c

_____ **21.** The channel of drug administration does not influence the amount of drug administered.
  a. True
  b. False

_____ **22.** Parenteral drug routes may include
  a. Intramuscular
  b. Intravenous
  c. Oral
  d. a and c
  e. a and b

_____ **23.** An abnormally rapid heartbeat is called
  a. Tachypnea
  b. Tachycardia
  c. Tetany
  d. Teratogenic

_____ **24.** A drug that increases the flow of urine is called a
  a. Derivative
  b. Diuretic
  c. Digestant
  d. Demulcent

25. Define _cumulative effect_ of drugs, _drug tolerance_, and _drug resistance_.

26. List the assessment questions that you as the radiographer must ask before your patient receives an iodinated contrast agent.

27. List precautions to be taken if iodinated contrast agents are to be administered.

28. Match the words with the most appropriate word or medical abbreviation below.
  1. The study of drug actions and interactions with living organisms
  2. Drugs with potential for abuse
  3. Interaction of drugs with body tissues
  4. Drugs metabolized and changed into water-soluble substances
  5. A change in normal physiologic function due to a drug

  a. Controlled substances
  b. Pharmacology
  c. Pharmacokinetics
  d. Pharmacodynamics
  e. Biotransformation

_____ **29.** Which of the following statements is not true regarding barium?
   a. It is an inert substance.
   b. It is a metal, so it will not dissolve.
   c. It is mixed in solution for the purpose of GI studies.
   d. It is suspended in solution.

_____ **30.** Which of the following is a false statement?
   a. Radiolucent contrast agents are in the form of liquids, powdersor tablets.
   b. Radiolucent contrast agents are also known as negative contrast agents.
   c. Positive contrast agents contain iodine.
   d. Ionic contrast agents are also known as high-osmolar contrast

_____ **31.** Nonionic contrast agents contain iodine.
   a. True
   b. False

_____ **32.** Ionic contrast agents (HOCM) differ from nonionic contrast agents (LOCM) only in the number of particles in solution.
   a. True
   b. False

_____ **33.** Reactions that are expected and predictable and are not detrimental to the health of the patient are
   a. Adverse reactions
   b. Side effects
   c. Unknown situations that the radiographer is not able to predicate
   d. Vasovagal reactions

_____ **34.** Signs of a vasovagal reaction include
   1. Pallor   a. 1 and 2 only
   2. Cold sweats   b. 2 and 4 only
   3. Rapid pulse   c. 1 and 4 only
   4. Bradycardia   d. All of the above

13

Drug Administration

Objectives

After studying this chapter, you will be able to:

1. List the precautions to be taken during drug administration.

2. Differentiate between the apothecary and metric systems of measurement and be able to quickly convert from one measure to the other.

3. List the components of a medication order and the method of documenting drug administration.

4. Describe your accountability as the radiographer in drug administration and your responsibilities if an adverse reaction occurs.

5. State the components of a patient's drug history.

6. Explain the procedure to be followed if a medication error is made.

7. Identify accurately the sites for administering by oral, buccal, and sublingual routes and for intradermal, subcutaneous, intramuscular, intravenous, and intradermal routes.

8. Accurately demonstrate in the school laboratory the administration of drugs by oral, buccal, sublingual, subcutaneous, intramuscular, intravenous, and intradermal routes.

9. List the symptoms that indicate infiltration or extravasation into the surrounding tissues by an intravenous injection or infusion, and list the radiographer's actions if either of these occurs.

10. Identify and define the common medical abbreviations used in medication administration.

Glossary

antipyretic: An agent that reduces fever

arrhythmia: An irregularity in or loss of rhythm of the heartbeat

cochlear: Pertaining to the bony structure of the inner ear; the bony spiral tunnel within the cochlea

enteric coated: A covering added to oral medications that is designed to be absorbed in the intestinal tract

extravasation: An escape of fluid into the body tissues, usually blood

gtt: Medical abreviation for drop

infiltration: Fluid passing into the body tissues

intra-articular: Within the joint

intrathecal: An injection into the spinal cord

percutaneous: Performed through the skin

periostitis: Inflammation of the periosteum of the bone

sclerosed: To become hardened

wheal: A localized area of edema of the body surface

All drugs (medications) are potentially harmful. You must never become casual or careless when administering drugs or assisting with drug administration. You must never give a drug that has not been specifically ordered by a physician, and you must understand the intended action, contraindications, side effects, and potential adverse reactions of any drug that you administer.

If you are not familiar with a drug that you are to administer, consult the pharmacist or an available literary source before administering the drug. All diagnostic imaging departments should have a current *Physician's Desk Reference* available for this purpose. There are addenda to this reference that include contrast agents. There is also detailed information packaged with drugs used commonly in diagnostic imaging. If you do not know and cannot find information about a drug, do not administer it. *The radiographer must remember that contrast agents are drugs and the precautions listed in this chapter pertain to these agents as well!*

You must adhere to the *five rights of drug administration* at all times: (1) the right patient, (2) the right drug, (3) the right amount or dose, (4) the right route, and (5) the right time (Display 13-1).

CALL OUT!

To help remember the five rights of drug administration, think PDART!

Patient

Drug

Amount

Route

Time

Other precautions that must be taken before administration of a drug are as follows:

1. Read the label carefully before pouring or drawing up a medication for administration. Check the strength, dosage, and name of the drug.

2. If a drug contains a sediment or appears to be cloudy, do not use it until the pharmacist has approved it. If in doubt, discard the drug.

3. The expiration date of each drug is written on its label. If that date has already passed, discard the medication.

4. Never use drugs from unmarked or poorly marked containers. Destroy these drugs.

5. Measure the exact amounts of every drug used. If medication is left over, do not replace it in the container; discard it according to the institutional policy.

6. Drugs must be stored in accordance with the manufacturer's specifications. No drug should be stored in an area where temperature and humidity vary greatly or are extreme. Low room temperature is advised.

7. If the medication is a liquid to be poured, always pour it away from the label of the bottle.

8. Do not combine two medications without verifying their compatibility with the pharmacist or a drug compatibility chart. If you have doubt, do not combine.

9. Before selecting a medication, check the label of the container three times: before it is taken from the storage area, before pouring or drawing it up for administration, and after it has been poured.

10. Take only one drug to one patient at one time. Stay with the patient while he or she takes the drug. Do not leave a medication at a patient's bedside to be taken later.

11. When approaching a patient who is to receive a drug, ask the patient to state his or her name. Do not accept the fact that a patient answers to what is thought to be the correct name. When a patient is anxious, he or she may not hear clearly or respond correctly.

12. After identifying the patient, explain what medication you are administering and how you wish him or her to take the drug.

13. A drug history of allergies must be taken before administering a drug. If the drug is to be administered intravenously, include allergies to iodine and latex in the history, since they will be used in the administrative process.

14. Do not leave unattended a patient who may be having a drug reaction.

15. The patient must not be allowed to drive him- or herself home after a drug reaction or after receiving a sedative, hypnotic, antianxiety, or narcotic analgesic medication.

16. A child who has received a medication and is sleeping may not leave the department until fully awake.

17. Patients must be observed for at least 1 hour before leaving the department alone after receiving any drug.

18. Do not administer a drug that you have not prepared.

The Five Rights of Drug Administration

PDART

1. The right Patient
2. The right Drug

3. The right Amount or dose
4. The right Route
5. The right Time

19. Report and document any drug that the patient refuses to take.

20. Document any drug that you administer immediately according to department procedure.

/// WARNING \\\

Patients who receive narcotic analgesics or hypnotics may suffer respiratory depression and shock. They must not be left alone.

Systems of Drug Measurement

The metric system of measurement has been adopted in most countries of the world as the official standard; however, its use is recommended but not required in the United States. It is used in most medical settings in this country, but the apothecary system of measurement is also used. This means that anyone who administers drugs must understand and be able to use the two systems interchangeably. Household measurements are not commonly used in medical facilities and only those most commonly used are mentioned. When you plan to administer drugs, you must learn to convert quickly from metric to apothecary measurement, depending on how the physician's order is written.

The basic unit of weight in the apothecary system is the grain. The fluid equivalent of 1 grain is the minim. Units derived from the grain are the dram, ounce, and pound. Units derived from the minim are the fluidram, fluidounce, pint, quart, and gallon.

The metric unit of measure is the liter (L), which contains 1000 milliliters (mL) or the approximate cubic metric equivalent of 1000 cubic centimeters (cc). The unit of weight is the gram (g). Kilograms (kg), milligrams (mg), and micrograms (mcg) are used in health care. The kilogram is 1000 g or, in nonmetric terms, 2.2 pounds.

You must have a conversion table at hand or memorize conversions so that you are able to use these measures interchangeably. You must also be able to compute dosages if required.

Medical symbols and abbreviations are used in health care on a daily basis, and any person who works in this arena is expected to understand them. A list of the most common abbreviations and equivalencies appears in Table 13-1. You must not make up your own abbreviations nor administer a drug unless you are certain that your understanding of the dosage is correct.

The Medication Order and Documentation

Licensed physicians, dentists, podiatrists, and, in some states, optometrists can prescribe, dispense, and administer drugs. Under specific circumstances that vary from state to state, registered nurses with specialized education, physician assistants, and pharmacists may legally order and dispense drugs.

No health care worker may take it on him- or herself to prescribe or administer drugs that are not ordered by a person licensed to do so. In health care settings, an order must be dated, written, and signed by the physician. If the patient is to be cared for in a hospital setting, such as a diagnostic imaging department, the order is written on an order sheet.

If a patient is to be discharged with a prescription, it will be written on the physician's personalized order form. The following information is required on a legal physician's order.

The patient's full name, the date, and the time the order is written

The date and time or times that the drug is to be administered

The generic or trade name of the drug

The dosage form and the route of administration

The physician's signature

An example of a physician's order for a hospitalized patient might be as follows:

June 3, 2002, 7 am

Give Valium, 5 mg PO at 8 am

J. Glucose, M.D.

TABLE 13-1

Measurements

HOUSEHOLD	APOTHECARY	METRIC
1 teaspoonful (tsp)	1 fluidram (f3)	4 or 5 mL
1 tablespoonful (tbs)	½fluidounce (f3)	15 mL
2 tablespoonfuls	1 fluidounce	30 mL
1 cup (c)	8 fluidounces	240 or 250 mL
1 pint (pt)	16 fluidounces	473 or 500 mL
1 quart (qt)	32 fluidounces or 30 fluidounces	1000 mL (1 L)

APOTHECARY	METRIC
15 grains (gr)	1 gram (g)(1000 mg)
10 gr	0.6 g, 600 mg
7½ gr	0.5 g, 300 mg
1½ gr	0.1 g, 100 mg
¾ gr	0.05 g, 50 mg
½ gr	0.03 g, 30 mg
¼ gr	0.015 g, 15 mg
1/60 gr	0.001 g, 1 mg
1/100 gr	0.6 mg
1/120 gr	0.5 mg
1/150 gr	0.4 mg
Other frequently used equivalents:	
1 cubic centimeter (cc) = 1 mL	
1 inch = 2.54 centimeters (cm)	
2.2 pounds = 1 kilogram (kg)	

An order may be given verbally or by telephone by a physician. Any person authorized to receive physician's orders may take such an order. If an order is given in this manner, it must be written on the prescriber's sheet in the chart and signed by the person receiving the order, followed by VO for a verbal order or TO for a telephone order.

John Glucose M.D. by Jane Terminal RN (VO) or (TO)

The physician giving such an order must sign the order in a designated period of time, usually within 24 hours.

There are also *stat* orders. This means that a physician gives an order for a medication to be administered immediately. This order must also be written on the order sheet and signed by the physician.

Another type of order is the *prn* (*pro re nata;* as the occasion requires order. This order is written for a drug to be taken or administered to the patient as necessary. Medications for relief of pain are frequently prn orders.

A *single order* is an order written for a medication to be given only once at a designated time. The order used as an example above is a single order. The med-ication ordered would be given once and would not be given again without a new physician's order.

In radiographic imaging, you will frequently assist with medication administration rather than actually give the drug. If this is the case, after receiving a verbal order from a physician to procure a drug for the physician to administer, you will proceed as follows:

1. Obtain the drug from the storage area.

2. Verify that it is the correct drug by checking the label before taking the drug from storage.

3. Obtain the correct supplies for the particular route of administration and prepare the drug; that is, draw it into a syringe or pour it into a medicine glass for oral administration as appropriate (this is discussed in later sections of this chapter), and read the label a second time.

4. Put the medication, the package from which it was taken, and other items that will be needed for administration on a tray and take them to the physician.

5. Hold the package (bottle, vial) at the physician's eye level, and state the name and dosage of the drug that you have prepared. Be certain that the physician reads and acknowledges that he or she has approved the drug.

6. Assist the physician in administering the drug to the patient.

7. Document the drug in the correct area of the patient's chart, and present it to the physician to sign.

CALL OUT!

Know medical abbreviations:

STAT: immediately

PRN: as necessary

SINGLE ORDER: give only once

Every institution has a slightly different manner of documentation. It is your responsibility as the radiographer to learn the correct method in the facility in which you are employed. Whatever the situation, you are obligated to document the following on the patient's chart, the department form, or the computer information system: the name of the drug, the dosage, the route, the time, and the patient's reaction to any drug that you administer. You must also sign your full name and title. It may also be your obligation to record the drugs administered by the physician and then have the physician sign the entry.

CALL OUT!

Remember that contrast agents are drugs.

Medication Errors

As a professional health care worker, you are responsible for your own actions. It is your legal and ethical obligation to be knowledgeable about any drug you feel competent to administer. If you administer a drug incorrectly or misinterpret an order from a physician, you are legally liable and may also have violated your code of professional ethics, since administering a medication without sufficient knowledge of its potential is not acting in the best interest of the patient.

You must be aware of the federal regulations pertaining to controlled substances. The Controlled Substances Act of the federal government restricts personnel who are legally permitted to administer narcotic and hypnotic substances and drugs that may produce dependency (as described in Chapter 12). It also restricts access to these drugs, which are always kept in a locked area. Documentation of use of these drugs is also carefully controlled. You must learn the methods of adhering to these regulations in the department in which you are employed and abide by them at all times.

Medication errors are an area of frequent litigation in diagnostic imaging. The radiographer who is administering or assisting with administration of drugs is frequently implicated in this type of litigation. If an error in medication administration is made (this includes contrast agents) or if the patient has an adverse reaction to a drug, as the radiographer involved you must assess the patient's condition and then notify the prescribing physician immediately. The error or adverse reaction must be included in the patient's chart. You must also write an incident report (sometimes called an *unusual occurrence report*).

Every detail of the incident must be included in the incident report, which becomes the property of the department and is not a part of the chart. Items to include in this report are the incorrect dosage of the drug, why it was given, the patient's reactions, and how the error was remedied. For instance:

3/3/02: 8 am Iopamidol 30 mL administered IV. Administered in error to this patient.

8:10 am BP 110/60, AO 70, R 16. Patient is alert and oriented to person, place, and time.

8:15 am Dr. J. Glucose notified of the error. (radiographer's signature)

8:20 am Dr. J. Glucose at pt's bedside, assessment of pt. performed by Dr. Glucose.

BP 120/80, AP 72, R 16. Pt. Reports no complaints.

The patient must be observed for an appropriate time interval and periodic reports on his or her condition are added to the chart until the patient is discharged from the department. Accurate documentation is the best defense to have if there is litigation.

Equipment for Drug Administration

Needles for parenteral drug administration range in length from 3/8 to 2 inches for average use. Longer needles are used for special procedures. Needles may come attached to a syringe of appropriate size, or they may come in various sizes packaged separately. Needles are made of stainless steel and consist of the following parts:

• The hub (the part that attaches to the syringe)

• The shaft (the elongated part of the needle)

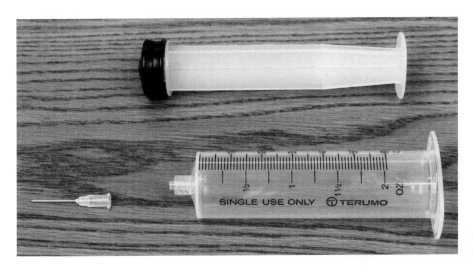

Figure 13–1. Parts of a syringe and needle.

- The lumen (the hollow tube that runs the length of the shaft)
- The bevel (the sharp, angulated tip of the needle)

Selection of the correct size of needle with which to administer a drug is very important. The size of the lumen of the needle can vary from very large to very small. The smaller the lumen, the larger the gauge of the needle (e.g., *a 30-gauge needle is much smaller than a 12-gauge needle*). The viscosity of the fluid to be injected determines the gauge selected. The area for injection and the condition of the patient determine the length of the needle chosen.

Syringes also vary in size depending on the amount of fluid to be injected. They generally range in capacity from 1 to 50 mL The parts of the syringe are as follows:

- The tip (the end of the syringe to which the needle is fastened)
- The barrel (the body of the syringe)
- The plunger (the interpart that fits into the barrel)

Syringes are calibrated in milliliters and minims (minim is the singular). One milliliter equals 15 or 16 minims. Syringes are packaged in treated paper or plastic wrappers to maintain sterility, and needles are often attached in the package. The size of the syringe and the size of the needle are printed on the package (Figs. 13–1 and 13–2).

Most health care facilities now use syringes with needles attached in a manner that protects the health care worker from needle-stick injuries. This is accomplished in a variety of ways depending on the manufacturer. Some syringes come encased in an extra plastic barrel that is outfitted with a safety lock; others have a plastic guard that is pulled down following the injection (Fig. 13–3). There is also a one-handed scoop technique that may be used to guard against needle-stick injuries. After injection, the needle cover is scooped over the used needle with the dominant hand and placed into the disposal container (Fig. 13–4).

Syringes and needles are disposable and must not be reused. They should be disposed of in a container

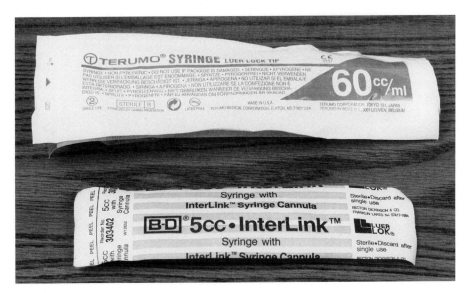

Figure 13–2. Needle and syringe packaging.

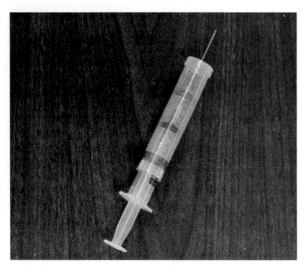

Figure 13–3. Syringe with safety lock.

prepared for this purpose. These containers are labeled "contaminated sharps" and are made of hard plastic material. You must consider all used needles as potentially lethal. A needle that has been injected into a person must not be recapped and, if it has a protective mechanism, it should be engaged after the injection. The used syringe should be held by the barrel and carried immediately to the receptacle for disposal, where it is deposited needle first. Never place a used syringe and needle back onto a tray to be disposed of at a later time. You must use great care to prevent needle sticks. This is considered a hazardous medical incident and must be reported as a "critical incident" and attended to immediately. HIV and hepatitis B, non-A, non-B, and C can be contracted in this manner.

Medicine glasses are used for oral drug administration. Most medicine glasses are made of disposable plastic. All are of 1-ounce (30-mL) size and are calibrated for household, apothecary, and metric measures (Fig. 13–5).

Packaging of Parenteral Medications

Drugs intended for parenteral administration are packaged to maintain sterility. If they are intended for intramuscular, subcutaneous, or intradermal injection, they are either in an ampule or a vial. Drugs to be administered intravenously may be contained in an ampule or a vial if the amount to be administered is small. If a large amount of fluid or drug is to be administered, it will be contained in calibrated glass or plastic container.

Vials

A vial is a glass container with a rubber stopper circled by a metal band; the band holds the rubber stopper in place. Vials are generally available in 5-, 10-, 20-, 30-, and 50-mL sizes. On the label is the name of the medication, the dosage per milliliter, and the route by which it may be administered (e.g., morphine sulfate—1 mL = 15 mg). Multidose vials are not usually used because of the hazards of contamination. If a multidose vial is used, a sterile needle must be inserted into the vial for each dose.

Cleanse the top of the rubber stopper thoroughly with an alcohol wipe. Then draw air equivalent to the amount of fluid to be withdrawn from the vial into the syringe. Insert the needle into the vial and inject the air in the syringe. The fluid in the vial will replace the air in the syringe rather quickly. The plunger of the syringe can be drawn back until the exact amount of drug needed is obtained (Fig. 13–6).

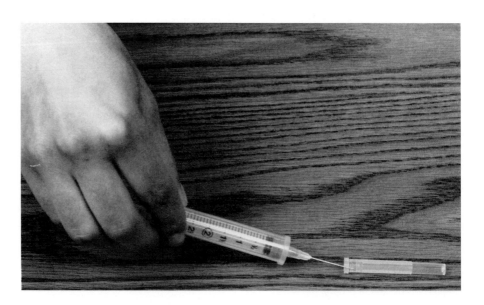

Figure 13–4. Needle scoop technique to prevent injury.

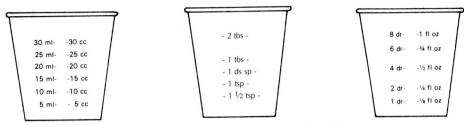

Figure 13–5. Calibrations on a medicine glass: metric and apothecary.

Ampules

An ampule is made of glass and contains a single dose of a drug. The indented area at the neck is opened by filing the neck with a small metal file (Fig. 13–7A). The top then easily snaps off the container. You must never attempt to snap the top off an ampule without protecting your hands with a sterile gauze pad, because the glass may break unevenly and cut your hand (see Fig. 13-7B). Like the vial, the ampule is labeled with the name of the medication, the dosage per milliliter, and the route of administration. If all the medication is not used, the remainder must be discarded, because it does not remain sterile after the ampule has been opened.

Packaging of Fluids and Medications for Intravenous Use

Fluids, contrast agents, and medications that are of a large volume (50 to 1000 mL) are packaged in either heavy plastic or glass containers. Plastic bags containing fluid for intravenous (IV) infusion collapse under atmospheric pressure as the fluid leaves it. Glass

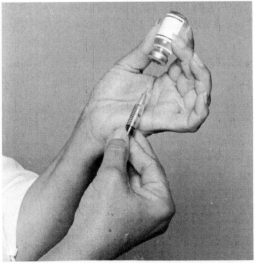

Figure 13–6. Insert a sterile needle through the rubber stopper in the vial.

bottles do not collapse; therefore, they are constructed with an air vent so that air can replace the fluid as it infuses into the vein.

Like the vial, the glass IV fluid container has a rubber stopper that is protected by a metal cap and a rubber diaphragm. There are two ports in the stopper, one for air and one for insertion of the IV tubing. The plastic bag has two ports, one for the IV tubing and one to use if other drugs are to be added to the infusion. The methods of proceeding with IV drug administration are discussed in a later section.

Methods of Drug Administration

Oral Route

Oral medications are available in liquid, tablet, or capsule form. Liquid drugs are most quickly absorbed into the systemic circulation. A solid form of a drug is absorbed more quickly if it is given with an adequate amount of fluid, usually water. If a tablet has an enteric coating, instruct the patient not to chew it, because its effect may be destroyed by gastric secretions. It must also not be crushed or cut. If a tablet is not scored, it should not be broken. Capsules must not be tampered with, since this may result in incorrect dosage.

Drugs given by the sublingual or buccal routes must be small, uncoated tablets. They disintegrate or dissolve very quickly and bypass the gastric mucosa to go directly into the bloodstream.

When the physician prescribes an oral medication, you must observe the five rights of drug administration(see Display 13-1) and follow the procedure outlined below:

1. Read the order or make certain that the order is correct.

2. Write the name of the patient, the name of the drug, and the dosage on a small identification ticket or paper.

3. Wash your hands.

4. Obtain a tray on which to carry the drug to the patient.

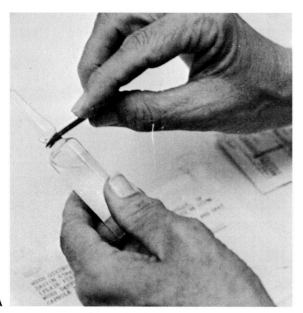
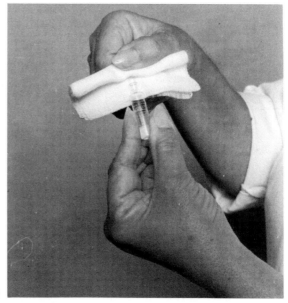

A   B

Figure 13–7. (**A**) Before attempting to snap off the neck of the ampule, file the indentation so it will break evenly. (**B**) Protect your hand with a sterile gauze pad.

5. Obtain the correct medication, a medicine glass, or pill cup in which to pour the drug.

6. If you are to administer the drug, pour it while reading the label. Make certain the drug is the correct one and the dosage is correct. Pour tablets into the cap of the bottle and then into the cup. Do not touch the tablet (Fig. 13–8).

7. Place the identification ticket on the tray, and carry the drug to the patient.

8. Ask the patient to state his or her name. Then, if the patient has an identiband, read the band to further check the identity.

9. If the drug is to be swallowed, give the patient the drug and direct him or her to swallow. Give the patient water to assist in swallowing the drug if it is permitted.

10. If the drug is to be absorbed by the buccal route, instruct the patient to hold the tablet inside the

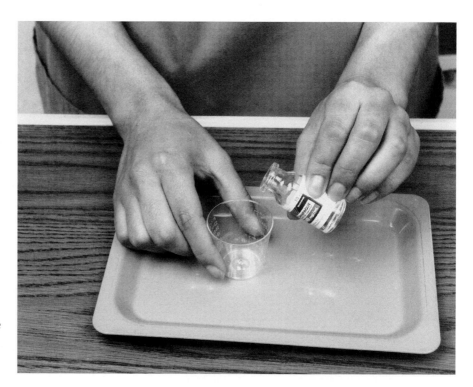

Figure 13–8. Pour medication into graduated medicine glass. Have the physician check the patient's name and the dosage.

lower cheek beside the gum toward the back of the mouth until it is absorbed. Do not give water with tablets administered by this route.

11. If the drug is a sublingual tablet, instruct the patient to hold the tablet under the tongue until it is absorbed. Do not give water with tablets administered by this route.

12. Stay with the patient until the drug has been taken.

13. Return to the area where the equipment is kept; clean and replace or discard the equipment and wash your hands.

14. Document that the drug was given, by what route, and at what time.

15. Observe the patient carefully to be certain he or she has no adverse reactions to the drug.

Parenteral Drug Administration

The methods of administering drugs by the parenteral route vary according to the route ordered by the physician. Intra-arterial, intrathecal, intraventricular, and intra-articular drug administration is performed by the physician and is not discussed here. Any health care worker who plans to administer parenteral medications to children requires special education beyond the scope of this textbook. All parenteral drug administration requires laboratory instruction and practice before administering drugs to actual patients. The procedures described in the following paragraphs pertain to the average adult patient. There are some rules that apply to all parenteral drug administration.

1. All equipment that penetrates the skin including needles, syringes, and the drug itself must be sterile.

2. The patient must be correctly identified, as described earlier.

3. The procedure is explained to the patient, and the medication to be administered is identified.

4. If the patient refuses the medication, document the refusal. Do not insist that the patient accept the drug.

5. The skin at the injection site is cleansed with an antiseptic solution to be as free of microorganisms as possible.

6. The antiseptic chosen for skin preparation varies from institution to institution, but isopropyl alcohol or povidone-iodine solution is frequently used.

7. All persons administering parenteral drugs must wear gloves during the procedure because exposure to blood is possible.

8. There must be a physician's order for all drugs to be administered. This includes contrast media.

9. The five rights of drug administration must be followed.

10. The drug administered must be documented according to the policy of the department.

11. The patient must be observed closely for 1 hour after drug administration for adverse or allergic reactions.

12. A patient who has had a sedative, tranquilizing, or hypnotic drug administered may *not* drive him- or herself home.

Intradermal Administration

Intradermal injections are also called *intracutaneous injections*. This type of injection is usually used for testing for sensitivity to a drug or antigen. Usually, less than 0.5 mL of medication is used. After the test dose is given, observe the patient carefully for an anaphylactic reaction. These injections are usually administered into the dermis on the inner aspect of the forearm. Areas with excessive hair or scarring must not be used because results may be difficult to detect.

Following is the equipment for intradermal injections:

A tuberculin syringe with a 25- to 27-gauge needle, 1/2 inch in length

An alcohol wipe

A pair of clean gloves

The drug to be injected

The procedure is as follows:

1. Cleanse the site with an alcohol wipe in a firm, circular motion.

2. Put on gloves.

3. Hold the skin at the area to be injected taut with the nondominant hand.

4. Insert the needle, bevel side up at a 5- to 15-degree angle.

5. Inject the drug. A small raised area, or wheal, should be seen at the injection site.

6. Withdraw the needle and do not massage or cleanse the site.

7. Instruct the patient concerning time to read the results of the test. Watch for a reaction.

Subcutaneous Administration

Medications are injected into the tissues beneath the dermis at a 45-degree angle. The following equipment is required:

A syringe of the correct size. A tuberculin syringe may be used for an amount of less than 1 mL; a 2- or 3-mL syringe may be used for administering 1 mL of a drug. *No more than 1 mL of fluid may be injected subcutaneously.*

A 23- to 25-gauge needle of 1/2 to 5/8 inch in length

2 or 3 alcohol wipes

The correct medication

A pair of clean gloves

Subcutaneous injections are given in the outer aspect of the upper arms, the abdomen, the scapulas, or the anterior thigh (Fig. 13–9). Only small amounts of the drug (1 mL) should be administered in these areas. Subcutaneous drugs should be highly soluble and non-

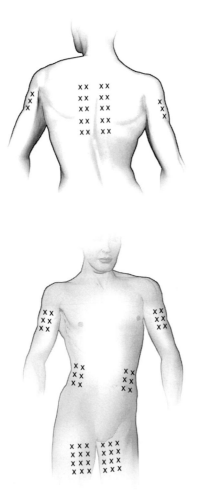

Figure 13–9. Appropriate sites for subcutaneous injection. (Walsh J, Parsons CB, Wieck L: Manual of Home Health Care Nursing. Philadelphia: JB Lippincott, 1987.)

irritating to the tissues into which they are injected. Since this is an invasive procedure, use sterile or surgical aseptic technique. Do not use edematous or scarred tissue and the 2-inch diameter of flesh around the umbilicus for injection. The procedure is as follows:

1. Identify the patient and expose the site for injection.

2. Cleanse the site with an alcohol wipe.

3. Put on gloves.

4. If the patient is very thin, grasp the skin in a slight fold or bunch.

5. Inject the medication at a 45-degree angle; do no aspirate.

6. Withdraw the needle. Do not rub the area after injection.

7. Correctly discard the needle and syringe, and make the patient comfortable.

Medications commonly administered by the subcutaneous route are heparin, epinephrine, insulin, and some vaccines.

Intramuscular Administration

The intramuscular (IM) route for medication administration is chosen when prompt absorption of drugs is desired, because there is a rich blood supply to muscles. It is the site chosen when a medication given subcutaneously would be irritating to the tissues and when a larger amount of a drug is needed. The amount of medication that can be given intramuscularly ranges from 1 to 5 mL; however, the person receiving the injection must be relatively large if more than 3 mL of medication is to be injected into a muscle.

You must to administer an injection into a muscle in a laboratory setting before actually performing it in the clinical setting, since incorrect technique can result in harm to the patient. Major blood vessels and nerves traverse muscles used for injection, and permanent damage can be done to a person who is given an injection incorrectly or in a site that is inappropriate for a given drug. The tissues around an injection site may also be damaged. Complications that may result from incorrect injection into a muscle are abscesses, necrosis, skin slough, nerve damage, prolonged pain, and periostitis.

Identifying Correct Sites for Intramuscular Injection

The radiographer who administers injections into muscles must be able to select a safe site. The sites commonly used to administer IM injections for adult patients are the dorsal gluteal, ventrogluteal, rectus femoris, and deltoid muscles. Avoid a site that is already sore, hardened from many injections, or extremely tense. Sites of IM injections must be rotated if the patient is to receive a series of drugs by that route. The following text discusses methods of identifying the correct sites for IM injection.

DORSOGLUTEAL

The patient may be placed in a prone position with toes pointed inward or in Sims' position with the entire gluteal muscle exposed. The posterior superior iliac spine and the greater trochanter are palpated, and an imaginary line is drawn between them. The site for injection is lateral and slightly above the midpoint of the imaginary line (Fig. 13–10A). Another method of identification of the correct site is to divide one buttock into four quadrants using the iliac crest and the gluteal fold as the superior and inferior boundaries. The injection is given into the upper outer quadrant of the buttock. Incorrect placement of the injection can result in damage to the sciatic nerve, which is located in the lower midline of the muscle.

VENTROGLUTEAL

The patient may be in a supine, Sims', or prone position. If the patient is in a prone position, encourage him or her to flex the knees if possible, since this relaxes the muscle. The health care worker giving the injection should place the palm of the hand on the greater trochanter and the index finger on the anterior superior iliac spine. Then, the middle finger is stretched as far as possible along the iliac crest. The injection should be given within the triangle that is formed by the spread fingers (see Fig. 13–10B).

VASTUS LATERALIS

The patient may be placed in a sitting or prone position. The thigh is then visually divided into thirds, both horizontally and vertically. The injection is given into the outer middle third of the muscle (see Fig. 13–10C). This is a relatively safe area for injection because the muscle is thick and there are no large blood vessels or nerves.

DELTOID

The patient may be placed in a sitting or supine position with the arm away from the body. This muscle, which is located in the lateral aspect of the upper arm, is relatively small and not frequently used for IM injections because it is not able to absorb large amounts of medication. No more than 1 mL of solution is recommended to be injected into this site. Damage to the radial nerve and artery are possible here. The deltoid

muscle may be located by identifying the lower aspect of the acromion process and forming an imaginary inverted triangle with the midpoint in line with the axilla on the lateral aspect of the arm (see Fig. 13–10D).

Administering an Intramuscular Injection

The following equipment is needed for an IM injection:

A 3- to 5- mL syringe

An 18- to 22-gauge needle 1 1/2 inches in length. A 1-inch long 22- or 23-gauge needle may be selected for use in the deltoid area or for use on a very thin patient.

Three alcohol wipes

A pair of clean gloves

The procedure is as follows:

1. Assess the patient to determine the length of needle that is appropriate; this depends on the site and the size of the patient.

2. Determine the gauge of needle that is appropriate. Use the smallest gauge possible to accommodate the viscosity of the drug.

3. Draw up the drug into the syringe. If the medication is an irritating substance such as hydroxyzine (Vistaril), change the needle after it is drawn into the syringe.

4. Proceed to the patient, position, and cleanse the area with an alcohol wipe. Put on clean gloves. Open a second alcohol wipe to have it available.

5. Place the nondominant hand on the muscle to be injected to support the patient. Quickly insert the needle into the muscle at a 90-degree angle.

6. When the needle is inserted, support the needle with the nondominant thumb and index fingers, and draw back (aspirate) the plunger slightly. If a blood vessel has been entered, blood will return in the syringe and you must withdraw the needle.

7. Assuming that no blood returns in the syringe, inject the fluid into the muscle and quickly withdraw the needle.

8. When the needle is withdrawn, gently wipe the area where the needle was inserted.

9. Make the patient comfortable, and follow procedures as described earlier.

Under normal circumstances, you will not be injecting irritating substances into the muscle with the exception of hydroxyzine. If there is an occasion for this to occur, a Z-track method of IM injection is used. This procedure varies as follows:

1. Draw a small amount of air into the syringe after the medication is drawn up (about 0.2 mL as an air

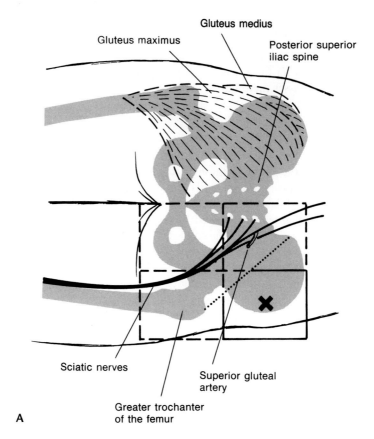

A

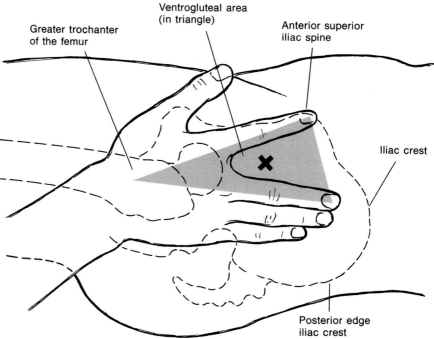

Figure 13–10. Sites for intramuscular injection: (**A**) Dorsal gluteal. (**B**) Ventrogluteal. (**C**) Vastus lateralis. (**D**) Deltoid. (Abrams: *Clinical Drug Therapy,* 4th ed. Philadelphia: JB Lippincott, 1995.)

B

lock). Change the needle to prevent irritating medication from gaining access to subcutaneous tissues.

2. The deltoid muscle is not appropriate for this purpose, nor is the ventral gluteal muscle.

3. The injection procedure is as described above. However, the skin is pulled to one side before the needle is inserted and held in this position with the nondominant hand as the medication is injected. Aspirate for blood. After the medication and the air in the syringe are injected, count to 10 (wait 10 seconds) before withdrawing the needle.

4. Withdraw the needle and release the skin simultaneously.

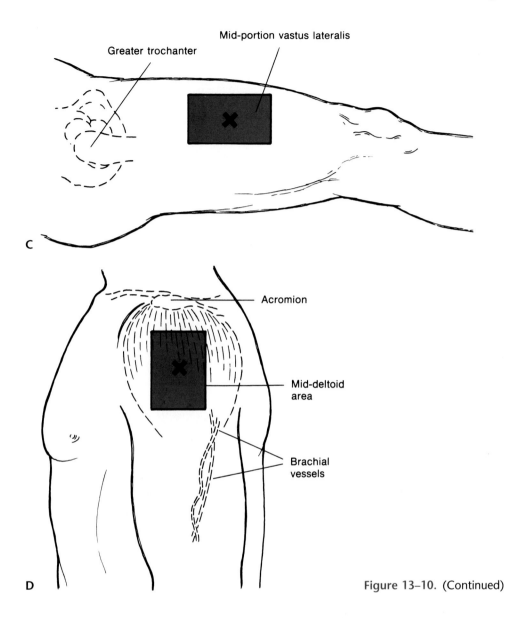

Figure 13–10. (Continued)

5. Do not massage the site after the injection. An alcohol wipe may be held in place over the site for a moment.

Peripheral Intravenous Drug Administration

The IV method of drug administration is selected when immediate effect of a drug is desired or when a drug cannot be injected into body tissues without damaging them. This can be one of the most hazardous routes of drug administration, because once a drug is injected directly into the circulatory system, reaction to it is instantaneous. Any health care worker who administers IV medications must be aware of the hazardous effects of the drug and its life-threatening potential. In many areas of the United States, official authorization is required of all persons administering IV drugs.

Most drugs given in diagnostic imaging are administered intravenously. You must not leave a patient receiving an IV drug or contrast agent alone; the patient must be observed continuously. Pulse rate and blood pressure should be taken before and at frequent intervals during IV drug administration. Report any change in the patient's vital signs or behavior to his or her physician immediately.

Because your primary experience will be with IV administration of contrast agents and drugs given by infusion or as a bolus, these methods will be discussed in some detail. Other IV methods are discussed only briefly.

Some drugs are given in small amounts through preexisting IV lines. They are of several types, and their use is not within your scope of practice as a radiographer. The heparin or saline lock and an IV piggyback, both commonly seen, as well as central venous lines, are discussed in Chapter 10.

A *heparin* or *saline lock* is a venous catheter that is left in place in the vein for a designated period of time but is not attached to IV tubing. It has a protective rubber cap over a reservoir at the top of the venous cannula into which a small amount of heparin is added after each drug administration to prevent blood from clotting in the cannula. If a medication is to be administered through this port, the rubber cap is cleansed with alcohol wipes, and it is irrigated first with 1 mL of sterile normal saline to ensure that it is not clogged. If the lock is clogged, it must be changed. Saline should not be forced through a clogged cannula.

An IV *piggyback* is another method of administering drugs though an established line (Fig. 13–11). A piggyback is a small IV infusion (usually 100 to 250 mL), which is attached to an adjoining or already existing line. This solution is attached to the preexisting line in such a manner that it flows into the vein at the intended rate. When it has been fully administered, the original IV solution is continued, and the piggyback is discontinued.

Medications (including contrast agents) may be given by bolus or infusion. A *bolus* is a designated amount of a drug that is administered at one time, usually over a period of several minutes. An *infusion* usually refers to a larger amount of a drug, fluid, or fluid containing a drug or electrolytes that is administered over a longer period of time ranging from hours to days. Both of these methods require venipuncture; each require different equipment and preparation.

WARNING

The radiographer must not leave a patient receiving an IV drug or contrast agent alone.

Site Selection and Preparation for Venipuncture

The area selected for venipuncture requires careful assessment before the procedure is begun. The type of drug, the purpose of its administration, and the age and condition of the patient all are factors influencing venipuncture site selection. Except in an extreme emergency or if no other vein is accessible, veins in the hands and arms should be selected over those in the lower extremities because of the greater hazard of embolus formation in the lower extremities related to IV infusion. Unless a drug is to be injected by bolus, do not select a vein located over a joint, because any movement will dislodge the needle or catheter and the arm or hand must be immobilized. The volar (palm) side of the wrist must not be used because the radial nerve is in that area, and the patient may feel extreme pain.

For infusions, veins in the lower arm recommended if they are not sclerosed or bruised. Veins in the

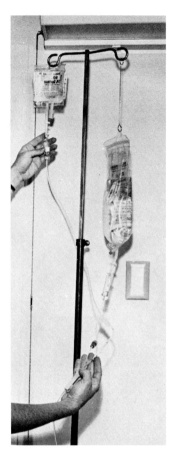

Figure 13–11. Giving intravenous medication using the piggyback method. The medication in the small container will enter the venous system before the solution in the larger container. (Walsh J, Parsons CB, Wieck L: *Manual of Home Health Care Nursing.* Philadelphia: JB Lippincott, 1987.)

hand may seem attractive, but many are small and the walls are thin and easily perforated. The basilic and cephalic veins are often good choices if available (Fig. 13–12). Veins must be palpated during the selection process to assess for elasticity, firmness, and engorgement. Veins should not be hard, bumpy, or flat.

After the site for venipuncture has been selected, prepare the area. Infection, tissue damage, pain, and discomfort all are hazards of IV drug administration. The radiographer participating in this procedure must make every effort to avoid each of these. Any jewelry or restrictive clothing is removed from the area. Hair is not removed because shaving may increase the possibility of infection.

Elderly patients must receive special consideration. Their veins are more fragile and have a greater tendency to "roll" as the needle or catheter is inserted. The tissues of the elderly patient are also more fragile, necessitating use of a smaller needle or catheter. The tourniquet is more apt to damage the skin and must be applied with less tension.

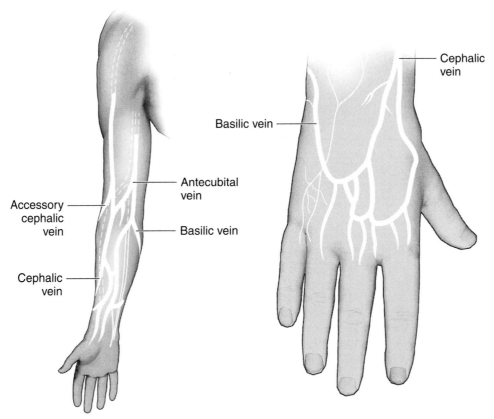

Figure 13–12. Sites recommended for insertion of venous cannulas.

Equipment needed for an IV bolus or infusion is as follows:

A tourniquet

A syringe of the correct size or an infusion set (choice depends on the IV to be administered)

An IV cannula of the correct type and size

A butterfly needle (also called a scalp vein needle or a winged needle) and a venous catheter are two of the common types of cannulas used for IV therapy (Fig. 13–13A and B). The butterfly needle is a short steel needle that is not recommended if it is to be in place for more than 2 or 3 hours because it is inflexible and is more apt to injure the vein or result in infiltration. A wing-tip needle is recommended for a bolus injection. The venous catheter with an over-the-needle plastic cannula (often termed an *angiocatheter)* of the correct size is most desirable for longer infusions. These catheters are available in several sizes as are other needles for injection. This device is easy to insert and is flexible once the needle is removed after insertion. Several venous catheters that assist in prevention of needle-stick injuries are on the market. If one of these is available, it is recommended. Once the vein is chosen, the size of the cannula is decided. The diameter and length of catheter must be as small as possible considering the viscosity of the fluid to be administered and the length and depth of

the vein. The smaller catheter does not interfere with blood flow and decreases the incidence of venous inflammation; however, contrast agents tend to be viscous and require a larger-gauge cannula than that for many other drugs.

CALL OUT!

A bolus injection of a drug is usually administered by a specially trained nurse because this is a potentially lethal method of drug administration. If you administer a drug by this method, you must be certified to do so! Drugs given by this method take effect immediately, and the patient must be monitored for adverse or allergic reaction!

Povidone-iodine or alcohol (if the patient is allergic to iodine) for skin preparation

Skin preparation before IV therapy is dictated by the policy of the institution in compliance with standards of practice and must be followed.

A pair of clean gloves

Tape or a clear adhesive dressing to be placed over the infusion site

The drug or fluid to be administered

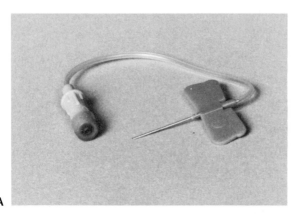

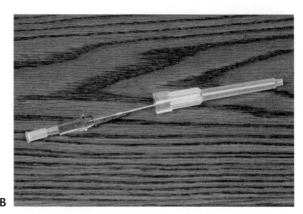

A   B

Figure 13–13. (**A**) A butterfly needle. (**B**) Angiocatheter or venous catheter

An IV standard must be on hand if an IV infusion is to be started. An infusion pump or controller may be required in some situations.

An IV infusion controller is an electronic system controlled by gravity. The amount of fluid infused is controlled according to the amount desired to be administered in a set time period. An alarm sounds if the desired rate is not met.

An infusion pump allows a more precise monitoring of the amount of fluid to be infused in a set time frame. It may pump more fluid than would be allowed by the gravity drip method (Fig. 13–14).

CALL OUT!

IV fluids must be infused at no lower than room temperature. They must be prepared beforehand so that they are not cold when administered!

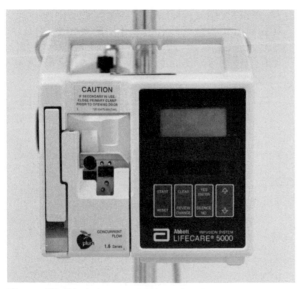

Figure 13–14. Intravenous pump.

IV infusion requires the following additional preparation:

1. Obtain the solution to be administered. If it is in a glass bottle, remove the metal cap and the rubber diaphragm (Fig. 13–15*A*).

2. Obtain an infusion set that includes IV tubing and a drip chamber.

3. Open the outer packaging from the infusion set, and remove the protective cover from the insertion tip of the drip chamber. Do not allow this tip to be touched or contaminated because it will be placed into the IV fluid and must remain sterile.

4. Place the tip into the opening in the rubber stopper that is marked for it until it is completely covered (see Fig.13–15*B*).

5. There is a clamp attached to the tubing. Close the tubing with the clamp.

6. Have a receptacle or a sink at hand. Invert the bottle of solution and hang it on the standard. Remove the protective cover from the end of the IV tubing, again being careful not to contaminate it (see Fig. 13–15*C* and *D*).

7. Open the clamp and allow fluid to run through the tubing until all the air in the tubing is displaced by fluid. Air must not remain because it may cause an air embolus.

8. When all air is removed from the tubing, replace the protective cover on the tip of the tubing using sterile technique, and proceed to the patient with the equipment.

If the solution is in a plastic bag, remove the container from its protective covering (Fig. 13–16A). Once the protective cap is removed from the port of the drip chamber on the IV tubing and the port of insertion on the bag, you can connect the drip chamber and tubing to the port (see Fig. 13–16B). You then follow the procedure for identification of the patient and documentation as discussed previously.

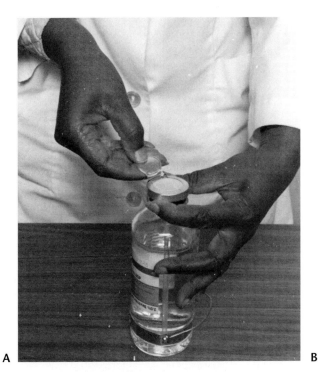

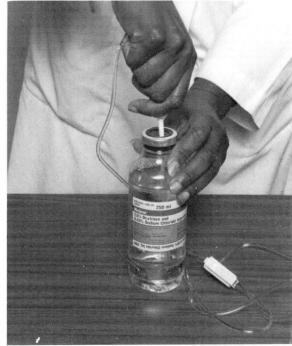

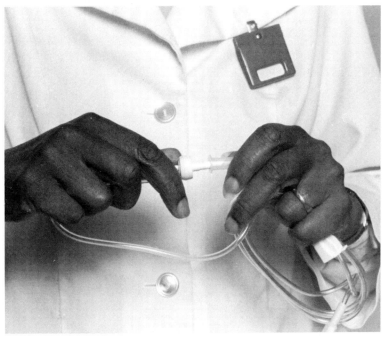

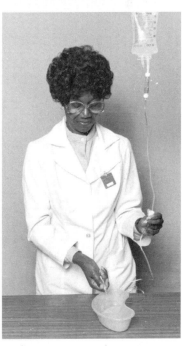

Figure 13–15. (**A**) Remove the metal cap and the rubber diaphragm from the vacoliter. (**B**) Insert the drip chamber into the rubber stopper. (**C**) The tips of the drip chambers that are inserted into the solution containers must be kept sterile. (**D**) Invert the bottle or bag of solution and allow the fluid to run through the tubing.

Venipuncture

The radiographer who performs venipuncture must be competent in the technique so that the patient is not subjected to the pain and threat of injury or infection. You must learn this skill in a classroom laboratory before actual practice. The procedure is as follows:

1. Obtain the order for the drug.
2. Identify the patient and explain and plan the procedure with the patient. Assess the patient's veins at this time. Assess for allergies to latex and iodine. If the patient's veins are difficult to palpitate, apply a warm compress to the area of intended injection to increase circulation.

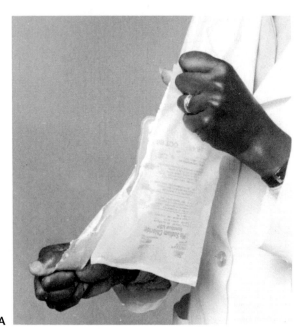

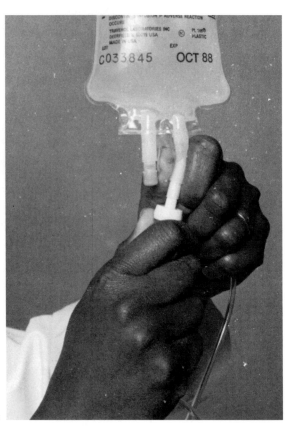

A   B

Figure 13–16. (**A**) Intravenous solutions in plastic bags must be removed from their outer covering. (**B**) Place the tip of the infusion tubing into the port.

3. Gather the equipment as described on previous pages. Displace the air in the tubing. You will need the following:
   a. The solution or drug to be administered, an IV drip set, and the correct-sized venous catheter
   b. An IV standard onto which to hang the solution if this is not a bolus
   c. Skin preparation items
   d. Clean gloves
   e. A tourniquet
   f. The tape to secure the cannula or needle
   g. A needle disposal container
4. Proceed to the patient.
5. Secure the tourniquet over the site selected. Do not secure so firmly that arterial circulation is impaired or skin is damaged. Secure the tourniquet so that it can be released by pulling one end (Fig. 13–17).
6. Have the patient make two or three tight fists as the tourniquet is applied. This forces more blood into the veins so that they are more visible.
7. Put on clean gloves. Gloves do not have to be sterile, but prep swabs and all items that enter the vein must be sterile.

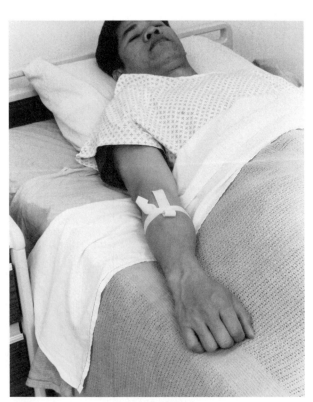

Figure 13–17. Secure the tourniquet so that it can be released by pulling one end.

8. Cleanse the area using at least three swabs to remove as many microbes as possible. Cleanse the site from the site of injection outward using firm strokes. Do not allow the solution to pool on the skin. Allow the area to dry.

9. Hold the skin taut above or below the insertion site, since this will be most effective. Insert the needle with the bevel up into the vein (Fig. 13–18). When the needle enters the vein, blood returns immediately into the flashback chamber. If no blood returns, the venipuncture was not successful. Use a new sterile needle to start the IV. If the second effort is not successful, call a member of the IV team or the anesthesia department to start the IV. *Do not subject the patient to multiple punctures.*

10. If an over-the-needle catheter is inserted, remove the needle and thread the catheter into the vein.

11. Release the tourniquet and attach the drug or infusion to be administered after ascertaining that all air is removed from the tubing. A bolus is administered at the speed required according to the drug order. An infusion is begun at the rate ordered by the physician.

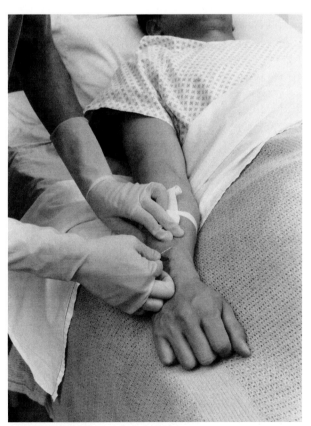

Figure 13-18. Hold the skin taut above or below insertion site. Insert needle with bevel up.

12. Tape the needle or venous catheter securely in place, and monitor the infusion to be certain that it maintains a safe rate of flow. A control pump may be attached at this time to monitor the rate of flow. Label the tape so that the date, time, size of the cannula, and the initials of the person inserting the IV are legible. Document the procedure.

To calculate rate of flow or drip rate, use this formula:

$$\frac{\text{Volume of infusion (in milliliters)}}{\text{Time of infusion in minutes} \times \text{drop factor in drops/mL}} = \text{drops/minute (gtts/min)}$$

Each company manufacturing IV fluid administration sets has a slightly different amount of fluid in drops per milliliter. The amount is stated on the package.

CALL OUT!

You must obtain an order from the physician for large-quantity IV infusions in rates of solution in milliliters per hour to avoid confusion.

Care of Patients with Intravenous Infusions in Place

If the IV infusion site is the antecubital vein, place the patient's arm on an arm board so that the elbow joint is immobilized. The arm may be attached to the arm board with plain or elasticized gauze. Check the arm frequently to be certain that the arm board is not applied so tightly that it interferes with circulation. The signs and symptoms of impaired circulation for a patient with a casted extremity listed in Chapter 4 may be used. Also, the infusion site must be checked for any signs of infiltration of the fluid into the surrounding tissues.

The IV standard should be placed 18 to 24 inches higher than the level of the vein, because the height at which the container of solution is suspended affects the rate of flow. If the bottle of solution is positioned lower than the vein, blood will flow into the tubing. The rate of flow of an IV infusion may also be affected by the position of the catheter or needle in the vein. If the bevel of either is positioned against the wall of the vein, it will slow or stop the infusion. Changing the position of the patient's arm often corrects the problem.

If there is a question about rate of infusion, a safe rule to follow is to allow the solution to infuse at 15 to 20 drips per minute. If a large amount of solution infuses too quickly, there is a danger of fluid intoxication or pulmonary edema. Unless the physician has ordered a rapid infusion, the IV solution that is flowing very rapidly should be slowed down. This can be done by simply tightening the control mechanism on the tubing slightly.

Some drugs are extremely irritating to the tissues. If these drugs are administered intravenously and allowed to infiltrate into the surrounding subcutaneous tissues, tissue necrosis and subsequent sloughing of these tissues can result. This is called *extravasation* and is to be avoided if at all possible. Dopamine hydrochloride and vasoconstricting drugs are apt to cause this problem. If extravasation occurs, notify the physician immediately so that antidotal therapy may be ordered. Stop the infusion immediately; remove the cannula, and elevate the affected arm. Ice packs or warm compresses are recommended. Document the incident naming the location, appearance of the area, the amount of solution infiltrated, and the palliative actions taken.

If a large amount of solution infuses too rapidly, there is a danger of fluid intoxication; this may lead to congestive heart failure or pulmonary edema. If an IV bolus of medication is delivered too rapidly, plasma levels of the drug being delivered may reach a toxic level resulting in headache, syncope, flushing of the face, feelings of tightness in the chest, shock, and cardiac arrest. This is termed *speed shock*. Dilution of a drug for a bolus is usually 10 mL, but must not exceed 25 mL, since this method of drug administration exerts additional pressure on a vein and also is a greater threat of infiltration. Never place pressure on the syringe when administering a bolus of drug; the fluid must be able to flow into the vein with ease.

Any complaint of pain or discomfort at the site of insertion of an IV needle should be heeded, and the site should be checked immediately. Swelling around the site or cold, blanched skin indicates that the needle or catheter has become dislodged from the vein and that the fluid or medication is infiltrating into the surrounding tissues. You should turn the IV off immediately, and notify the physician in charge of the patient. Severe tissue damage may result from infiltration of IV drugs and fluids. Drugs administered intravenously act very rapidly. Any complaint of itching or feeling of congestion or fullness in the chest or throat is cause to discontinue administration of an IV drug. You should not wait for further evidence of complications. Stop the infusion immediately, and then notify the patient's physician.

A warm or cold compress may be applied to the site of an infiltration. The temperature of the compress depends on the medication that has infiltrated. The physician or a pharmacist must be consulted.

Discontinuing Intravenous Infusions

An infusion is not discontinued without a physician's order to do so. The patient who must receive IV drug therapy endures varying amounts of discomfort to begin the procedure, because venipuncture can be painful. You must be certain that the procedure is to be discontinued so that the patient does not have to endure such discomfort a second time as a result of carelessness or misunderstanding.

To discontinue an IV, you need the following equipment:

A pack of dry, sterile, 2- by 2-inch gauze sponges

Clean, disposable gloves

Scissors to cut the tape

Tape

A tourniquet

The following procedure should then be observed:

1. Go to the patient and carefully identify him or her.

2. Clamp off the IV solution and prepare two strips of tape; place them where they can be reached easily later.

3. Loosen the tape that holds the venous catheter or needle in place so that the hub is clearly visible and free of tape.

4. Open the sterile gauze sponges, being careful not to contaminate them.

5. Put on clean gloves.

6. Gently withdraw the needle or catheter from the vein until it is completely removed (Fig. 13–19).

7. Immediately after the catheter is removed, apply pressure to the site of withdrawal with a dry, sterile sponge until bleeding stops—approximately 2 minutes.

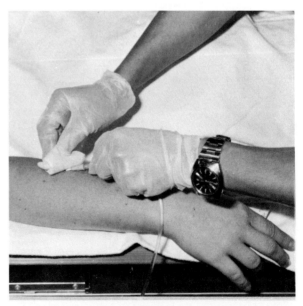

Figure 13–19. Gently withdraw the needle or catheter from the vein before applying pressure.

8. Inspect the needle or catheter that has been removed from the vein to make sure that it has emerged intact. If there is a possibility that a portion of it has broken off and remains in the vein, immediately apply the tourniquet above the insertion site, place the patient on the left side with head lowered, and prepare to administer oxygen. Immediately notify the physician. Do not leave the patient alone.

9. When the bleeding stops, use another sterile gauze pad, fold a sterile dry sponge, and tape it in place over the insertion site with some pressure applied. A small adhesive bandage (Band-Aid) may be used for this purpose.

10. Explain to the patient that this dressing may be removed in 1 or 2 hours.

11. Place the used syringe and needle into the "contaminated sharps" disposal container. Do not recap the needle. Remove your gloves.

12. Dispose of the vacoliter, and wash your hands.

13. Document the procedure.

Summary

All drugs are potentially harmful; therefore, you must never become casual or careless when administering or assisting with drug administration. Any drug administered to a patient must be ordered by the physician. There are several methods of obtaining an order for a drug to be administered, including written and verbal orders, as well as standing orders and telephone orders. The radiographer's responsibility is to understand and obtain a legal order before preparing or administering any drug. You must also be able to document the medication correctly after it is administered.

Remember that contrast agents are drugs and that all precautions pertaining to other drugs also pertain to them. You must always abide by the *five rights of drug administration* and follow all precautions pertaining to drug administration.

There are basically three methods of measuring drugs: household, apothecary, and metric systems. Although the metric system is followed exclusively in most of the world, apothecary and household measurements are used at times in the United States; therefore, as a radiographer, you are compelled to use each system interchangeably. You must also be able to understand common medical abbreviations.

Only persons licensed to prescribe and dispense drugs may do so. As the radiographer, you must understand the components of a legal prescription and how to correctly document medications given. You must also be able to follow the correct procedure if a medication error is made. You must be aware of and follow the federal regulations pertaining to controlled substances.

Each route of drug administration requires its own particular equipment and procedure. You must learn the lengths and gauges of needles and cannulas necessary for each route of drug administration. You must also learn the correct sites for all routes of drug administration. As with all invasive procedures, the rules of surgical asepsis apply to all drugs administered by parenteral routes.

A number of precautions must be taken when drugs are administered. This is particularly true for IV drug administration because these drugs travel immediately into the systemic circulation. As the radiographer, you must learn how to prepare the equipment and the site for IV drug administration. You must learn the precautions to be taken when IV drugs are administered to the elderly patient.

If a drug administered intravenously infiltrates into the surrounding tissue, it must be discontinued immediately. You must be able to recognize when this is occurring and take the necessary precautions to prevent tissue damage.

If a bolus of a drug is ordered, it must be administered by a person who is certified to do so. Each institution has its own policy concerning this. You must remember that this is the most potentially lethal method of drug administration, and you must be alert for adverse or anaphylactic reactions when this method of administration is used.

If an IV infusion is to be discontinued, you must receive an order to do so. You must then disconnect the IV using the correct procedure. Waste must be disposed of correctly during drug administration, and universal blood and body fluid precautions must be adhered to at all times.

Chapter 13 Test

1. Match the following:
   1. 0.4 mg _____
   2. gr 1/120 _____
   3. 1 g _____
   4. 1 kg _____

    5. gr 1/12   _____
       a. 2.2 lbs
       b. 0.5 mg
       c. gr 1/150
       d. 60 mg
       e. gr 15

2. Match the following:
    1. Give immediately   _____
    2. Give one time only   _____
    3. Give as necessary   _____
    4. Written and signed by the physician   _____
    5. To be signed within 24 hours   _____
       a. prn order
       b. Verbal order
       c. Stat order
       d. Single order
       e. Written order

3. Match the following:
    1. IM   _____
    2. SC   _____
    3. IV   _____
    4. Intradermal   _____
    5. PO   _____
       a. Buccal
       b. Scapulas
       c. Abdomen
       d. Vastus lateralis
       e. Ventrogluteal

4. List the equipment necessary to administer an IV infusion.

5. List the potential adverse effects of an IM injection

6. List the patient care precautions to which you must adhere as the radiographer when a patient is receiving an IV contrast agent.

7. List the factors to consider when assessing a patient for a site for an IV infusion.

_____ **8.** You are requested to administer hydroxyzine (Vistaril), 50 mg IM before a special radiographic procedure. You plan to administer this drug by
    a. Oral route
    b. IM
    c. Z track
    d. SC
    e. Intradermal

9. Match the word, phrase, or symbol with the most appropriate word or medical abbreviation below.
    1. Short needle, 5/8 inch long, 23 to 25 gauge   _____
    2. Needle, 1 1/2 inches long, 18 to 22 gauge   _____
    3. Needle, 1 inch long, 18 to 20 gauge   _____
    4. Needle, 31/2 inches long, 20 to 22 gauge   _____
    5. Needle, 1/2 inch long, 26 gauge   _____
       a. IM
       b. IV
       c. Subcutaneous
       d. Intrathecal
       e. Intradermal

10. Match the following:
    1. prn _____
    2. gtt _____
    3. stat _____
    4. bid _____
       a. immediately
       b. before meals
       c. twice a day
       d. whenever necessary
       e. drop

11. All drugs given by parenteral routes are given by which of the following?
    a. Medical aseptic technique
    b. Surgical aseptic technique

12. List the five rights of drug administration.

13. List the potential adverse events when administering an IV medication by infusion or by bolus.

14. List the equipment needed to start an IV infusion.

14

Patient Care During Urologic Procedures

Objectives

After studying this chapter, you will be able to:

1. Explain the need for infection control when working with patients who have urologic diagnoses.
2. Demonstrate the correct method of inserting a straight catheter and a retention catheter into the urinary bladder.
3. Explain the correct method of transporting a patient who has a retention catheter in place.
4. Demonstrate the correct method of removing a retention catheter from the urinary bladder.
5. Describe the patient care precautions that you must take as the radiographer when a patient is receiving

cystography, a retrograde pyelogram, or placement of a ureteral stent.

6. Define the term *autonomic dysreflexia,* and explain the actions that you must take if symptoms of this reaction are suspected.
7. Describe alternate methods of catheterization of the urinary bladder, and explain your patient care responsibilities as a radiographer when these catheters are in place.

Glossary

Cerebral hemorrhage: A profuse amount of blood flowing into the cerebral spaces in the brain from the rupture of a blood vessel, usually an artery

Cystoscope: An instrument used for examining the urinary bladder and the ureters, which is equipped with a light, a viewing obturator, and a lumen for passing catheters

Glans: A gland on the head of the penis containing the urethral orifice

Incontinence: The inability to refrain from yielding to the normal impulse to defecate or urinate

Lithotomy position: A posture in which knees are flexed and thighs abducted and rotated externally

Penoscrotal junction: The area of the male penis that meets the scrotum

Perineal: Pertaining to the area between the anus and the scrotum in the male and the vulva and the anus in the female

Reflux: Backward flow; usually unnatural, as when urine travels back up the ureter

Retrograde: Moving in the direction that is the opposite of what is normal

Sphincter: A circular band of muscle constricting an orifice, which contracts to close the opening

Ureteral catheter: A firm catheter inserted into a ureter attached to a cystoscope

Urologic: Pertaining to the study of the urinary tract

Void: The action of emptying urine from the bladder

Infections of the urinary tract are the most common nosocomial infections. A common cause of these infections is poor infection-control practices by health care workers during placement of catheters in the urinary bladder or during care for patients who have indwelling catheters in place. As a radiographer, you will frequently work with patients who have urinary catheters in place. In some institutions, you will be responsible for inserting a catheter into the patient's urinary bladder before radiographic imaging procedures.

Catheterization of the urinary bladder refers to the insertion of a plastic, silicone, or rubber tube through the urethral meatus into the urinary bladder. Catheters are inserted into the urinary bladder for a number of reasons: to keep the bladder empty while the surrounding tissues heal after surgical procedures; to drain, irrigate, or instill medication into the bladder; to assist the incontinent patient to control urinary flow; to begin bladder retraining; or to diagnose disease, malformation, or injury of the bladder.

Cystography, retrograde pyelography, and placement of ureteral stents all involve radiographic imaging. These procedures are performed frequently in the special procedures area of the radiographic imaging department or in the cystoscopy laboratory. As part of the health care team, you will actively participate in these diagnostic examinations and treatments because fluoroscopy and radiographs are required while they are in progress.

Preparation for Catheterization

The urinary bladder is sterile, and urinary catheterization requires sterile technique. Since the urinary bladder is easily infected, any object or solution that is inserted into it must be free of bacteria and their spores. Poor technique when performing catheterization of the urinary bladder or when caring for a patient who has an indwelling catheter in place may result in infection or injury.

Catheterization is not performed without a specific order from the physician in charge of the patient, and you must not perform the procedure by yourself until you have been adequately supervised and are certain that you understand the technique required. It is less stressful for some patients if male nurses or technologists catheterize male patients, and female nurses or technologists catheterize female patients.

When a physician requests that you catheterize a patient, you must establish which type of catheter is to be used. Depending on the reason for the radiographic procedure, a straight catheter or an indwelling catheter (usually a Foley) is chosen. An indwelling catheter is inserted and left in place to allow for continuous drainage of urine. A straight catheter is used to obtain a specimen or to empty the bladder and is then removed. Most hospitals provide prepared sterile trays for catheterization with the desired type and size of catheter and the necessary equipment included. A tray set is chosen according on the type of catheter to be inserted. The equipment needed to perform a catheterization is as follows:

A straight or indwelling catheter (14F or 16F for an adult female; 16F to 20F for an adult male)

Antiseptic solution

Cotton balls for cleansing

Water-soluble lubricant

A specimen bottle

A receptacle for draining urine for a straight catheterization

A closed-system drainage set for an indwelling catheterization

Sterile gloves

Sterile drapes

Sterile forceps

The antiseptic solution most frequently used for cleansing the penis or the female perineum before catheterization is a povidone-iodine solution. The patient must be assessed for allergic response to iodine before this solution is used for cleansing purposes. A drape sheet and an extra means of casting light on the perineal area are also needed. Do not attempt to catheterize a female patient unless adequate lighting is provided. Catheter size and tips vary and are graded according to lumen size, usually on the French scale. The size of the catheter is listed on the prepared catheterization set (Fig. 14–1).

A straight catheter is a single-lumen tube (see Fig. 14–1A). Indwelling catheters have a double lumen with an inflatable balloon at one end. One lumen is attached to a urinary bag to allow for continuous urinary drainage; the other lumen is a passageway controlled by a valve that serves as a portal for instilling sterile water into the balloon. The balloon holds the catheter in place after it is inserted into the bladder (see Fig. 14–1B). You may occasionally see a third type of catheter, known as the Alcock catheter, which has three lumens. The third lumen provides a passage for irrigation solution and is used for patients in need of continuous bladder irrigation.

Female Catheterization

The female urethra is usually 3 to 5 cm (11/2 to 2 inches) in length and smaller in diameter than the male urethra. A smaller catheter than that used for

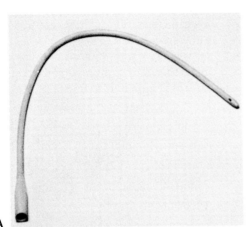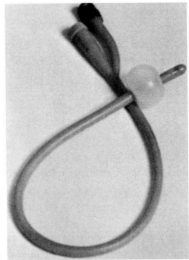

Figure 14–1. (**A**) A plain French-tipped, or straight, catheter. (**B**) A Foley catheter with the balloon inflated.

male catheterization is necessary for the female patient. Catheters are sized by the French scale. The smaller the number, the smaller the lumen size of the catheter. A 14F (used for an adult female) is smaller in diameter than a 20F (used for an adult male).

When you receive an order to perform a catheterization, you must determine the type of catheter to be inserted. Then assemble the equipment necessary, wash your hands as described for 2 minutes, and approach the patient, identify her, and explain what is to be done. Patients are often embarrassed and apprehensive about this procedure, so a good explanation and reassurance that there will be little, if any, pain are vital to the success of the procedure. Inform the patient that there will be a slight sensation of pressure when the catheter is inserted. Provide privacy for her by using a screen or by closing the door to the procedure room. Assess the patient's ability to maintain a position that allows for adequate exposure of the perineum. Assess the perineal area for soiling at this time. If the perineum is soiled, obtain washcloths, soap, warm water, and clean disposable gloves and cleanse the area before beginning the procedure. Then proceed with the steps for catheterization.

1. Position the patient on her back; have her flex her knees and relax her thighs so as to externally rotate them. This is called the *dorsal recumbent* (lithotomy) position.

2. Drape the patient with a sheet so that only the perineum is exposed. If she is disabled and cannot maintain this position, be prepared to assist her to maintain adequate exposure.

3. Adjust the light so that it shines directly on the perineal area (Fig. 14–2*A*). It is difficult to locate the urinary meatus in many women unless adequate lighting is available.

4. Open the sterile pack, which may be conveniently placed between the patient's legs if she is cooperative and will not contaminate the sterile field. If this is not the case, open the tray on a Mayo stand at the side of the table. You may use the outer plastic veering of the pack as a waste receptacle or provide an impermeable waste bag. Place it in a convenient spot away from the sterile field and in a place where your hand will not cross the sterile field as you place soiled items into the bag.

5. Put on the sterile gloves. The gloves are usually the uppermost item in the sterile pack and are cuffed for putting on by means of the open-gloving technique for sterile gloving.

6. Pick up the first sterile drape. Cover your hands with the drape to protect your gloves from contamination. Place the drape slightly under the patient's hips extending it to the front of the buttocks to cover the table (see Fig. 14–2*B*).

7. Place the second drape, which is a fenestrated drape allowing for only perineal exposure. This drape is frequently omitted.

8. If the catheterization to be done is an indwelling type, the syringe containing sterile water will be attached to the inflation valve at this time. You may test the balloon by pushing the plunger down and instilling 2 or 3 mL of solution to be certain that the balloon will not leak. After determining this, withdraw the water. Leave the syringe tip connected to the valve to be used later.

9. Open the container of sterile, water-soluble lubricant, and lubricate the catheter tip (about 1/2 inch [1.2 cm] for the female patient) (see Fig. 14–2*C*).

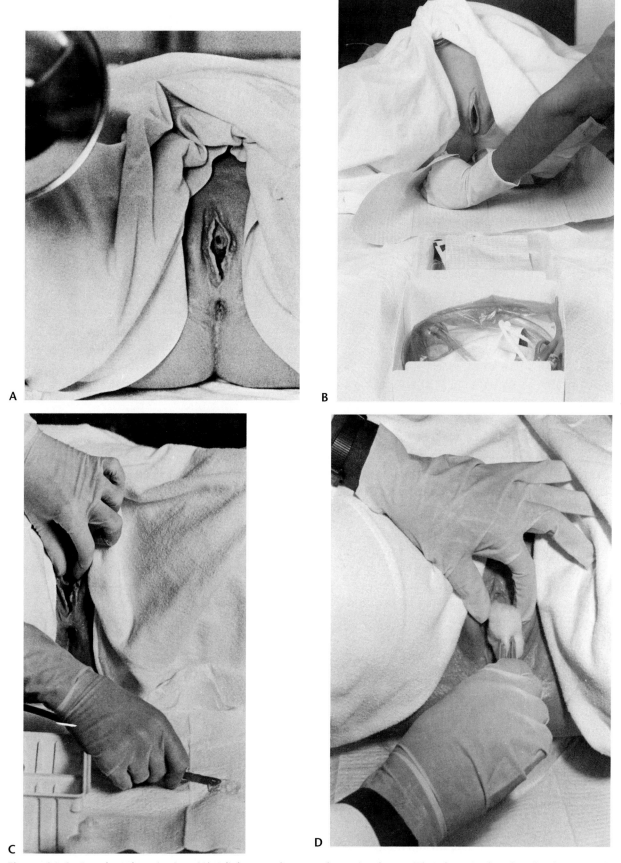

Figure 14–2. Female catheterization. (**A**) A light must focus on the perineal area. (**B**) A drape is placed under the patient's hips. (**C**) Lubricate the tip of the catheter. (**D**) Cleanse the meatus with single downward strokes. (**E**) Insert the lubricated catheter into the urethral meatus. (**F**) Instill the water in the syringe into the balloon if the catheter is the indwelling type.

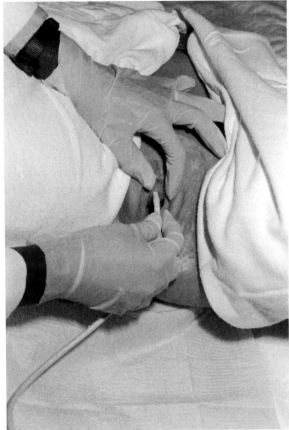

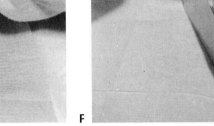

E   F

Figure 14–2. (Continued)

10. An iodophor solution is usually included in the sterile catheterization set. Open it at this time. If the kit contains solution and cotton balls, pour the solution over all except two of the cotton balls. Keep one or two cotton balls dry to wipe away the excess antiseptic. If the kit contains swabs, tear open the top of the package and set aside in the upright position.

11. Inform the patient that you will be cleansing her perineum with a solution that may feel slightly cold.

12. With the nondominant hand, separate the labia minora until the urethral meatus is clearly visible. This glove is now contaminated and will be maintained in this position to maintain exposure until the procedure is complete.

13. With the forceps, pick up one of the antiseptic-saturated cotton balls. If using swabs, pull one out of the package, leaving the rest in place.

14. Cleanse the distal side of the meatus with a single downward stroke (see Fig. 14–2D). Drop the contaminated cotton ball (swab) into the waste receptacle prepared earlier. Be careful not to cross over the sterile field with the contaminated article.

15. Pick up a second cotton ball (swab) that is saturated with antiseptic solution and wipe down the proximal side of the labia and meatus. Discard this appropriately. Next, using the third saturated ball (swab), wipe down the center directly over the meatus. Discard this without crossing the sterile field. If there is excess solution, use one of the dry cotton balls (or one of the provided dry cotton swabs) to make a single downward stroke over the center of the meatus.

16. Inform the patient that you will be inserting the catheter, and ask her to take a deep breath as you insert the catheter.

17. Keep the contaminated, nondominant hand in place; with the dominant hand, which is sterile, pick up the lubricated catheter and insert it into the urethra. As the patient exhales, the sphincter will relax, allowing the catheter to pass unobstructed into the bladder. If you feel definite resistance despite slight pressure on the catheter, do not continue with the procedure. When urine begins to flow from the catheter, the catheter has passed through the sphincter and into the bladder. When this occurs, insert the catheter about 1 inch more, then remove your

hand from the perineum, continuing to hold the catheter in place until the bladder is emptied.

18. If a straight catheter is being used, place the drainage basin so that it will catch the urine. If a urine specimen is required, allow a small amount of urine to pass through the catheter. Clamp the catheter, remove the drainage basin and replace it with the specimen container. Release the clamp and allow approximately 30 mL of urine to drain into the sterile specimen container. Reclamp the catheter so that the lid of the specimen container can be closed. After removing the specimen, allow the remaining urine to drain into the drainage basin.

19. If an indwelling catheter is being used, a drainage tube may be attached at the distal end of the catheter, and the urine will flow into the tubing and on into the drainage bag that is attached. Insert the catheter 1 inch more (2.5 cm), and then you may remove your hand from the perineum.

20. If the catheter is to be indwelling, pick up the syringe, which you have already attached to the valve, and push in the plunger until all of the water in the syringe has been injected into the balloon. It is most often filled with 5 to 10 mL sterile water (see Fig. 14–2F). Pinch the valve portal with the nondominant hand while you remove the syringe from the valve. Most indwelling catheter valves are self-sealing, so when the syringe is removed, the procedure is complete.

21. Gently tug on the catheter to be certain that it will be retained. If you feel resistance, the balloon is properly inflated and seated against the urethral opening inside the bladder.

22. Remove the soiled equipment and make the patient comfortable. Remove your gloves and wash your hands.

23. If the catheter is to remain in place for some time, tape it to the patient's inner thigh to prevent it from becoming dislodged. Make certain that there is no tension placed on the catheter as you tape it. Arrangements for urinary drainage must be made, depending on the procedure that is to follow.

Male Catheterization

The equipment needed for catheterizing male patients is much the same as for female patients; however, because the male urethra is considerably longer than that of the female, a slightly larger catheter is usually required. The male urethra is 5.5 to 7 inches (14 to 18 cm) in length; therefore, a 16F

to 20F catheter is required. The patient is placed in a supine position with his legs slightly abducted. His torso and legs are covered to the pubis so that exposure is minimal. Make certain that the patient's pubic area is clean. If he is not circumcised, withdraw the foreskin of the penis, and clean the urethral meatus. Wear clean disposable gloves to do this, and remove them on completion. Have good lighting available. Then begin the procedure by washing your hands as for medical asepsis.

1. Open the sterile pack on a Mayo stand beside the patient or between the patient's thighs if he can be depended on not to contaminate the sterile field.

2. Prepare the pack as in steps 4 through 10 for female catheterization. Place the first sterile drape over the thigh up to the scrotum and the fenestrated drape over the pubic area, leaving the penis exposed.

3. Pick up the catheter and lubricate it heavily from the tip down about 7 inches, since more lubricant is required to facilitate passage of the catheter for males than for females.

4. Inform the patient that you will be cleansing him with an antiseptic solution; then grasp the penis firmly at the shaft with the nondominant hand, retract the foreskin, and keep it retracted until the procedure is complete. Slightly spread the urinary meatus between the thumb and forefinger. If the penis is not firmly held, an erection may be stimulated. This hand is now contaminated and continues to hold the penis in position until the procedure is complete.

5. Pick up the forceps and a cotton ball saturated with antiseptic solution (or a swab). Cleanse from the urethral meatus to the glans using a circular motion. Do not go over an area already cleaned. Drop the cotton ball (swab) into the waste receptacle.

6. Repeat this procedure two more times.

7. Inform the patient that you are going to insert the catheter. Pick up the lubricated catheter with the sterile hand. Ask the patient to bear down as if he were trying to urinate, since this action will relax the sphincter.

8. With the nondominant hand only, extend the penis forward and upward. Stretching the penis into a slight angle will straighten the urethra and make insertion of the catheter into the bladder easier.

9. Using gentle, constant pressure, insert the catheter (Fig. 14–3). Too much force may cause a spasm of the sphincter and delay insertion. Do not try to proceed if there is an obstruction; withdraw the catheter and notify the physician.

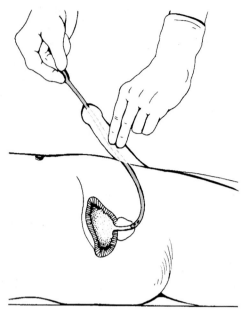

Figure 14–3. Using gentle, constant pressure, insert the catheter into the bladder.

10. When the urine begins to flow, you will know that the catheter is in the bladder; insert the catheter slightly farther (another 1/2 inch or 1.2 cm).

11. Depending on the type of catheter used for the procedure, follow steps 16 through 20 as for female catheterization listed previously. Replace the foreskin over the glans.

12. If the indwelling catheter is to be in place for some time, tape it to the lower abdomen using nonallergenic tape, with the penis directed toward the patient's chest. Allow slack so that there is no tension on the catheter. This position minimizes trauma to the urethra by straightening the angle of the penoscrotal junction.

Removing an Indwelling Catheter

A physician's order is needed before an indwelling catheter may be removed. Equipment needed will be a 10-mL syringe or a calibrated medicine glass, several thicknesses of paper toweling, a nonpermeable disposable bag, and clean, disposable gloves.

When you receive an order from the physician in charge of the patient to remove an indwelling catheter, collect the equipment necessary and wash your hands. Identify the patient, and explain the procedure to him or her. There is usually little, if any, discomfort with this procedure.

1. Uncover the patient just enough to see the insertion point of the catheter. Ask the female patient to

separate her legs slightly. Remove the tape that holds the catheter in place. Put on the clean gloves, and place the paper toweling under the catheter.

CALL OUT!

When removing an indwelling catheter, remember to deflate the balloon!

2. Insert the tip of the syringe into the valve port and pull back on the plunger until all the sterile water from the retention balloon is removed; then disconnect the syringe from the valve (Fig. 14–4).

3. When the water is completely removed from the balloon, wrap the paper toweling around the catheter and gently withdraw it from the bladder. If you feel any resistance, stop the procedure and notify the physician. The catheter should come out easily.

4. Wrap the catheter in the toweling, and place it and the drainage set into the nonpermeable bag.

5. If urine output measurement is required, do this after removing the catheter. This allows urine to drain from the catheter and tubing into the bag. Record the total amount of urine in the chart.

6. Place the soiled equipment into a contaminated-waste receptacle. Remove your gloves and wash your hands.

7. Return to the patient to make certain that he or she is comfortable.

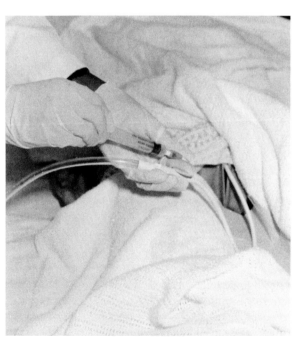

Figure 14–4. Remove the water from the balloon with a syringe attached to the valve port.

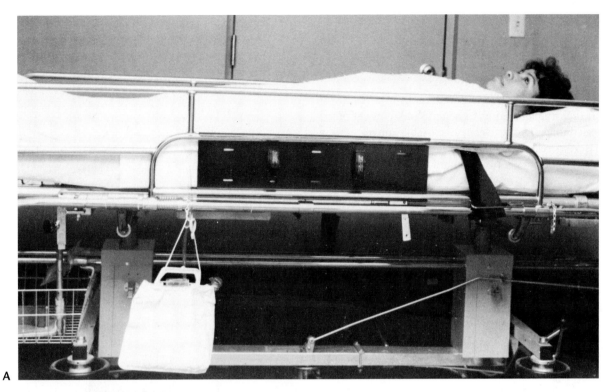

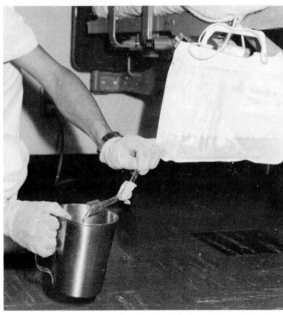

Figure 14–5. (**A**) The drainage bag from an indwelling catheter must be positioned below the level of the urinary bladder. (**B**) To empty the drainage bag, release the clamp that closes the spout, and allow the urine to drain into a graduated flask.

Catheter Care in the Radiographic Imaging Department

Often patients must be transported to the diagnostic imaging department with indwelling catheters in place. If this is the case, you must keep the drainage bag below the level of the urinary bladder. This maintains gravity flow and prevents contamination due to backflow of urine. If urine is allowed to flow back into the bladder or if drainage is obstructed, a urinary tract infection may result (Fig. 14–5A). The drainage tubing must be placed over the patient's leg and coiled on the gurney or table top, not below the level of the patient's hips. If the drainage bag is to be lifted above the patient during a move, the drainage tubing should be clamped and the drainage bag emptied before the move is begun to prevent a backflow of urine. Be sure to check with the patient's nurse before emptying the drainage bag because the patient may be having the urine output measured.

> ## CALL OUT!
> Always keep the level of the drainage bag lower than the level of the patient's bladder.

If the drainage bag is to be emptied, you will need six alcohol sponges, clean, disposable gloves, and a measuring receptacle. The emptying spout should be withdrawn from its housing and wiped several times with alcohol sponges from top to bottom. The clamp that keeps the spout closed is then released, and the urine is allowed to drain into the graduated receptacle (see Fig. 14–5B). When the drainage bag is empty, the spout is reclamped, cleaned again with alcohol wipes, and replaced in the housing.

Throughout the procedure, be watchful of the tubing so that kinks do not occur. When moving a patient with a catheter in place, take care to avoid undue tension on the catheter. Pulling on the catheter can cause the patient great discomfort or injury if it becomes dislodged.

If the patient with an indwelling catheter is transported by wheelchair, attach the drainage bag to the underside of the wheelchair. The tubing must be coiled at the level of the patient's hips. Take care not to allow the tubing or drainage bag to become entangled in the wheels of the chair or to touch the floor. Never place a drainage bag on the patient's lap or abdomen during transport, because this may cause a reflux of urine into the bladder.

Avoid disconnecting the catheter from its closed drainage system. Maintenance of a closed urinary drainage system is essential if infection is to be prevented. Once the closed drainage system has been invaded, it should not be reconnected. The patient must have a new catheter with new closed-system drainage reinserted if catheter drainage of the bladder is to be continued.

Alternative Methods of Urinary Drainage

There are two common methods of dealing with urinary drainage on a temporary or permanent basis. These are the suprapubic catheter (also called a cystocatheter) and the condom, or Texas, catheter. You must recognize both methods.

The *suprapubic catheter* is placed directly into the bladder by means of an abdominal incision. This method is sometimes chosen to divert the flow of urine from the urethral route after gynecologic surgery, urethral injuries, or prostatic obstructions, or for chronic incontinence or loss of bladder control.

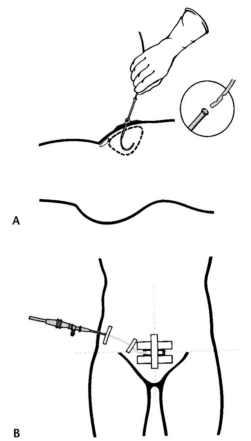

Figure 14–6. (**A**) Introduction of the suprapubic catheter. (**B**) The body seal and catheter are taped to the abdomen. (Brunner L, Suddarth DM: *Lippincott Manual of Nursing Practice.* Philadelphia: JB Lippincott, 1986. Courtesy of Dow Corning Corp.)

Suprapubic catheters are believed to reduce the risk of infection as a long-term method of bladder drainage and to facilitate normal urination after surgical procedures. The catheter is attached to a closed urinary drainage system and is secured with sutures, tape, or a body seal system (Fig. 14–6).

When you are caring for a patient with a suprapubic catheter, you must guard against placing tension on the catheter. Also, follow the same rules of asepsis as for patients with other closed-system urinary drainage. That is, the drainage bag must be kept below the patient's bladder level at all times and not lifted over the patient. The bag must be emptied before moving the patient under the direction of the nurse in charge of the patient.

The *condom catheter* is an externally applied drainage device used for male patients who are susceptible to urinary tract infections or are incontinent or comatose and whose bladder continues to empty spontaneously (Fig. 14–7). If the patient is not prone to urinary tract infections, a Foley indwelling catheter is most likely to be used.

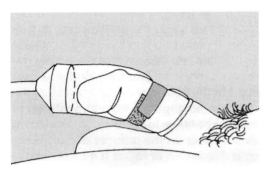

Figure 14–7. A condom catheter. (Taylor C, Lillis C, LeMone P: *Fundamentals of Nursing: The Art and Science of Nursing Care.* Philadelphia: JB Lippincott, 1989.)

The condom catheter is a soft rubber sheath that is placed over the penis and secured with a special type of adhesive material. The distal end of the condom has an opening that fits onto a drainage tube and terminates in a drainage bag that attaches to the patient's thigh. The drainage bag can be emptied easily when necessary.

The condom catheter is changed every 24 to 48 hours. This helps to reduce the possibility of acquiring a urinary tract infection. When you are caring for patients who have condom catheters in place, you must guard against dislodging the catheter from the drainage tube or twisting the condom and causing pain or skin irritation.

Cystography

Cystography is radiographic imaging of the urinary bladder. Using fluoroscopy and radiography, the urinary bladder is visualized as it fills and empties. This procedure is done to diagnose pathological changes in its function. The pathology may be due to tumors inside or outside the bladder, trauma, or vesicoureteral reflux (abnormal backflow of urine into the ureters). Cystography also demonstrates anatomic changes in the bladder floor, the posterior urethrovesical angle, and the angle of the urethra in female patients when stress is applied to the bladder wall. It also determines cystoureteral reflux due to incompetent ureteral valves.

Cystographic procedures that may be scheduled are cystourethrography (radiography of the urinary bladder and urethra), voiding cystography (radiography of the patient's ability to empty the urinary bladder), and voiding cystourethrography (the urethra is studied as the patient voids upon removal of the catheter). Metallic bead chain cystourethrography examines the cause for stress incontinence in women. The patient may be scheduled for any one or combination of these procedures.

Patient Education Before Cystography

The patient is usually advised to restrict intake of liquids for several hours before the procedure. This helps to prevent the dilution of the contrast by urine in the patient's bladder. Inform the patient that he or she will be catheterized and an iodinated contrast agent and possible air will be instilled into the bladder. The patient should be prepared to expect some discomfort and a feeling of the need to void. Instruct the patient not to move unless directed to do so during the examination. Assess the patient for allergic reactions to drugs and iodinated contrast agents, as well as for other health problems. However, note that the incidence of anaphylactic reaction to an iodinated contrast medium is not as great in this examination, since the contrast agent is administered into the bladder, not intravenously. Pregnancy is generally a contraindication to having this procedure, and patients with urinary tract infections must have special consideration. It is possible to spread the infection to other pelvic organs by inserting the catheter and instilling a contrast medium. Usually, an informed consent is required to be signed.

Care During Cystography

When the patient arrives in the examining room, instruct him or her to disrobe and put on a patient gown. You may ask the patient to urinate before the catheterization to empty the bladder as much as possible. The patient is placed in a supine position and preliminary (scout) images are taken. The patient is then catheterized with a retention catheter as described earlier in this chapter and as directed by the physician. In some institutions, you will be responsible for performing catheterization. A gonadal shield protects male patients during the procedure. Female patients are not able to have this protection, since the bladder would not be visualized with such a shield in place.

All patients are draped to maintain privacy. To prevent infection, follow strict surgical aseptic technique while the examination is being performed.

The bladder is filled with a contrast agent (200 to 300 mL for an adult; 50 to 100 mL for a child). Air may be used to provide contrast on some occasions. Take films of the patient in varying positions. The bladder is drained, or the patient is asked to urinate so that you can examine his or her ability to empty the bladder in a normal manner. The catheter is removed, and more films may be taken as the patient voids and the contrast agent passes through the urethra. This is called a *voiding cystourethrogram.*

This procedure may cause a great deal of stress and embarrassment for the patient. You must take great care to preserve the patient's dignity and privacy while it is in progress.

Care Following Cystography

After cystography, the patient is told that he or she may resume normal activities as the physician prescribes. Instruct the patient to report any symptoms of chills, fever, excessive blood in the urine, any changes in the ability to urinate, or pain on urination to the physician immediately.

Also instruct the patient to increase fluid intake for 24 hours to aid in elimination of contrast agent from the bladder. Inform him or her that some burning may occur on urination and that there may be a small amount of pink-tinged urine for a few hours after the examination.

Cystourethrography may be performed on patients who are paralyzed owing to spinal cord injury or disease. These patients are susceptible to a condition called *autonomic dysreflexia.* This is a condition in which a stimulus, such as a full rectum or an overdistended bladder, creates an exaggerated response by the sympathetic nervous system. In such cases, the patient may complain of a sudden, severe headache that results from hypertension. Other symptoms of this condition include sweating and flushing of the face while other areas of the body may be cold and pale, tachycardia or bradycardia, nasal stuffiness, and a feeling of apprehension.

If a paralyzed patient, especially a patient with paraplegia or quadriplegia, is being cared for and complains of a sudden headache, you must take the following action:

1. Stop the procedure and notify the physician; prepare to call the emergency team, and have the emergency cart at hand.

2. Place the patient in Fowler's position.

3. Monitor the patient's blood pressure and apical pulse.

4. Remove the source of the stimulus; if the bladder is distended with contrast agent or urine, empty it immediately.

5. Hydralazine hydrochloride or diazoxide are administered by the physician cautiously to prevent hypertension.

6. Propantheline bromide may be administered to prevent or treat nausea.

Failure to respond to these symptoms may result in myocardial infarction or cerebral hemorrhage.

Retrograde Pyelography

Retrograde pyelography is a radiographic technique performed to visualize the proximal ureters and the kidneys after injection of an iodinated contrast agent. This procedure is usually performed in a cystoscopy suite, routinely located in the surgery area under the direction of a urologist. As the radiographer, you must be present to take necessary radiographic images and to provide fluoroscopic examinations of the patient as ordered. Retrograde pyelography is performed to assess the ureters for obstruction resulting from strictures, tumors, stones, scarring, or other pathological processes when other methods are contraindicated. Since this procedure is a filling of the renal collecting system through a catheter, renal function is not studied.

Patient Education and Preparation

To ensure adequate visualization during this procedure, the patient may be instructed to have enemas to clear the bowel just before the procedure is to be performed. The procedure may be performed under a light general anesthesia or under local anesthesia. If general anesthesia is to be given, the patient will be instructed to have no food or fluids by mouth after midnight the night before the procedure. For local anesthesia, the patient may have a liquid breakfast. The patient must be informed that he or she may receive a mild sedative and a drug to reduce bladder spasm during the procedure. An informed consent must be signed, and the patient must be screened for pregnancy and allergies to drugs and iodinated contrast media. Because of the nature of the procedure, the preparation of the patient is generally the responsibility of the surgery staff, the urologist, and the anesthesiologist; however, you should still make sure that the radiology request and informed consent are in order.

The Procedure

The patient may be placed in a modified lithotomy position. To prevent impaired circulation, take care to keep pressure off the legs while the patient is in this position. You will be responsible for fluoroscopy and radiographs during this procedure, and a nurse and the physician will monitor the patient.

A contrast medium is injected through a catheter inserted into the ureter from the bladder by means of a cystoscope. Retrograde pyelography is normally performed on one side. However, it is possible that both kidneys must be studied. When this is the case, each side is catheterized and examined independently of the other. Images are taken to demonstrate the proximal ureters and the structure of the renal pelvis. The catheter is withdrawn, and more contrast agent is injected to visualize the remaining portion of the ureter. The procedure takes approximately an hour.

After the procedure is completed, the patient is instructed to notify the physician if he or she observes bleeding, fever, chills, or other signs of infection. If the patient has had a general anesthetic, he or she will be observed in a recovery area until awake and alert and the vital signs are stable. The patient may resume a regular schedule as soon as the physician gives permission. Fluids should be increased for 24 hours to aid in elimination of the contrast agent.

Ureteral Stents

If the patient has an obstructed ureter due to a stricture, edema, or an advanced malignant tumor, a stent may be inserted into the ureter on a temporary or permanent basis to relieve the problem. Stents are made of soft, pliable silicone (Fig. 14–8) and may be placed surgically or during a retrograde pyelogram.

There are complications associated with the presence of any foreign body in the ureter, stents included. These are infection and obstruction from encrustation and clot formation. You will be responsible for the radiographic aspects of this procedure, and patient care and instruction will be the responsibility of the physician and the nurse. The patient usually receives a general anesthetic for this procedure and is allowed to recover in the recovery suite.

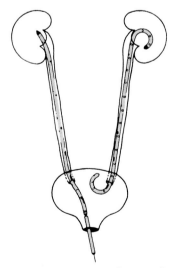

Figure 14–8. Retrograde passage of ureteral stent. The double-J ureteral stent is shaped to resist migration. The proximal J hooks into the lower calix or renal pelvis, and the distal J curves into the bladder. (Courtesy of Medical Engineering Corporation, Racine, WI.)

Summary

All health care workers have the responsibility to practice infection control when inserting catheters into the urinary bladder and caring for patients with catheters in place. As the radiographer, you will not only work with patients who have catheters in place, but on some occasions you will be responsible for performing the catheterization procedure. You must be able to maintain surgical aseptic technique when performing this procedure, and you must learn appropriate catheter care when the patient has a retention catheter.

Catheterization of the urinary bladder is the process of inserting a plastic, rubber, or silicone tube through the urethral meatus into the urinary bladder. There are two types of catheters: the straight catheter and the indwelling catheter. Catheter insertion and removal require a physician's order.

The same type of equipment is required for catheterization of both male and female patients, although the procedure varies slightly because of anatomic differences. (A larger catheter is required for the adult male.) Before a catheterization procedure, the patient must be given adequate explanation, reassurance, and privacy to reduce embarrassment and anxiety.

Correct care of the indwelling catheter while the patient is being transported to the diagnostic imaging department is necessary for the prevention of urinary tract infection or injury. You must be certain that the drainage bag remains lower than the level of the urinary bladder to ensure gravity flow of urine. Closed-system drainage of the urinary bladder should not be broken, and tension on the catheter must be avoided.

As the radiographer, you are a member of the health care team when cystography, retrograde pyelography, and placement of ureteral stents are being performed. You must learn your obligations concerning patient education and care during these procedures and must take all precautions to maintain infection control and patient safety while these procedures are in progress.

Caution should be used when cystourethrograms are performed it the patient is paralyzed. *Autonomic dysreflexia,* a life-threatening complication, may result from the stimulus of a full urinary bladder. You must familiarize yourself with the symptoms of this problem and be prepared to respond if these symptoms occur.

Alternative methods of urinary drainage are by suprapubic catheter and external condom catheter. Patients who have these types of urinary drainage require precautionary care to prevent urinary tract infections and injury.

Chapter 14 Test

_____ 1. The most common nosocomial infections are
   a. Bloodborne infections
   b. Respiratory tract infections
   c. Wound infections
   d. Urinary tract infections

_____ 2. The best way to prevent urinary tract infections during catheterization of the urinary bladder is
   a. By maintaining strict surgical aseptic technique
   b. By increasing the patient's fluid intake
   c. By requesting that the physician initiate antimicrobial therapy
   d. By keeping the patient isolated

_____ 3. When performing a urethral catheterization, how will you know whether the catheter is in the bladder?
   a. The patient will relax.
   b. There will be a mucoid discharge.
   c. Urine will start to flow.
   d. There is no way of knowing.

_____ 4. When inserting a retention catheter, after you have placed the sterile drape, pre-pared the lubricant, and poured antiseptic solution over the cotton balls, the next step is to
   a. Insert the catheter
   b. Inflate the balloon
   c. Cleanse the meatus
   d. Put on sterile gloves

_____ 5. When removing a retention catheter, the most important consideration is to
   a. Deflate the balloon
   b. Cleanse the meatus
   c. Maintain privacy
   d. Explain the procedure to the patient

_____ 6. When transporting a patient with a retention catheter with closed-system drainage in place, you must remember
   1. To keep the drainage bag below the level of the bladder
   2. To prevent tension on the catheter
   3. To keep the excess tubing coiled at the level of the patient's hips, not below
      a. 1 and 2
      b. 1 and 3
      c. 2 and 3
      d. 1, 2, and 3

_____ 7. You may disconnect the catheter from the closed-system drainage before transporting the patient.
   a. True
   b. False

_____ 8. If a urinary drainage bag must be lifted over a patient to prepare for transport, you must
   1. Empty the drainage bag   a. 1 and 2
   2. Disconnect the drainage bag   b. 2 and 3
   3. Raise the bag quickly   c. 1 and 4
   4. Clamp the drainage tube   d. 1, 2, 3, and 4

_____ **9.** If a retention catheter is to be taped onto a male patient, it must be taped
    a. To the inside of the leg
    b. To the scrotum
    c. To the lateral aspect of the thigh
    d. To the lower abdomen

_____ **10.** During a cystogram, you must assist in maintaining

1. The patient's privacy	a. 1 and 2
2. The patient's dignity	b. 2 and 3
3. The patient's comfort	c. 1 and 3
	d. 1, 2, and 3

_____ **11.** Patient care instruction after cystourethrography includes
    a. Discouraging fluid intake for 24 hours
    b. Informing the patient of possible bleeding and to disregard this
    c. Informing the patient to increase fluid intake for the next 24 hours
    d. Instructing the patient in measuring intake and output

12. Describe the rules of asepsis that must be followed when caring for a patient with a suprapubic catheter.

13. List your responsibilities as the radiographer before and during retrograde pyelography.

14. List the symptoms of autonomic dysreflexia, and explain your response if these symptoms occur.

15. List the precautions you must take if the patient has a condom catheter.

15 Basic Electrocardiogram Monitoring

Objectives

After studying this chapter, you will be able to:

1. Explain the cardiac conduction system.
2. Correctly apply the three lead cardiac monitoring electrodes.
3. Identify electrocardiogram waveform components.
4. Interpret a basic electrocardiogram rhythm strip.
5. Recognize ominous cardiac arrhythmias.
6. Explain you role as a radiographer role in responding to ominous arrhythmias

Glossary

Acidosis: A pathological state characterized by higher than normal concentration of hydrogen ions in the arterial blood

Arrhythmia: An irregularity in or loss of rhythm of the heartbeat

CODE: A term used in hospitals to describe an emergency, requiring situation-trained members of staff; the signal to summon team

Deflection: In the electrocardiogram, a deviation of the curve from the isoelectric base line

Dyspnea: Shortness of breath

Hypoxia: Lower than normal levels of oxygen in inspired gases, arterial blood, or tissue

Oscilloscope: An oscillograph in which the record of oscillation is continuously visible

In the mid-1880s, it was discovered that the heart's electrical activity could be measured externally by placing an electrode on a person's skin. In 1901, Dr. Willem Einthoven improved on this initial discovery and devised a means of measuring the heart's electrical activity with a timed record. He named these measured waves or rhythmic movements the P, QRS, and T waves. And he named the tracing of these movements an *electrokardiogram*. In many circles, it is still known as an EKG. In the English language, we spell *cardiogram* with a *c* and call this measurement of the electrical activity of the heart an ECG. It will be known in this text as an ECG; however, EKG and ECG are the same.

You will participate as a radiographer in many diagnostic procedures that require continuous cardiac monitoring. In some institutions, you may be expected to prepare the patient for cardiac monitoring. In others, you may observe the patient who is being monitored and recognize ominous ECG patterns as they appear on the screen of an oscilloscope.

An ECG records the electrical activity of the heart, thereby providing a record of the heart's electrical activity and information concerning the heart's function and structure. As the heart is monitored, a tracing of its electrical activity is made on electrically sensitive paper or on the screen of an oscilloscope. This tracing is used to detect abnormal transmission of cardiac impulses from the heart through the surrounding tissues to the skin surface. When the impulses reach the skin, electrodes that have been placed in standardized anatomic positions transmit them to the ECG machine, and the impulses are then recorded in graphic form.

You must understand that ECG readings that seem abnormal are not necessarily indicative of heart disease. Conversely, a normal ECG pattern is not always an indication that the heart is healthy. The ECG cannot detect all cardiac pathology conditions.

There are several types of ECG testing. They require that electrodes be placed in varying numbers on the exterior body. A radiographer who must learn this subject in detail must plan to enroll in a special class for this purpose, which includes clinical practice in learning to read ECG rhythm strips.

Continuous monitoring with the patient connected to a cardiac oscilloscope is the type of ECG testing to which you will most often be exposed. An *electrocardiograph* is the instrument that measures, records, and prints on electrocardiographic paper an electrocardiogram. It detects patterns of cardiac impulses and displays them on a monitor so that the patient's status is readily observable during special procedures in imaging and for other medical purposes. Blood pressure, respiratory rate, and oxygen saturation are also continuously monitored and displayed on the oscillo-scope. If the patient's heart rate, rhythm, or other vital signs deviate from the normal rate or rhythm, an alarm sounds to alert the team caring for the patient. In this manner, life-threatening problems are detected instantly. A printout of the ECG pattern is made at specified times to keep for the patient's record and to compare the current pattern with previous patterns on each patient.

A Review of Cardiac Anatomy

The heart is a fist-sized muscular organ that is located in the left side of the body between the lungs and the mediastinum. It is a double pump. Its purpose is to pump deoxygenated blood through the heart to the lungs for reoxygenation and then to pump reoxygenated blood back through the heart into the aorta and to all body tissues. You will recall that the heart has four chambers: the right and left atria and the right and left ventricles. The apex of the heart is at the lowest aspect of the organ, and the base of the heart is the upper aspect. The right and left ventricles of the heart are separated by the interventricular septum. The chambers of the heart are protected from re-entry of blood that has been pumped from one chamber of the heart to another by a series of valves. The walls of the atria and ventricles are composed of three layers: the epicardium (the thin outer layer), the myocardium (the middle muscular layer), and the endocardium (the thin inner layer). The muscular layer of the atria is thinner than that of the ventricles.

Deoxygenated blood flows into the right atrium from the inferior and superior vena cava and veins draining into the heart. It is then pumped through the tricuspid valve into the right ventricle. The contraction of the right ventricle sends deoxygenated blood through the pulmonic (semilunar) valve into the lungs for re-oxygenation through the pulmonary artery. The oxygenated blood then flows through the pulmonary veins into the left atrium. The contraction of the left atrium pumps the blood from the left atrium through the mitral (bicuspid) valve into the left ventricle. With the contraction of the left ventricle, the oxygenated blood is pumped into the aorta and then circulates to all parts of the body (Fig. 15–1).

The myocardium (the heart muscle) is supplied with oxygenated blood via the right and left coronary arteries and their branches. The branches of the left coronary artery supply the interventricular septum, the walls and surfaces of the atria and ventricles, and the sinoatrial (SA) and atrioventricular (AV) nodes. The right coronary artery supplies the remainder of the myocardial blood supply (Fig. 15–2).

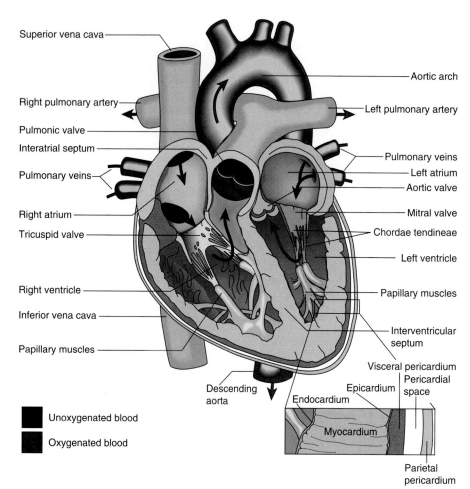

Superior vena cava

Right pulmonary artery

Pulmonic valve

Interatrial septum

Pulmonary veins

Right atrium

Tricuspid valve

Right ventricle

Inferior vena cava

Papillary muscles

Descending aorta

Endocardium

Aortic arch

Left pulmonary artery

Pulmonary veins

Left atrium

Aortic valve

Mitral valve

Chordae tendineae

Left ventricle

Papillary muscles

Interventricular septum

Visceral pericardium

Epicardium

Pericardial space

Myocardium

Parietal pericardium

■ Unoxygenated blood

■ Oxygenated blood

Figure 15–1. Structure of the heart. Arrows show the course of blood flow through the heart chambers. (Smeltzer SC, Bare BG: *Brunner and Suddarth's Textbook of Medical-Surgical Nursing,* 9th ed. Philadelphia: Lippincott Williams & Wilkins, 2000.)

The Cardiac Conduction System

The ECG reports the electrical activity of the heart, particularly the contraction of the myocardium. It also supplies information concerning the heart's rate and rhythm. Electrical stimulation results in contraction of the heart. The cells of the heart muscle (*myocytes*) are influenced by sodium, calcium, and potassium ions. At rest, myocytes are polarized, and the interior of the cells are negatively charged. When they are depolarized, the interior of the myocytes become positive. When an electrical impulse is initiated, potassium rushes out of the myocytes and sodium rushes in. Calcium also enters the cells at this stage but at a slower rate and acts as a regulator of cardiac contraction. This initiates depolarization and converts the electrical charge of the cell into a positive charge. Depolarization acts as a wave throughout the myocardium and results in contraction of the heart. Repolarization takes place as the cells return to a resting state.

The conduction system of the heart has myocardial cells that have the properties of automaticity, conductivity, excitability, and contractility. The SA node, located in the upper posterior wall of the right atrium, is the dominant pacemaker of the heart. At rest under normal conditions, the SA node initiates 60 to 100 impulses per minute. It is responsible for the rate and rhythm of the cardiac cycle or the *automaticity.*

From the SA node, the wave of depolarization is carried through to the right atrium to the left atrium and results in nearly simultaneous contraction of the right and left atria. The atrial conduction system has three internodal tracts in the right atrium (anterior, middle, and posterior) and one conduction tract in the left atrium called *Bachmann's bundle,* which depolarizes the left atrium. Depolarization is then conducted to the AV node. The AV node is located in the right atrial wall near the tricuspid valve and coordinates the incoming electrical impulses from the atria. After a brief delay during which the atria contracts and completes filling the ventricles, the impulse is conducted to the bundle of His.

The bundle of His is a group of cells that travels through the ventricular septum. It divides into the right and left bundle branches and conducts impulses to the right and left ventricles. The left bundle branch bifurcates into the left anterior and left posterior bundle branches to reach the terminal point in the conduction system, the Purkinje fibers. At this point, the myocardial cells are stimulated and result in ventricular contraction. This cell-to-cell passage of impulse is the *conductivity.* When the impulse spreads to all areas of the heart the

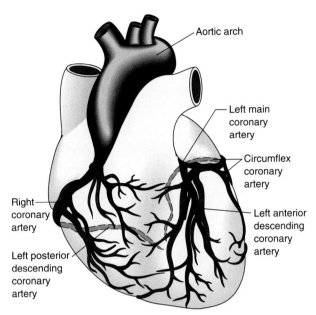

Figure 15–2. Coronary arteries (red vessels) arise from the aorta and encircle the heart. Coronary veins are shown in gray. (Smeltzer SC, Bare BG: *Brunner and Suddarth's Textbook of Medical-Surgical Nursing,* 9th ed. Philadelphia: Lippincott Williams & Wilkins, 2000.)

action potential is called *excitability*. This leads to the shortening of the myocardial cells and *contractility*. The heart rate is determined by the myocardial cells with the most rapid firing rate (Fig. 15–2).

Electrophysiology of the Cardiac Cycle

The depolarization-repolarization cycle goes through five phases, which can be seen as it registers on the ECG monitor. They phases are as follows:

- *Phase 0:* The cardiac cell receives an impulse from a neighboring cell and is depolarized (sodium ions move across the cell membrane into the cell; calcium ions follow). The ECG records a P wave as the impulse from the SA node spreads through the right and left atria and depolarizes them, resulting in their simultaneous contraction. There is a slight pause while the blood from the atria fills the right and left ventricles, which is registered on the ECG as a short baseline. THE P WAVE RECORDS THE CONTRACTION OF THE ATRIA (atrial depolarization).

  This is followed by the depolarization of the right and left ventricles and results in the QRS complex as the electrical impulse travels slowly through the AV node and more rapidly through the bundle of His into the right and left bundle branches to the Purkinje fibers. THE QRS COMPLEX RECORDS VENTRICULAR CONTRACTION.

- *Phase 1:* Repolarization begins. Sodium ions decrease in number entering the cell, and the positive charge within the cells become less positive.

- *Phase 2:* The cell membrane is neutral in electrical charge. The ST segment is recorded on the ECG at this time.

- *Phase 3:* Repolarization proceeds. The T wave is recorded on the ECG at this time. THE R WAVE REPRESENTS REPOLARIZATION OF THE VENTRICLES. A U wave may follow the T wave and is associated with repolarization of the Purkinje fibers in the ventricles. It is not always present but is pronounced with hypokalemia and other pathological conditions.

- *Phase 4:* Sodium ions move outside the cell, and potassium ions move inside. The *refractory period* begins with depolarization at Phase 0 following the recording of the QRS complex and ends with depolarization. At this time, no stimulus can excite the cell. At the end of Phase 4, the resting phase, the cell is prepared for another stimulus (Fig.15–3).

Recall that the autonomic nervous system also has a marked effect on the activity of the heart. The parasympathetic fibers affect the atria and ventricles primarily. The sympathetic fibers enhance myocardial excitability and increase pacemaker firing rate, conduction speed, and contractility of the heart.

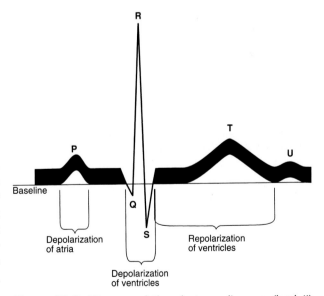

Figure 15–3. Diagram of the electrocardiogram (lead II) and representative depolarization and repolarization of the atria and ventricles. The P wave represents atrial depolarization; the QRS complex, ventricular depolarization; and the T wave, ventricular repolarization. Atrial repolarization occurs during ventricular depolarization and is hidden under the QRS complex. (Patrick ML, Woods SL, Craven RF et al: *Medical-Surgical Nursing.* Philadelphia: JB Lippincott, 1986.)

The parasympathetic fibers slow excitability, automaticity, and conduction speed but do not affect contractility.

Interpreting the ECG

The recorded ECG is printed on electrographic paper that moves through the recorder at 2.5 mm per second. The ECG paper is divided into 1 mm × 1 mm squares (Fig. 15–4). These squares are grouped together in 5 mm × 5 mm darkly lined boxes. Each millimeter represents 0.04 second and each 5 mm represents 0.20 second (Fig. 15–5). Five of the 5 mm divisions equal 1 second. There is a vertical line at the top of the ECG paper every 75 mm or every 3 seconds. This method of dividing the electrographic paper allows one to measure the heart rate and the time intervals in the PQRST complex.

An upward deflection on the graph is positive, and a downward deflection is negative. A straight line (*an isoelectric line*) on the graph indicates no electrical activity or activity too slight to measure. To identify the isoelectric line on a cardiac rhythm strip, draw a line connecting the area of each complex that immediately follows the P wave before the Q wave. If there is a deflection above this line, it is positive; below the line

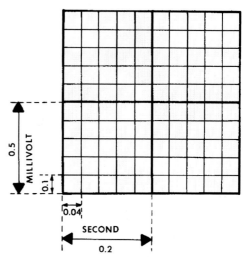

Figure 15–5. Time and voltage lines on ECG paper, *Vertically*: 1 mm = 0.1 mV; 5 mm = 0.5 mV; 10 mm = 1.0 mV. *Horizontally*: 25 small boxes = 1 second; 1500 small boxes = 60 seconds. (Patrick ML, Woods SL, Craven RF et al: *Medical-Surgical Nursing.* Philadelphia: JB Lippincott, 1986.)

is negative. The ECG waveform consists of the P wave, the QRS complex, an ST segment, a QT interval, and occasionally a U wave (Fig. 15–6). Display 15-1 describes the characteristics and timing of the ECG.

Lead Placement

There are several methods of placing electrodes to monitor the electrical activity of the heart. You will rarely be called on to place the electrodes for a 12-lead ECG or to monitor this method. The lead placement does not change the heart's electrical activity, but it does change the angle from which the activity is recorded. When a depolarization wave moves toward a positive electrode, the deflection on the ECG will be upward.

The two leads most often used for continuous monitoring are lead II and a modification of V_1 (midclavicular 1 or MCL_1) (Fig. 15–7). Lead II best demonstrates atrial depolarization, and MCL_1 demonstrates ventricular activity. If a third electrode (a ground electrode) is used, it may be placed anywhere on the upper anterior chest.

To prepare a patient for cardiac monitoring, approach the patient, explain the procedure, and provide for privacy. Inform the patient that the monitor does not detect chest pain or dyspnea and that, if these symptoms occur, the patient must immediately inform you or the person who is caring for him or her.

Wherever the electrodes are to be positioned, the patient's skin must be prepared by removing the dirt and oils present with soap and water or alcohol. Hair in those areas is sometimes removed by physician's

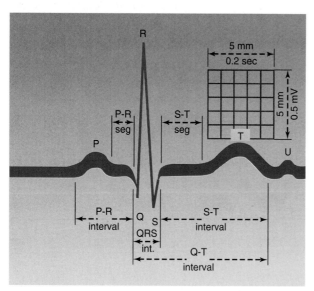

Figure 15–4. ECG graph and commonly measured complex components. Each small box represents 0.04 second on the horizontal axis and 1 mm or 0.1 millivolt on the vertical axis. The PR interval is measured from the beginning of the QRS complex; the QRS complex is measured from the beginning of the Q wave to the end of the S wave; the QT interval is measured from the beginning of the Q wave to the end of the T wave. (Smeltzer SC, Bare BG: *Brunner and Suddarth's Textbook of Medical-Surgical Nursing,* 9th ed. Philadelphia: Lippincott Williams & Wilkins, 2000.)

DISPLAY 15–1

COMPONENTS OF THE ECG

P wave: precedes the QRS complex = atrial depolarization; first deflection above or below the isoelectric line

Normal amplitude = 2 to 2.5 mm in height

Normal duration = 0.06 to 0.12 second

PR interval: the time from the beginning of the P wave to the beginning of the QRS complex

Normal interval = 0.12 to .20 second

Configuration and deflection not measured

QRS complex: depolarization of the ventricles

Follows the P wave

Normal configuration = 0.04 to 0.11 second

Configuration consists of three waves. Deflection depends on the lead and may be positive with most of the complex above the baseline or negative with most of the complex below the line.

ST segment: begins at the end of the QRS complex and ends at the beginning of the T wave

Indicates that the myocardial cells is in a neutral phase at beginning of repolarization

Configuration—usually isoelectric but may vary slightly; normally not more than 1 mm; configuration and deflection not measured

T wave: repolarization of the ventricles

Follows QRS and ST segment

Normal amplitude = 5 mm or less; follows same deflection as the QRS complex

Duration of T wave not measured

QT interval: time required for ventricular depolarization and repolarization to take place

Extends from the beginning of the QRS complex to the end of the T wave and includes all of these in the measurement

Normal duration = no more than 0.38 second in men and 0.42 second in women.

U wave: associated with repolarization of the Purkinje fibers in the ventricles

Not always seen but more pronounced in hypokalemic, hyperkalemic, and digitoxin toxicity states

Follows the T wave; deflects upward

Amplitude and duration not measured

---

order to reduce skin resistance. Place the electrodes on flat areas of the skin. The electrodes used for continuous monitoring usually come prelubricated in a prepared package. If the electrodes are not prelubricated, apply an electroconductive paste to each electrode before placement. Once the electrodes are in place, set an alarm on the ECG machine for 30% above and 30% below the patient's baseline heart rate. Then the monitor and the electrocardiograph are activated. Any deviation from the settings or the cardiogram itself activates the alarm.

Reading ECGs

The reading process can be complex; however, you must remember that you have to be able to quickly observe the monitor, perhaps run an electrocardiograph strip, and be able to identify normal sinus rhythm and any adverse configuration or deflection on the monitor or strip. You are not educated to make diagnoses. You must only be alert for ominous symptoms. This can be done simply. Display 15-2 describes the method.

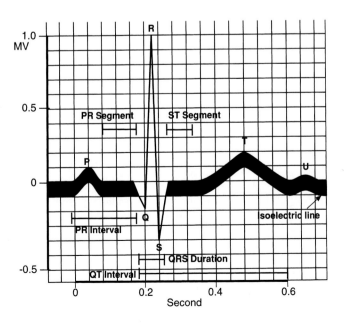

Figure 15–6. The ECG wave form.

Normal ECG Parameters and Normal Sinus Rhythm Criteria

Scanning the ECG Strip

1. Calculate the atrial rate: rate = P waves per 6 second strip x 10 = atrial rate. There must be a P wave for each QRS complex.

2. PR interval? Normal PR interval is 0.12 to 0.20 second.

3. QRS duration? Normal duration is less than 0.12 second and all QRS complexes must be present.

4. Ventricular rate = QRS complex x 10 = ventricular rate.

5. P wave to P wave regular?

6. R to R regular?

7. ST segment flat on the isoelectric line?

8. T wave rounded and above the isoelectric line?

Normal Sinus Rhythm Criteria

1. P waves are present, and there is one P wave for each QRS complex. P wave is always in front of QRS complex, normal and consistent in shape.

2. The PR interval is 0.12 to 0.20 second.

3. QRS complexes must be present, and the QRS duration less than 0.12 second.

4. Rate is 60 to 100 per minute.

5. Rhythm is regular.

P wave and QRS complex, and T wave will be upright in leads I, II, III, and aVF. If these criteria are met, the interpretation is normal sinus rhythm (Fig. 15–8).

To calculate the heart rate on an ECG, you will need a 6-second rhythm strip. Count the number of complete R-to-R cycles on the 6-second strip and multiply by 10 to obtain the cardiac rate.

$$6 \text{ seconds} \times 10 = 60 \text{ seconds}$$

$$\text{Cycles/6 second strip} = \text{cycles/minute}$$

Cardiac rhythm is measured for regularity. Cardiac arrhythmia or *dysrhythmia* describes any disturbance or variation in normal sinus rhythm. It is not possible to describe the many types and causes of each rhythm in this brief chapter. A simple means of observing for irregular rhythm is by measuring the distance between R waves on a strip or, if no R waves are present, by measuring the distance between the QS waves. This is more conveniently done with calipers set at the peaks of two successive R waves, but it may also be done with a ruler. If the distances are the same, the rhythm is regular. To assess atrial regularity, the distance

between P waves may be measured in the same manner. Some of the pathological cardiac rhythms are displayed in the following section.

Analyzing ECG Rhythm Strips and Assessing the Patient

The ECG is used to detect cardiac dysrhythmias, conduction disorders, myocardial ischemia, injury, and infarction. As a radiographer, you must be able to determine normal sinus rhythm. Any deviation from this that may indicate a pathological condition that is immediately ominous. You may be the first person to observe a change in the patient's ECG rate and/or rhythm. You must also observe the patient's observable or reported signs and symptoms and report them immediately to the physician directly in charge of the patient's care. Cardiac dysrhythmias affect the heart's

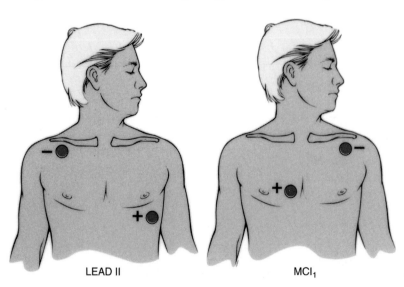

LEAD II   MCI₁

Figure 15–7. Two leads (views of the heart) commonly used for continuous monitoring. To monitor lead II, the negative electrode is placed on the upper right chest; the positive electrode is placed on the lower left chest. To monitor MCI₁, the negative electrode is placed on the upper left chest; the positive electrode is placed in the V1 position. If three electrodes are used, the third electrode, which is the ground electrode, can be placed anywhere on the chest. (Smeltzer SC, Bare BG: *Brunner and Suddarth's Textbook of Medical-Surgical Nursing,* 9th ed. Philadelphia: Lippincott Williams & Wilkins, 2000.)

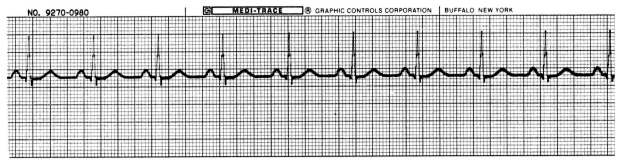

Figure 15–8. Normal sinus rhythm. (Smeltzer SC, Bare BG: *Brunner and Suddarth's Textbook of Medical-Surgical Nursing,* 9th ed. Philadelphia: Lippincott Williams & Wilkins, 2000.)

ability to pump adequate blood throughout the body, thus diminishing the supply of oxygen needed by body organs and tissues. Signs and symptoms that may be observed or reported by the patient are as follows.

CLINICAL MANIFESTATIONS

- Anxiety
- Lightheadedness
- Syncope
- Reports of chest pain
- Altered level of consciousness
- Neck vein distention
- Pallor
- Cool skin
- Shortness of breath
- Altered rate and rhythm of apical pulse
- Altered blood pressure

RADIOGRAPHER'S RESPONSE

You must maintain a calm and reassuring attitude with the patient and prepare the following:

1. Oxygen administration
2. Intravenous administration of medications
3. Emergency cart at hand
4. Potential necessity of calling a CODE

Several ECG arrhythmias that may be observed are as follows.

Sinus Bradycardia (Fig. 15–9)

Note!

- Ventricular and atrial rates are less than 60 in the adult.
- Ventricular and atrial rhythms are regular.
- QRS complex shape and duration are usually normal but may be regularly abnormal.
- P wave normal and consistent in shape and always in front of the QRS complex.
- PR interval should be at consistent intervals between 0.12 and 0.20 second.
- QRS ratio = P wave in front of every QRS 1:1.

Potential Problems: Sinus bradycardia may result in significant hemodynamic changes, that is, decreased level of consciousness, angina, hypotension, shortness of breath, and ST-segment changes.

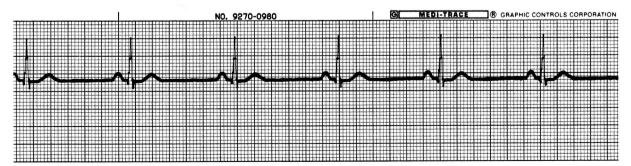

Figure 15–9. Sinus bradycardia. (Smeltzer SC, Bare BG: *Brunner and Suddarth's Textbook of Medical-Surgical Nursing,* 9th ed. Philadelphia: Lippincott Williams & Wilkins, 2000.)

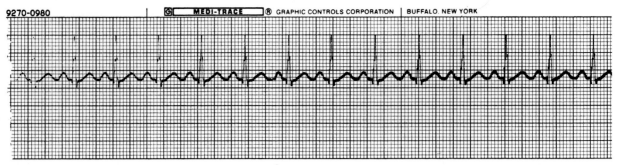

Figure 15–10. Sinus tachycardia. (Smeltzer SC, Bare BG: *Brunner and Suddarth's Textbook of Medical-Surgical Nursing,* 9th ed. Philadelphia: Lippincott Williams & Wilkins, 2000.)

Sinus Tachycardia (Fig. 15–10)

Note!

- Ventricular and atrial rate are more than 100 in the adult.
- Ventricular and atrial rates and rhythm are regular.
- QRS shape and duration are usually normal; may be regularly abnormal.
- P wave is normal and consistent in shape and always in front of the QRS complex but may be buried in the preceding T wave.
- PR interval is consistent between 0.12 and 0.20 second.
- P to QRS ratio is in front of every QRS 1:1.

Potential Problems: Sinus tachycardia may result in reduced cardiac output due to decreased diastolic filling time. This may lead to decreased blood pressure and syncope. If tachycardia continues, the heart cannot compensate, and the decreased ventricular filling may lead to pulmonary edema.

Atrial Flutter (Fig. 15–11)

Note!

- Atrial rate is between 250 and 400 times per minute.
- Not all atrial impulses are conducted into the ventricle resulting in a therapeutic block at the AV node; therefore, ventricular rate usually ranges between 75 to 150 per minute.
- QRS shape and duration are usually normal, but may be abnormal or absent.
- P waves are saw-toothed in shape (referred to *as F waves or fibrillatory waves*).
- PR interval is not possible to determine.
- P:QRS ratio may be 2:1, 3:1, or 4:1.

Potential Problems: The patient may have signs and symptoms of chest pain, shortness of breath, and decreased blood pressure. Electrical conversion may be necessary. This may result in atrial fibrillation that is a life-threatening dysrhythmia.

Atrial Fibrillation (Fig. 15–12)

Note!

- Atrial rate is between 300 and 600 per minute.
- Ventricular rate is usually 120 to 200 per minute.
- Ventricular rhythm and atrial rhythm are highly irregular.
- QRS shape and duration are often normal but may be abnormal.
- P waves are not visible or are irregular and seen as F waves.

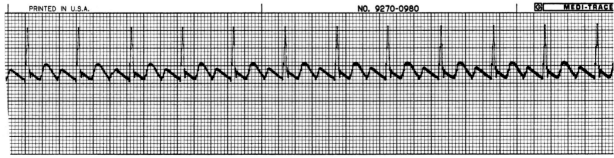

Figure 15–11. Atrial flutter. (Smeltzer SC, Bare BG: *Brunner and Suddarth's Textbook of Medical-Surgical Nursing,* 9th ed. Philadelphia: Lippincott Williams & Wilkins, 2000.)

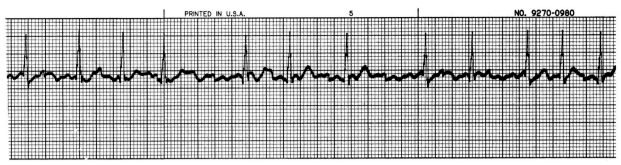

Figure 15–12. Atrial fibrillation. (Smeltzer SC, Bare BG: *Brunner and Suddarth's Textbook of Medical-Surgical Nursing,* 9th ed. Philadelphia: Lippincott Williams & Wilkins, 2000.)

Potential Problems: This rhythm results in the atria and ventricles contracting at different times and in inefficient ventricular filling. Coronary artery perfusion is diminished, and erratic atrial contraction may lead to the formation of thrombi. This may lead to increased risk of stroke.

Ventricular Fibrillation (Fig. 15–13)

Note!

• Ventricular rate is more than 300 per minute.

• Ventricular rhythm is highly irregular with undulating waves and no particular pattern.

• QRS complex is irregular and undulating in appearance.

Potential Problems: This life-threatening event is an immediate emergency. Basic life support now calls for and provides immediate defibrillation and places calling for emergency medial team assistance a priority before initiating CPR in the adult patient (automated external defibrillation is discussed in Chapter 8). The heartbeat is not audible, the pulse is not palpable, and respirations are not detectable.

Idioventricular Rhythm (also called an escape rhythm) (Fig. 15–14)

Note!

• Ventricular rate ranges between 20 and 40 beats per minute.

• The ventricular rhythm is regular.

• The QRS complex is bizarre in shape, and the duration is 0.12 second or more.

• The electrical impulse begins below the AV node, and the Purkinje fibers discharge an impulse.

Potential Problems: The patient has symptoms of reduced cardiac output and may lose consciousness. Immediate medical care is necessary.

Third-Degree AV Block (Fig. 15–15)

Note!

• The ventricular and atrial rates depend on the escape and underlying atrial rhythm.

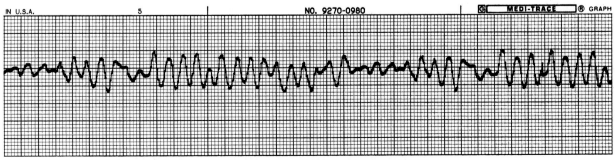

Figure 15–13. Ventricular fibrillation. (Smeltzer SC, Bare BG: *Brunner and Suddarth's Textbook of Medical-Surgical Nursing,* 9th ed. Philadelphia: Lippincott Williams & Wilkins, 2000.)

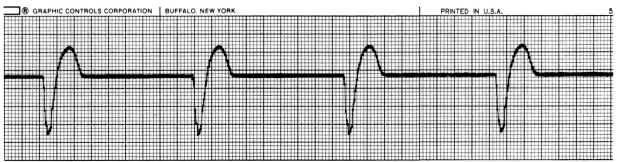

Figure 15–14. Idioventricular rhythm. (Smeltzer SC, Bare BG: *Brunner and Suddarth's Textbook of Medical-Surgical Nursing,* 9th ed. Philadelphia: Lippincott Williams & Wilkins, 2000.)

- The PP interval is regular and the RT interval is regular, but the PP interval is not equal to the RR interval.
- The QRS shape and duration are usually normal in the junctional escape and usually abnormal in the ventricular escape.
- P waves depend on the underlying rhythm.
- The PR interval is irregular.
- There are more P waves than QRS complexes.

Potential Problems: The patient with third-degree AV block may or may not have symptoms. If the symptoms such as shortness of breath, chest pain, lightheadedness, and low blood pressure are present, treatment is necessary. Initial treatment is with atropine. If the patient has an acute myocardial infarction, transcutaneous pacing and possibly a permanent pacemaker will be called for.

Ventricular Asystole (Fig. 15–16)

Note!

- Often called *flat line*.
- There is no QRS complex.

- P wave may be briefly visible and then disappear.
- There are no heartbeat, no palpable pulse, and no apparent respirations.

Potential Problems: This is a life-threatening emergency. Without immediate treatment, ventricular asystole is a fatal arrhythmia. CPR and emergency service are critical. Rapid assessment to identify the cause is urgent. The cause may be hypoxia, acidosis, severe electrolyte imbalance, drug overdose, or hypothermia.

If ventricular asystole occurs in your presence, you must call a CODE and prepare to administer IV medications and oxygen. The patient is intubated. If emergency efforts fail, the resuscitation efforts are terminated except in special circumstances.

You must be aware of the many useful cardiac drugs that are used to treat cardiac arrhythmias of all causes. Many of these are on the emergency cart and are used to treat cardiac emergencies. Your role is to assist in monitoring the patient and in being able to respond to the patient's needs rapidly in an emergency situation.

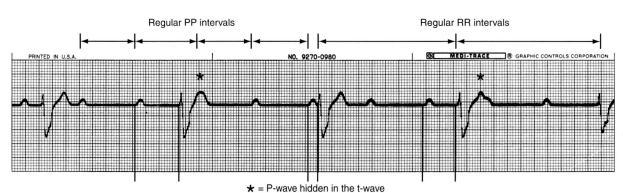

★ = P-wave hidden in the t-wave

Figure 15–15. Sinus rhythm with third-degree AV block and idioventricular rhythm; note irregular PR intervals. (Smeltzer SC, Bare BG: *Brunner and Suddarth's Textbook of Medical-Surgical Nursing,* 9th ed. Philadelphia: Lippincott Williams & Wilkins, 2000.)

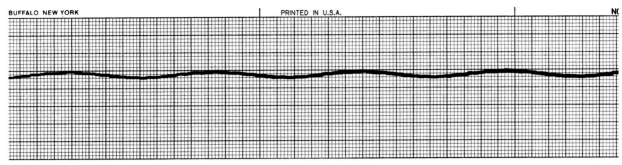

Figure 15–16. Asystole. (Smeltzer SC, Bare BG: *Brunner and Suddarth's Textbook of Medical-Surgical Nursing,* 9th ed. Philadelphia: Lippincott Williams & Wilkins, 2000.)

ECG Artifacts

You must be aware that there may be artifacts on the ECG that must be attended. Often seen as ominous or bizarre signs, they are simply errors in electrode connections or patient movement. Before calling a CODE, assess the patient's condition. If the patient is alert and without signs or symptoms of distress, reassess the electrode placement and connections. Be certain that an artifact is not the cause of an ominous or bizarre ECG because the electrocardiograph will record any muscle movement.

Summary

As a radiographer, you will participate in and care for many patients who are receiving cardiac monitoring. You may be called on to observe patients who are being monitored, and you must be able to recognize ominous ECG patterns as they appear on the screen of the oscilloscope. All ECG recordings that appear to be abnormal are not life threatening, and some malfunctions of the heart may not be demonstrated on the ECG.

You need to understand the anatomy and the electrical conduction system of the heart before learning to interpret a basic ECG. The ECG reports the electrical activity of the heart, particularly the hearts automaticity, conductivity, excitability, and contractility. The electrolytes involved in this process are sodium, potassium, and calcium. The cells of the heart muscle are polarized at rest, and the interior of the cells are negatively charged. As an electrical impulse is initiated (automaticity), the potassium in the cells rushes out, sodium and calcium enter, and depolarization is initiated (cardiac contraction) and spreads through the normal myocardium.

The depolarization-repolarization cycle goes through five phases that are seen on the ECG. They are registered as the P wave, the QRS complex, the T wave, and occasionally a U wave. The autonomic nervous system has a marked effect on the activity of the heart. The sympathetic fibers enhance myocardial excitability, and the parasympathetic fibers slow excitability, automaticity, and conduction speed but do not affect contractility. To interpret an ECG strip, you need to understand the components of the ECG graph. You also need to be able to interpret the configuration, intervals, and duration of the ECG deflections.

Preparing a patient for ECG monitoring requires explaining the process to the patient and providing privacy and skin preparation. The lead placement depends on the reason for the monitoring. You will most commonly be associated with the three-lead ECG. Place the leads on the anterior chest on flat areas of the skin. Remove dirt, oils, and hair before placing the lubricated leads. After the leads are placed, the electrocardiograph is activated. Any deviation from the settings of the cardiogram will activate the alarm. Before calling a CODE, assess the patient's condition and be certain that the deviation is not artifact.

Reading an ECG may be a complex process. You must be able to quickly observe the monitor and notify the physician directly in charge of the patient if an adverse rhythm is displayed on the monitor. Criteria for normal sinus rhythm are as follows: P waves are present and there is a P wave for every QRS complex; P waves are in front of the QRS complex and are consistent in shape; the PR interval is 0.12 to 0.20 second; the QRS complexes must be present and the duration is 0.12 second; the rate is 60 to 100 per minute; and the rhythm is regular. Cardiac rhythm is measured for regularity, and cardiac dysrhythmia describes any disturbance or variation in normal sinus rhythm. Your role as a radiographer is to assist in monitoring the patient and in being able to respond to the patient's needs rapidly in an emergency situation.

Chapter 15 Test

1. List the route of the electrical impulse activity through the heart.

_____ 2. Match the following:
   a. Excitability   1. Depolarization begins in the AV node
   b. Conductivity   2. Shortening of the myocardial cells
   c. Automaticity   3. Cell-to-cell passage of impulse
   d. Contractility   4. Action potential of the heart

3. Explain the role of sodium, calcium, and potassium in the electrical activity of the heart.

_____ 4. The P wave on the ECG represents:
   a. The repolarization of the ventricles
   b. The excitability of the parasympathetic fibers
   c. The contraction of the atria
   d. The refractory period of the atria
   e. Repolarization of the atria

_____ 5. The QRS complex on the ECG represents:
   a. The potassium ions entering the myocytes
   b. The repolarization of the atria
   c. The end of the resting phase
   d. The contraction of the ventricles
   e. The abundance of calcium in the myocardium

_____ 6. Each darkly lined box on the ECG graphic paper designates:
   a. 0.12 second
   b. 3 seconds
   c. 0.20 second
   d. 2.5 seconds
   e. 1 second

7. Each normal ECG waveform consists of _____, _____, _____, and occasionally a _____.

8. Match the following:
   a. Time required for ventricular   1. U wave
      depolarization and repolarization to occur
   b. First deflection above or below the   2. PR interval
      isoelectric line
   c. Associated with repolarization of the   3. P wave
      Purkinje fibers in the ventricles
   d. The time from the beginning of the P wave   4. ST segment
      to the beginning of the QRS complex
   e. Begins at the end of the QRS complex and ends   5. QT interval
      at the beginning of the T wave

9. List the five components of normal sinus rhythm on an ECG strip.

10. List your responsibilities as the radiographer in analyzing an ECG.

11. List your responsibilities in assessing the patient who is being monitored with an ECG.

12. List the signs and symptoms that may indicate alteration of a patient's condition while receiving ECG monitoring.

16

Care of Patients During Special Procedures

Objectives

After studying this chapter, you will be able to:

1. Describe the potential medical complications, emotional implications, and the patient care and teaching needs for the patient undergoing cardiac catheterization, angiography, and percutaneous transluminal angioplasty.

2. Describe the patient care and teaching needs of the patient for computed tomography.

3. Describe the patient care and teaching needs of the patient before and during ultrasonography.

4. Describe the patient care and teaching needs of the patient before and during magnetic resonance imaging.

5. Explain your responsibilities as the radiographer to the patient for positron emission tomography.

6. List the patient care considerations and teaching responsibilities for the patient receiving nuclear medicine imaging.

7. Explain the teaching and care needs of the patient receiving proton therapy.

8. List the potential side effects, emotional implications, and care and teaching needs of the patient receiving radiation therapy.

9. Describe the patient care considerations and teaching needs before and during mammography.

10. Describe the patient care considerations and teaching needs of the patient having arthrography or bone density imaging.

11. Explain the radiographer's role in patient care during lithotripsy.

12. Identify the patient care considerations and teaching needs of the patient during myelography.

Glossary

Anaphylactic: Manifesting extremely great sensitivity to foreign protein or active material

Dementia: The loss, usually progressive, of cognitive and intellectual functions

Doppler: A diagnostic instrument that emits an ultrasonic beam into the body; the ultrasound that reflects from moving structure changes

Gadolinium: The paramagnetic properties of the element used in contrast media for magnetic resonance imaging

Occlusion: The act of closing or the state of being closed

Patients undergoing special radiographic imaging procedures require special consideration. Many of these patients have been informed that they may have life-threatening illnesses and that the procedure that they are about to undergo will either confirm or rule out this threat. Special imaging procedures are not without pain and risk, and most patients find them anxiety provoking. Even something as innocuous as the diagnostic setting can cause the patient distress.

The atmosphere into which the patient is received is often forbidding. The chamber resembles an operating room, and the health care team is either masked and gowned or is hidden behind protective screens, which requires that they address the patient by microphone. This, combined with the prospect of a shortened life span, often elicits from the patient feelings of helplessness, vulnerability, and fear.

Patients receiving radiation or proton therapy may be in various stages of the grieving process. They know that they have a potentially terminal illness and that the prescribed treatment is being administered in an attempt to prolong their lives or provide them some relief from pain during their final days. As the radiographer working in these diagnostic and treatment areas, you must have exceptional technical skills and superior communication and patient-teaching skills. In these areas of patient care, the physician, the registered nurse, the radiographer, and other health care specialists work together as an interdependent team. Each depends on the other for safe and successful diagnostic and treatment outcomes. All patient care skills presented in the previous chapters of this text need to be applied in these areas.

As the radiographer who assists with special procedures, you must understand the properties of the contrast agents and be acquainted with basic cardiac monitoring, since many patients will be monitored continuously during these procedures. Most will also receive contrast agents to aid in visualization of organs and tissues.

Expertise in advanced radiologic and special imaging techniques is required to work in most departments discussed in this chapter. The intent of this text is to give the radiologic technology student an overview of patient care in these areas so that he or she may benefit from observational experiences and preview potential areas of specialization. Detailed technical discussion of these procedures is beyond the scope of this text and is mentioned only when relevant to patient care instruction.

Cardiac Catheterization and Coronary Angiography, Arteriography, and Nonsurgical Interventions

Cardiac catheterization and coronary angiography are performed by a cardiologist to diagnose coronary artery patency and, if indicated, treat atherosclerosis of the coronary arteries by nonsurgical means. These procedures are performed in a cardiac catheterization laboratory. As a radiographer, you will be a member of the health care team assigned to care for patients undergoing these invasive diagnostic and treatment procedures.

Your role as a member of this highly technical team is to participate in the patient's education, assessment, and general care. You also perform the fluoroscopy and digital subtraction angiography after injection of the contrast medium with an automatic power injector. One member of the team, either a radiographer or a nurse, performs a surgical scrub, dons gown and gloves, and prepares the sterile instruments. Another member of the team performs a sterile skin prep and drapes the patient for the procedure. All members of the team must be alert to any symptoms of respiratory or cardiac distress; be able to monitor vital signs accurately; assist with drug and contrast agent administration; apply surgical aseptic technique; and communicate with the patient in a therapeutic manner. Each member of the team must have special education in the problems and potential complications that may result from the procedure. The patient and the medical team must wear shields to protect themselves from unnecessary exposure to radiation during these lengthy procedures, which involve use of fluoroscopy and digital subtraction angiography.

The most common sites for insertion of the arterial catheter are the right and left brachial and femoral arteries.

The area surrounding the site of catheter insertion is surgically prepared, usually with an iodophor antiseptic as described in Chapter 5. This area is injected with a local anesthetic, and the artery is accessed with a large-bore needle containing a stylet to prevent return blood flow. When the artery has been accessed, the stylet is removed. A guidewire is then inserted through the needle into the artery, and the needle is removed. A catheter is passed over the guidewire into the artery with fluoroscopic guidance. The guidewire is removed, and the catheter is left in place and manipulated to visualize all vessels desired to diagnose potential areas of cardiac pathology.

A low-osmolar contrast agent is injected through the catheter, and the cardiac vessels are observed to assess cardiac output; locate and assess the severity of occlusive coronary artery disease; and diagnose congenital heart abnormalities, aneurysms, or other cardiac abnormalities. Treatment of diseased arteries may be performed at the time of the cardiac catheterization. If the coronary arteries are occluded and would benefit from percutaneous transluminal coronary angioplasty or if the patient has an evolving myocardial infarct, a balloon-tipped catheter is introduced through a guidewire. After the site of occlusion is reached, the balloon is inflated to compress the plaque that is causing the occlusion.

If there is reason to believe that vessel re-stenosis will occur, a stent may be used to maintain patency of the vessel. A stent is an object that provides support and structure to a vessel. It is introduced in the same way that the balloon is introduced and is left in place when the catheter is removed. Some of the potential complications from these procedures are cardiac arrhythmias, embolic stroke, allergic reactions to the iodinated contrast agent, and infection or hemorrhage at the catheter insertion site.

Arteriography

Arteriography uses the same technology and the same surgical aseptic technique as cardiac angiography to observe major blood vessels throughout the body. The kidneys, adrenal glands, brain, and abdominal aorta are the most common organs to be assessed by this method. The aorta is the typical route to access the vessels of the lower extremities for diagnosis of circulatory impairment of the lower extremities. Potential complications from arteriography are also much the same as with coronary angiography. If the kidneys are the focus of the procedure, renal failure is an added potential problem. If the adrenal glands are the focus, fatal hypertensive crisis may occur if the patient has the disease, pheochromocytoma. Medication to prevent this is administered several days before the procedure.

Patient Care Before and During Cardiac Catheterization, Angiography, or Arteriography

Nurses in a preoperative area perform most patient care in the hours before these procedures; however, you must carry out patient teaching and assessment immediately before the procedure. The process varies somewhat depending on the body organ to be assessed, but the process is largely similar, as follows:

1. An informed consent is signed after the patient receives instruction from the physician about all that is involved in the procedure, including all potential adverse effects.

2. Inform the patient before cardiac catheterization of the possible immediate need for coronary bypass surgery if complications or outcomes from the catheterization indicate.

3. For angiography of the heart, the patient must abstain from food and fluids for 4 to 8 hours before the procedure; however, for angiography in areas other than the heart, the patient is often asked to be well hydrated before the examination.

4. Instruct the patient to empty the bladder; to remove dentures, jewelry, and clothing; and to put on a patient gown.

5. When the patient enters the catheterization laboratory, you must explain all that will transpire so that he or she will be prepared for the procedure.

6. Allow the patient to express any anxieties or concerns about what is to occur.

7. Assess the patient for allergies to iodine or any medications to be administered.

8. The peripheral pulses are often identified and marked with a pen so that they may be quickly assessed during and after the procedure.

9. If ordered, medication is administered to alleviate anxiety.

10. The patient is transferred to the procedure table and placed in a supine position.

11. The area of catheter insertion is shaved and scrubbed with an antiseptic solution.

12. A peripheral IV line is started for access and to facilitate administration of drugs as needed. The leads for monitoring the heart rate are placed and connected to the oscilloscope.

13. It the patient is a child, he or she may be allowed to bring a CD or tape to play to ease feelings of fear and anxiety.

14. Inform the patient that he or she may be asked to cough or take deep breaths during the procedure to ease feelings of nausea or lightheadedness. Coughing may also correct arrhythmias.

15. A local anesthetic may be administered before arterial puncture.

16. The artery is accessed, the guidewire is inserted, and then the catheter is placed over the wire.

17. The patient is informed that the contrast agent is about to be injected and is told that he or she will feel a burning or flushed feeling from this and must not be concerned.

18. If the angiography is of the adrenal glands, the blood pressure must be monitored continually to assess for evidence of a malignant hypertensive crisis.

19. Serial images are taken in a timed sequence to demonstrate the arterial and venous blood blow to the organ being studied.

20. Nitroglycerin to dilate blood vessels and other drugs may be administered during the procedure.

Patient Care and Teaching After Cardiac Catheterization, Angiography, and Arteriography

Patient care after angiography and cardiac catheterization is relatively uniform and must be carried out meticulously to prevent circulatory deficit, thrombus formation, or hemorrhage. In most instances, the patient is transported to the hospital postanesthesia recovery area or to an intensive coronary care area to be monitored after cardiac catheterization or angiography. You must understand the monitoring and care required after these examinations so that you can instruct the patient and so that you can begin to monitor the patient before he or she leaves the diagnostic imaging area.

The patient may be extremely fatigued, and any movement required after the procedure must be done with adequate assistance so there is little demand on the patient. Monitor the patient's pulse rate on the side of the invasive procedure every 15 minutes for 1 hour and then every hour until an 8- to 12-hour period is complete and no complication has been detected. The blood pressure is monitored on the side opposite the invasive procedure at the same time intervals. The pulses distal to the site of catheter insertion must also be monitored at frequent, regular intervals for 24 hours after the procedure. After femoral catheterization, the patient should be instructed to move the toes and dorsiflex the feet frequently. Also instruct the patient to keep the legs straight and still. Assess the extremities for coldness, cyanosis, pallor, numbness, size of one extremity compared with the other extremity, and tingling. Instruct the patient to inform the nurse if he or she has any of the latter symptoms. If a circulatory deficit occurs, surgical intervention may be necessary to correct the problem. The patient should also inform the nurse of any feeling of wetness at the site of the catheter insertion; this may indicate hemorrhaging.

If a femoral artery was used for the catheter insertion, inform the patient that he or she must remain at bedrest for 10 to 12 hours after the procedure to prevent hemorrhage. A weight or sandbag is often placed over the site of catheter insertion to apply pressure. The patient should also be told to apply pressure at the insertion site when coughing or sneezing. Do not raise the patient's head more than 20 degrees during the immediate postcatheterization period.

If the brachial site was used for catheter insertion, the arm on the side of insertion is kept straight with an armboard for several hours, but the patient may be up as soon as the vital signs are stable. Regardless of the site of insertion, the patient must be monitored for 24 hours for external bleeding or for bleeding into the tissues surrounding the catheter insertion site.

Instruct the patient who has received iodinated contrast media to increase fluid intake to prevent dehydration and hypotension. This may be contraindicated in some patients with congestive heart failure. Patients are often given intravenous fluid replacement therapy during these procedures, but they should be made aware of the need for increased fluid intake.

Record the time that the procedure began and ended, any drugs or contrast agents administered, and the patient's tolerance of the procedure on the patient's chart. Also record the instructions given to the patient after the procedure.

Computed Tomography

Computed tomography (CT) is a diagnostic imaging procedure that can be used to scan body tissues and organs combining radiologic and computer technology. CT produces multiple cross-sectional images of body organs. It is a highly effective method of diagnosing intracranial and organic pathology, although other imaging modalities are more effective in some situations.

Iodinated contrast agents are used to increase tissue density for body and brain scans. Barium solutions may be used to increase organ density of the gastrointestinal organs.

Patient Care and Instruction Before Computed Tomography

In preparation for CT of the brain, instruct the patient not to eat or drink for 2 to 3 hours before the examination. The patient may take only medications that he or she routinely takes. If the patient has diabetes mellitus, his CT should be arranged so that the regular meal pattern and insulin administration are maintained. The patient will be receiving an iodinated contrast agent, so all precautions and questioning that precede administration of that drug are included in pre-CT patient care.

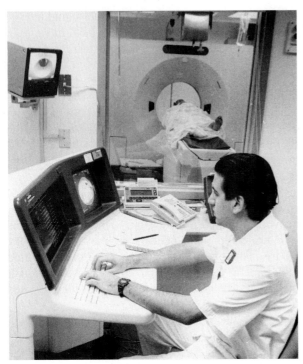

Figure 16–1. CT scanner.

You must spend a few moments explaining the procedure to the patient in order to alleviate anxiety. Tell the patient that he or she is expected to lie very quietly to ensure clear images. Allow the patient to inspect the equipment and to express any feelings of claustrophobia or fear of the procedure. You must inform the patient that he or she may communicate with you through a microphone placed above the machine portal. Show the patient that you will be sitting behind the glass window and tell him or her that you can observe, hear, and communicate with the patient at all times (Fig. 16–1).

You must establish a feeling of trust in the patient. It is very frightening for patients to feel that they are in a room alone, receiving an intravenous drug to which they may have a reaction, with nobody in close proximity on whom they can rely for help. The extremely anxious patient who is in pain and unable to lie quietly may need an analgesic or sedative medication if this can be prescribed.

Inform the patient that he or she may have feelings of nausea, warmth, flushing, and a metallic taste after the iodinated contrast agent is administered. Place an emesis basin near the patient, where he or she can pick it up easily if need be. Instruct the patient to inform you immediately if he or she has any feelings of pain during the procedure. Inform that patient that the procedure usually takes about 1 hour to complete. The patient must sign an informed consent before receiving a CT scan. The patient's medical history and history of allergies must also be taken before this procedure is begun.

Computed Tomography of the Body

Patients who are to have CT of the bowel and abdominal organs are allowed nothing to eat or drink after midnight the night before the examination. They may receive a barium contrast agent mixed in orange juice to drink the night before the examination and more (1000 mL) immediately before the scan. An iodinated contrast agent is also injected intravenously immediately before the CT scan begins.

You must spend the same amount of time explaining the procedure to the patient before beginning this examination as for the head CT scan. For the bowel and abdominal CT scan, instruct the patient to listen carefully for instructions to breathe, hold the breath, and release the breath. Tell the patient to expect many of these instructions.

Whichever area of the body is being scanned, you should pause from time to time and ask the patient how he or she is feeling and inform the patient of the time remaining for completion of the examination. If the patient is made to feel like the major focus of the procedure and is kept informed, he or she will be more cooperative and relaxed while the examination is in progress.

Patient Care After Computed Tomography

Patients who have come from their homes and plan to return home should be accompanied by a person who can drive them or assist them to get there safely. Patients who have received sedative or antianxiety medication may not drive themselves.

When the procedure is complete, the intravenous contrast agent is discontinued by order of the physician, as described in Chapter 13. The patient is then allowed to sit up with assistance. He or she should sit quietly on the table for several minutes before being assisted back to the dressing room, wheelchair, or gurney. If the patient is hospitalized, he or she may be returned to the hospital room with assistance. If going home, assist the patient to the dressing room, and help him or her get dressed, if needed. Observe the patient for at least 1 hour for adverse reaction to drugs and for general instability before discharging the patient from the department.

Instruct the patient who has received an iodinated contrast agent to increase fluid intake to at least 3000 mL for the next 24 hours to aid in excretion of the agent from the body and to prevent dehydration. If the patient has had barium, he or she should follow the instructions in Chapter 10 concerning post-barium administration.

Any adverse reactions that occurred during the CT and any medications that the patient received must be recorded on the patient's chart. Record the time that the procedure began and ended, the patient's tolerance of the procedure, and the instructions that the patient received for post-procedure care.

Ultrasonography

Ultrasound is a method of visualizing the soft tissue structures of the body for diagnosis of diseases without the use of radiation or contrast media. It is a noninvasive, painless procedure that requires the skill of a specially educated technologist, usually a radiographer with additional education. Ultrasound uses high-frequency sound waves to search for pathological changes in body organs. "After passing through tissue then the sound waves reflect back to the transducer, where they're converted into electrical impulses. Then these impulses are amplified and displayed on a screen. Because the densities of the tissues differ, sound waves pass through them at different speeds. The image on the display screen reflects this difference" (Springhouse, 2001).

The use of Doppler imaging has increased the imaging potential of ultrasound. Doppler examinations make it possible to study in a noninvasive manner the movement of body structures such as blood flow and a beating heart and to identify areas of occlusion and malformation.

While the ultrasound examination is in progress, images are displayed on a cathode ray tube. Permanent copies of the images are produced either as Polaroid pictures or on a sensitized paper with recordings somewhat like those from an ECG reading (Fig. 16–2).

This form of imaging is useful in obstetrics for fetal monitoring; in neurology for diagnosing brain disorders; and in urology for diagnosing urinary blad-der, scrotal, prostatic, and renal pathological conditions. It is also used to diagnose vascular aneurysms, as well as pancreatic, gallbladder, thyroid, venous, parathyroid, lymph node, eye, and breast pathological conditions. This is not an all-inclusive list, and new uses for ultrasonography continue to be found. The radiographer who is not trained as an ultrasonographer must have an awareness of the process of ultrasound to correctly schedule imaging procedures to the patient's best advantage.

Patient Care for Ultrasonography

Patient care considerations for ultrasound include instruction in preparation for the procedure, an explanation of the procedure itself, and correct scheduling to prevent unsatisfactory examinations. Little post-examination instruction is needed.

If a patient is to have barium studies as well as an ultrasound examination, the ultrasound examination should be scheduled to precede the barium studies because residual barium in the gastrointestinal tract will interfere with effective ultrasound examinations. If a patient has a tendency to have large amounts of gas in the bowel, the gas will interfere with visualization. A patient with this problem should be instructed to eat low-residue foods for 24 to 36 hours before the examination and be scheduled at a time when the bowel will be relatively gas-free, as is the case in the early morning before breakfast.

CALL OUT!

If a patient is to have barium imaging as well as an ultrasound examination, the ultrasound examination must be scheduled to precede the barium examination because residual barium will interfere with effective ultrasound results!

Active children or patients who are unable to remain quiet because of pain, emotional illness, or anxiety must be scheduled at a time when they can be accompanied by a person who can keep them calm and relaxed. Use of sedative drugs may also be recommended by the physician.

Patients should be informed that this is a painless, noninvasive procedure. A lubricating gel is used as the conductive agent. The ultrasonographer will apply the gel. A tap water enema may be required during the procedure for ultrasound of the pelvic area.

A transducer is held by the sonographer and is moved over the surface to be examined as the screen is watched and images are produced. The patient must be shown the transducer and reassured that it will cause no pain.

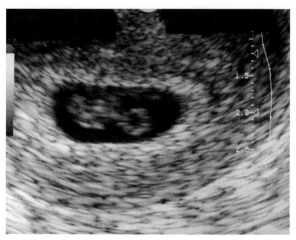

Figure 16–2. Ultrasound picture of fetus in utero.

Some examinations require a preparatory cleansing enema and fasting for several hours before the scheduled time. Other ultrasound procedures require the bladder to be filled with fluid. If either of these is required, you or the sonographer must explain the preparation to the patient.

Wound dressing, scars, and obesity all are factors to be considered when ultrasound is the imaging technique prescribed. Dressings must be removed, and lubricating gel cannot be applied over an open wound. Scars and obesity prevent good visualization. A clear sterile patch may be worn over wounds if ordered by the physician.

Patient care after ultrasonography is the same as thoughtful patient care after any diagnostic imaging procedure. The lubricating gel must be carefully removed so that the patient's clothing is not soiled by it. If the patient was immersed in water, he or she must be provided with towels and a private area in which to dry and dress. Patients who are in a weakened condition must not be left alone, and any assistance the patient needs must be provided. Patients who have had sedative medication must not be allowed to drive home or return to their hospital room unattended.

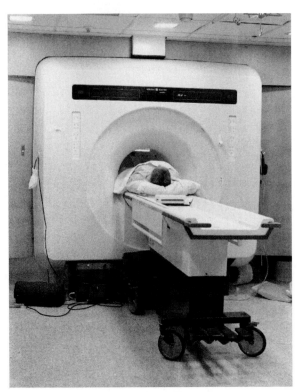

Figure 16–3. Patient on MRI pallet.

Magnetic Resonance Imaging

Magnetic resonance imaging (MRI) is a noninvasive procedure used for diagnosing neoplasms as well as vascular, soft tissue, bone and joint, and central nervous system pathological conditions. Gadolinium is the contrast agent that may be injected intravenously for some MRI procedures.

MRI is performed by placing the entire body, or a body part, in a magnetic field with radiofrequency waves to produce computerized images of body organs and tissues. These images are replayed on a video screen for diagnosis. MRI has many diagnostic advantages. Among them is the absence of radiation that may harm body cells. It also eliminates the need for iodinated contrast agents and decreases the possibility of anaphylactic reactions.

If a limb or limbs are being diagnosed to measure the blood flow to the extremities, the patient may sit or lie quietly while the limb being examined by MRI is placed in a cylinder. The limb or limbs are moved in and out of the cylinder as the extremity images are completed. If both legs and arms are to be examined, the legs are usually examined first.

If entire body imaging is ordered, the patient is placed on a pallet that moves slowly through a large magnetic cylinder (Fig. 16–3). If the patient's head is to be scanned, a large magnetic cylinder is placed over the head. If no contrast agent is administered, the MRI of the head only may be completed in a very short time.

Patient Care and Education for MRI

Patient education is the key to successful imaging when MRI is the diagnostic procedure selected. Inform the patient that the procedure may take from 1 to 2 hours to complete. Claustrophobic fears are common and emerge when the patient is faced with spending 1 hour or more in a close cylinder, in a large room, alone. Accurate information and instruction help to alleviate these fears. Anti-anxiety medication is often prescribed to assist in relieving the anxiety of the patient. These medications may not be given if blood flow is to be assessed because they may interfere with normal blood flow. Inform the adult patient that he or she will need to lie in a supine position with no movement. Also inform the patient that he or she will hear a pounding noise during the entire examination. The patient may wear earplugs to quiet the sound.

Explain to the patient that, although he or she may feel completely alone, at least two persons will be just on the other side of a glass window. They will be constantly observing the patient, and they can and will be communicating with the patient frequently during the procedure. Show the patient that there is a microphone through which to communicate to the staff. The patient should be allowed to examine the MRI equipment and ask any questions that he may have before beginning the procedure. If the patient is a child, a parent may be allowed to sit beside the cylinder and talk to the child during the MRI. Infants should be fed shortly before being placed in the cylinder.

You can help decrease the patient's anxiety by speaking to him or her frequently and letting the patient know how much time is left before the examination is completed. You must remember that many patients who are having MRI are anxious and fearful because of possible ominous diagnostic outcomes, as are the parents of children who are having this procedure. Patients may focus on their claustrophobic feelings in an attempt to deny the possibility of a threatening diagnosis. You must be patient, sensitive, and nonjudgmental when communicating with these patients and their family members. Making the patient's feelings seem foolish or offering reassuring cliché responses only increases anxiety. Time must be spent discussing the process and the patient's or the parents' feelings and concerns before beginning MRI. If this is not done, the patient may be unable to remain as quiet as is necessary for successful imaging.

A medical history, as previously described, must be taken before MRI. History of allergies must be included. The gadolinium-based contrast agent has been reported to have resulted in an occasional allergic reaction. If the patient is to receive a contrast agent, the institution may require the patient to sign an informed consent. The patient should be informed that this procedure does not expose him or her to radiation and is relatively painless. The patient who has metal dental work may feel some tingling sensations.

Instruct patients to remove all metal jewelry, dental bridges, clothing with metal closures, belts, metal-containing prostheses, hair clips, and shoes before entering the scanner room. Purses and wallets containing credit cards must be left outside in a secure place because magnetic resonance will deactivate credit cards. You will be responsible for placing the items safely away and for informing patients where their belongings are being kept.

Patients who receive anti-anxiety or sedative drugs before MRI and those who have a history of asthma and receiving a contrast agent should be monitored during the procedure. There are pulse oximeters made for use in the MRI chamber.

MRI is contraindicated for people who have internal pacemakers, implanted heart valves, metal orthopedic implants, or surgical clips. It may be contraindicated for pregnant women because the effects of MRI on pregnancy are unknown at present. Patients on life-support equipment or infusion pumps or who are critically ill may not receive MRI because monitoring equipment cannot be used in the scanner room. Other items that prevent MRI are an implanted insulin pump, bone-growth stimulator, internal hearing aid, cochlear implant, neurostimulator, metal eye prostheses, vena cava clot filter, an intrauterine device or diaphragm in place, some surgeries, claustrophobia, regular need for oxygen administration, and any metal device.

For persons with severe claustrophobia, open MRI is available is some medical centers. In open MRI, the patient is not completely enclosed in a chamber, which decreases the feeling of being closed in a small space. The disadvantage of this unit is that because it is a low-field unit, the image quality may not be as clear as with regular closed MRI. For accurate diagnosis of small body parts or the cervical spine, open MRI is not recommended at present.

Patient Care After MRI

There are no special patient instructions or teaching responsibilities after MRI unless the patient has received medication or a contrast agent. If the patient has received drugs or a contrast agent, the instructions are the same as for other invasive imaging procedures.

Children are sometimes sedated for this examination. If this is the case, the patient is monitored throughout the examination and until fully recovered from the drug by a nurse proficient in this field. Sedating children requires special evaluation that will not be discussed in this text.

Positron Emission Tomography

Positron emissions tomography (PET) combines the qualities of radionuclide imaging with CT to study blood flow and volume and protein metabolism. The body organ studies using this technique that have had great success to date are those of the brain, the heart, and the lungs. PET is able to assist in diagnosis of Alzheimer's disease, brain tumors, cardiac disease, and, most recently, the physiologic changes in psychiatric diseases. It is one of the most innovative techniques currently used. Unfortunately, it is a very expensive procedure that requires sophisticated technology such as a cyclotron, a specialized chemical laboratory, computerized equipment, and a team of scientists and health care specialists to carry out the diagnostic procedures. PET is available only at university medical centers, but it is expected to become a widely used diagnostic imaging technique in the future. The patient inhales or is injected with a radioisotope of an element that occurs naturally in the body such as oxygen, nitrogen, carbon, and fluorine. These isotopes emit subatomic particles called *positrons* (positively charged electrons). When a positron encounters an electron, which it does just after emission, both are destroyed and two gamma rays are released (Smeltzer and Bare, 1996). These rays are recorded on a computer to be reconstructed as an image on a cathode ray screen.

Patient Care for PET

The patient or caregiver must have a clear explanation of the PET procedure. The patient or caregiver must understand that there will be radiation exposure that is minimal and that he or she will receive the radioactive material either by injection or inhalation, depending on the organ to be studied. The examination will take from 60 to 90 minutes. An informed consent form is required by most institutions.

There is usually no food or fluid restriction before the examination; however, the patient should take no caffeine, nicotine, or alcohol for 24 hours. The patient should also receive no sedative or tranquilizing drugs. All these interfere with the examination. Diabetic patients may receive insulin 3 to 4 hours before the procedure. Patients who are pregnant or breastfeeding may be restricted from this examination. Immediately before the examination, the patient must be instructed to empty the bladder.

The patient receiving a brain scan must understand that he or she may be asked to perform an activity such as a recitation of a simple proverb or the pledge to the flag. This is so that brain activity during recall or cognitive processes can be assessed. The patient may also be blindfolded and wear earplugs to screen out external stimuli.

After the examination, instruct the patient to change positions slowly, and assist him or her to rise or leave the examining table because of possible dizziness due to orthostatic hypotension. Instruct the patient to increase fluid intake for 24 hours and to urinate frequently to eliminate the isotope from the body.

The patient receiving PET is often elderly and may have symptoms of dementia. If this is the case, you must recognize that the patient is unable to follow directions and may need to be closely guided through every aspect of the procedure. The strangeness of the environment may be frightening to a person with symptoms of dementia. Because excessive anxiety may affect the results of the examination, a family member or a familiar caretaker may need to remain with the patient to decrease his or her anxiety.

Radionuclide Imaging

Radionuclide imaging is frequently the diagnostic imaging technique of choice to detect or rule out malignant lesions or to produce images that are not visible on standard radiographs. It may be used to visualize pathological conditions of the kidneys, heart, bones, thyroid, and other body organs.

Before the radionuclide imaging examination, the patient may need to abstain from eating or drinking for several hours. The person who is to receive radionuclide imaging must sign a special consent form and must be informed that he or she will receive a small amount of a radioisotope and will be exposed to a minimal amount of radiation. He should be informed that the isotope will be excreted within 24 hours and there will be no residual radiation effects. Depending on the organ to be diagnosed, the patient may receive an intravenous injection of the isotope. He may also be given a radioactive tracer compound by inhalation or oral route. They should be told to expect to feel flushed for a short time after receiving the isotope.

Patients who are pregnant, have renal or hepatic disease, or who are allergic to iodine should be carefully screened before being scheduled for this diagnostic procedure. Only one radionuclide procedure should be scheduled on one day because one may interfere with another.

CALL OUT!

The patient must not receive more than one radionuclide procedure on one day. Other contrast media may interfere with this examination!

After initial preparation, the patient is taken to the nuclear medicine department for either dynamic or static scans, depending on the clinical symptoms. A tracer isotope and the contrast media are administered. The patient is placed on an examining table and expected to lie quietly while the test is in progress. This can be a problem for the elderly patient or for a person in pain.

The isotope accumulates in areas of pathology that are called "hot spots." If this is a bone scan, an area of decreased uptake of the radionuclide may indicate circulatory impairment and is called a "cold spot" (Fig. 16–4). If the total concentration of the radionuclide is less than normal, a diagnosis of a generalized renal disorder must be considered.

The standard imaging device in nuclear medicine is called the gamma camera. It does not move and produces a two-dimensional image. The newest nuclear imaging camera is three-dimensional. The third dimension has been achieved in gamma cameras through single photon emission computed tomography (SPECT). This has greatly increased the diagnostic ability of nuclear medicine imaging.

After radionuclide imaging, if an intravenous agent has been administered, assess the area for redness and

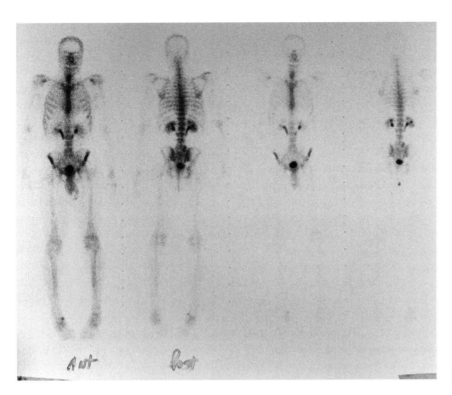

Figure 16–4. Normal bone scan.

swelling before discharging the patient. The patient must be cautioned to rise slowly to prevent postural hypotension. Do not allow the patient to leave the laboratory until the scintigraphs are reviewed for clarity.

Instruct the patient to resume his or her usual dietary and medication pattern unless contraindicated by the physician. Remind the patient that the radionuclide will be excreted within 24 hours and that the only precaution to be taken is to flush the commode immediately after each use.

Bone Scan

Bone scan images the skeleton by means of a scanning camera in order to diagnose malignant lesions of the skeletal system, degenerative bone infection, and unexplained bone pain. The scanner is able to detect "hot spots," as in radionuclide imaging. A radioactive tracer compound is administered intravenously approximately 3 hours before the scan. The patient is instructed to drink large amounts of water and to urinate immediately before the scan. You must explain this procedure in detail to the patient and alleviate any feeling of anxiety that the patient may have. This is particularly important if the scan is being performed to rule out cancer.

There should be no other radiographic examinations scheduled for 24 to 48 hours before or after this scan. A medical history, a history of allergic reactions, and a consent form must be signed.

After the bone scan, the patient must be instructed to increase fluid intake and notify the physician immediately if there is any sign of warmth, redness, or swelling at the site of injection. The physician may prescribe pain medication if it is indicated.

Radiation Therapy

At least half of the patients with a diagnosis of cancer will receive external radiation therapy during the course of the disease. This form of treatment is used to cure the disease, to control malignant tumors that cannot be removed, to prevent spread of the tumor to the brain and spinal cord, and to decrease pain when the cancer metastasizes to the bones, brain, or soft tissues. Radiographers who work in the area of radiation therapy should receive specialized education; however, the radiography student may rotate to this area in the course of his or her education and must have some understanding of patient care in radiation therapy.

The intent of therapeutic radiation is not to kill all tumor cells immediately. All cells react differently, and some may repair the radiation-induced damage and begin to reproduce again. For this reason, radiation for treatment of cancer is administered in a series of divided doses for an established period of time. In this manner, tumor cells that survive initial radiation are eventually destroyed. "Ionizing radiation breaks the strands of the DNA helix, leading to cell death" (Smeltzer and Bare, 2000).

The size, location, and degree of sensitivity of the tumor to radiation are the deciding factors when the plan of therapy is devised. The sensitivity of the cells surrounding the tumor is also a factor in the plan.

When a patient's physician prescribes external radiation therapy, the patient is sent to the radiation treatment area for preparation known as treatment simulation. During this simulation, the patient is evaluated, and treatment is mimicked with machines that determine the exact treatment field, the volume of tissue to be radiated, and the radiation dosage necessary to accomplish the treatment purpose. When these decisions have been made, the patient's external skin is marked with indelible pen so that the same area of tissue receives the radiation therapy with each treatment. A plan of treatment is outlined for the patient, which usually extends daily for several weeks. The patient is instructed to refrain from removing or altering the markings. If they are accidentally removed, patients are asked not to redraw them, but to notify the radiation team so that they can reconstruct them according to plan.

At the time that the treatment plan is made, show the patient the treatment room and he or she should be allowed to ask any questions concerning the treatment. The treatment rooms are large and impersonal, and the patient must remain alone during the radiation treatment. Inform the patient that he or she can communicate by microphone with the radiation team and vice versa. Also inform the patient that the treatment table is somewhat uncomfortable and hard. If the patient is in pain, suggest that he or she receive pain medication 30 minutes before each treatment. Also explain to the patient that the radiation treatments themselves are painless and that there is no danger of the patient carrying radiation out of the treatment area.

Patient Care for Radiation Therapy

As the radiographer caring for patients receiving radiation therapy, you must be aware that these patients are in various stages of the grieving process. They have received a diagnosis of a disease from which they may or may not recover. Some have hope of recovery and perhaps are in a phase of denial of the seriousness of their problem. Patients who are in this phase must never be confronted with their denial, since this may be their only means of coping with the problem. Others are in the later stages of the grieving process. Many have had radical surgical procedures that have altered their body image. This is particularly the case for a man or woman who has had reproductive organs or external genitalia altered by surgery during reproductive years.

Some patients receiving external radiation therapy are in the terminal stages of cancer and have metastasis of the disease to their bones. When this occurs, the structure of the bone weakens and becomes very fragile. There is a high incidence of pathological fractures with this condition. If you are caring for a person in the terminal stages of cancer, remember this and allow the patient to move at his or her own pace with as much assistance as necessary. You must be extremely cautious when lifting or moving cancer patients. Be certain to have adequate assistance to prevent abrupt, jarring, or pushing movements because this may cause fractures and a great deal of unnecessary pain for the patient. Allow the patient to direct all moves at his or her own pace.

Patients with cancer often have weakened immune systems. This must be taken into consideration because these patients are highly susceptible to infections. Radiographers must practice judicious medical asepsis and, when the occasion calls for it, meticulous surgical asepsis during patient care.

You must also remember that the patient undergoing a course of radiation therapy has localized toxic reactions to the treatment. This toxicity usually affects only the tissues surrounding the area being radiated, since the cells in the treatment area are destroyed by radiation. However, generalized systemic reactions may also occur. Some of the local reactions that may occur, depending on the irradiation site, are alopecia (loss of hair), erythema (redness and inflammation of the skin or mucous membranes), loss of appetite, alterations in oral mucous membranes (xerostomia and stomatitis), decreased salivation, difficulty swallowing, chest pain and cough, esophageal irritation, nausea and vomiting, diarrhea, and blood dyscrasias.

Generalized systemic side effects include fatigue, nausea, vomiting, and headache. Reassure the patient that all these effects will subside when the treatments are completed. Some changes in the area of the radiation treatment are called fibrous tissue formation (scar tissue). This is due to the destruction of the blood supply in the area of radiation, and that tissue will not regenerate.

Use of therapeutic communication techniques by radiographers caring for patients having external radiation therapy is of utmost importance. You should make yourself available to answer questions that you can answer and assist patients to find answers when you do not know. Allow patients to express their concerns and explore their feelings with the use of simple reflective statements.

Proton Therapy

Proton therapy is a recent innovation in the treatment of patients with cancer. Since this procedure requires CT scans and frequent radiographic films, the radiographer is directly involved in this therapy.

The benefit of proton therapy for treatment of malignant tumors is based on the fact that the proton works at the end of its desired pathway with very little effect on tissues that surround the area. In other words, the "scatter effect" that is such a problem in external radiation therapy is markedly decreased. This allows the dose to the tumor to be increased with no harmful effects to surrounding tissues. Proton therapy is currently being used in only a few isolated medical centers, but it is expected to become the treatment of choice for prostate, head and neck, and spinal cord tumors. Protocols for use of proton therapy are being added at this time for use in the treatment of tumors of the cervix, lungs, urinary bladder, and esophagus, and for melanomas. It is also used as a palliative measure in metastatic disease.

Patient Preparation for Proton Therapy

The patient preparation for proton therapy is preceded by a diagnostic workup that includes a CT scan to determine the area of treatment. After this, a "pod," or shell, is made to fit the contour of the patient's body. The pod is made by placing a patient in a semicircle of warm-malleable foam that quickly solidifies to his or her body contour. If the head and neck are the areas of treatment, a form-fitted mask of the same material is made to fit the treatment area. A beam-shaping device is created for each patient, depending on the treatment area.

Meticulous preparation is made at each treatment time, including re-determining the patient's area of pathology, because the proton beam must be directly aligned with the treatment area. This is done by a radiographic image taken as the patient lies in the pod made for him.

Instruct the patient to lie perfectly still during treatment because any movements will change the direction of the proton beam. If this occurs, the treatment must be stopped and the alignment process repeated.

No metal can be worn by the patient in the treatment room. Inform the patient that he or she will be alone in the room but that the therapist will be in contact with him or her by microphone just outside. If claustrophobia or pain is a problem for the patient, a mild antianxiety or analgesic drug may be prescribed 20 to 30 minutes before treatment. Each treatment lasts approximately 15 minutes.

As the radiographer caring for patients having proton therapy, you must understand that these patients, like patients receiving external radiation therapy, are in a stage of the grieving process because they have had a diagnosis of life-threatening illness. Their care requires extra sensitivity from the health care team, as described in the previous section.

Mammography

Mammography is an imaging modality that is performed on a routine basis for prevention or early diagnosis of breast cancer and on an acute-care basis if a lesion, lump, or nodule found in the breast is suspected of being cancerous. "The American Cancer Society [ACS] recommends that all women have a screening mammogram between ages 35 and 39 as well as a clinical physical examination of the breast every 3 years from ages 20 to 39. For women age 40 and older, the ACS recommends a yearly mammogram and a yearly physical examination of the breasts" (Springhouse, 2001). Men do not usually receive routine mammograms for prevention of disease; however, if there is a family history of cancer of the breast or if any abnormality of the male breast is discovered, a mammogram is ordered.

A medical history is taken before an initial mammogram and updated each year that follows. If a patient has breast implants, the radiographer must be informed prior to the procedure.

No iodinated contrast agent is used for routine mammography. You should instruct the patient to wear an item of clothing that can be easily removed to the waist. Deodorant or powders in the axillary region should not be used before the examination because they may prevent adequate visualization. The patient's breasts are exposed and positioned between an image receptor and a compression device. Radiographic images are taken from two views. During the procedure, the breasts are compressed tightly, to remove skin folds and air pockets. It is usually known by women presenting for mammogram that the procedure is most uncomfortable. They are therefore in a state of anxiety when they arrive for examination. If the patient is having the mammogram because of suspected pathology, you must ask the patient to identify the area that is suspect so that additional care is taken to obtain optimum images of that area. You must make every effort to preserve patient privacy and minimize anxiety.

The patient may be asked to wait until the radiographic images are checked. The patient is notified of any need for follow-up care necessary.

Arthrography

Arthrography is the diagnostic imaging examination of a joint. The indications for this procedure are continual complaints of incapacitating joint pain. The joints of the shoulder, knee, ankle, wrist, or hip can be visualized by this diagnostic imaging procedure. Abnormalities that can be diagnosed are joint capsule abnormalities, synovial cysts, and joint and ligament pathological conditions. MRI is often the preferred method of diagnosing some joint conditions.

There is no restriction of food or fluids for arthrography. The patient's history of allergies to local anesthetics, iodine, and contrast agents must be taken. Pregnancy is a contraindication to having this procedure, since fluoroscopy is used. Explain the procedure to the patient and adequately answer any questions. A consent form is usually required to be signed.

The area where the joint will be punctured for instillation of contrast media must be cleansed as for surgical prep. The puncture area is anesthetized with a local anesthetic. The patient and staff wear protective clothing to shield them from radiation. A radiopaque contrast or air contrast or both are used to visualize the joint in question fluoroscopically while it is put through the range of motion and the contrast media fill the joint space. After administration of the contrast, the needle is removed and the puncture may be sealed with collodium. Standard radiographs are taken during this time. If fluid is removed from the joint, it is collected in a sterile specimen tube and sent to the laboratory for analysis. You are responsible for its correct identification and safe arrival at the laboratory.

After arthrography, instruct the patient to rest the involved joint for several hours. If it is a knee or ankle joint, an Ace bandage may be applied to the site, and the patient should be instructed in the method of application and told to keep an Ace bandage on the site for several days. The patient should also be told that there may be some swelling or discomfort and there may be some crackling noise heard as the contrast is absorbed. The patient may be told to use ice applications for the swelling, and the physician may prescribe pain medication. Advise the patient to see the physician immediately if there is redness, warmth, or drainage at the site of needle insertion.

Lithotripsy

Extracorporeal lithotripsy is a relatively new method of removing gallstones (biliary calculi, cholelithiasis), renal calculi (kidney stones, urolithiasis), and salivary stone (sialolithiasis). This is a noninvasive procedure that uses shock waves directed at calculi in the gallbladder, the common bile duct, the renal calyx, and the submandibular gland. The radiographer is a part of the team that conducts these procedures because radiographic films and fluoroscopy are a part of the procedure.

For lithotripsy procedures performed for removal of biliary or renal calculi, the patient is immersed in a water bath or positioned on a fluid-filled cushion, and shock waves generated by electric, piezoelectric, or electromagnetic discharge are directed at the stones that are meant to be fragmented. The waves are transmitted through the water without being absorbed as long as solid body tissues such as the lungs, bones, or gastrointestinal tract are avoided. The calculi are broken into fragments and are then passed in the urine or dissolved in bile acid or saliva. Ultrasound may be used to visualize the calculi.

The patient who receives extracorporeal shockwave lithotripsy is usually treated on an outpatient basis, because there is no surgical incision or pretreatment care. If high total shock wave energy is used during the procedure to disintegrate the stones, the patient may receive a light anesthesia with a medication such as fentanyl or midazolam (Versed). The patient is usually discharged after the procedure, but he or she should be instructed to plan to be transported home by another person because he or she will be unable to drive.

A second type of lithotripsy procedure, called *intracorporeal lithotripsy*, is used to remove stones from the gallbladder or kidney after percutaneous insertion of an endoscope or nephroscope with visualization provided by use of a contrast agent and fluoroscopy. The stones are then fragmented with ultrasonic waves transmitted by an ultrasound probe placed near the stone. Another method of removing the pulverized stones is with a forceps or stone basket. The advent of laparoscopic cholecystectomy has reduced the use of this procedure.

Many of the patients who receive lithotripsy are in a weakened state, since they have undergone severe pain from the symptoms of their illness. They will also be anxious because of the unusual aspects of this treatment and will require additional time for reassurance and instruction. Explain the treatment to patients in some detail. If there will be a contrast agent or other drugs administered, the usual drug history is required. Informed consent forms must also be signed. Pregnancy and the presence of a cardiac pacemaker are contraindications to having a lithotripsy procedure of any kind.

After the procedure, instruct patients to inform their physician of any excessive blood in the urine, decreasing urine output, fever, or increasing pain. They may eat and drink according to physician's orders. If the procedure was for renal calculi or if the patient received a contrast agent, fluid intake must be increased.

Myelography

Myelography (myelogram) is a radiographic examination of the spinal cord in which an iodinated contrast agent, and, on some occasions, air is injected into the subarachnoid or epidural spaces of the spinal cord.

This examination is done to detect pathological conditions of the spinal cord such as a herniated intravertebral disc, tumors, malformation, and arthritic bone spurs. Other procedures that are less taxing often replace this diagnostic imaging procedure, and it is used less frequently than in the past.

Patient Care and Education Preceding Myelography

A consent form must be signed by the patient or an appointed person before this procedure is begun. Assess the patient for potential allergic reaction to iodinated contrast media. Instruct the patient to increase clear fluid intake and omit solid food for 4 hours before the examination to be well hydrated and to not become nauseated because of food in the stomach. Food and fluid restrictions may vary depending on the contrast agent used. The patient should empty the bladder and bowels before this examination.

Also instruct the patient to stop taking all drugs 24 hours before the examination. Drugs that may enhance the possibility of seizure activity are particularly important to omit. This includes phenothiazines, tricyclic antidepressants, central nervous system stimulants, and amphetamines. Monoamine oxidase inhibitors must be discontinued 2 weeks before a myelogram. Patients with a diagnosis of diabetes mellitus must be instructed by their physician on how to prevent a hypoglycemic or hyperglycemic reaction during preparation for myelography.

Myelography should not be performed on patients with multiple sclerosis, inflammation of the meninges, Pott's disease, infections or bloody subarachnoid fluid, increased intracranial pressure, or a recent myelogram. Iodinated contrast agents are used for this procedure, so all precautions taken when these drugs are administered apply. Myelograms may also be contraindicated in patients who are prone to seizures. Seizure-prone patients may receive medication to reduce the possibility of seizures before the examination. Physicians may order medication to reduce the patient's anxiety in preparation for this procedure.

The area into which the iodinated contrast agent is to be injected intrathecally is shaved, if necessary, and prepped as for other sterile invasive procedures. You should inform the patient that the table will be tilted during the examination but that a footrest and shoulder harness will prevent a fall. The patient's privacy must be protected by having him or her wear pajamas or by taping a drawsheet in place to prevent it from sliding off during the table movement.

Baseline vital signs should be taken before the myelogram begins and then monitored during the examination. Inform the patient that the examination will take from 1 to 2 hours to complete.

Intrathecal Drug Administration

Intrathecal (intraspinal) injections are given with a needle that is 3.5 inches long with a 16- to 25-gauge lumen. A stylet within the needle remains in place until the physician has completed the spinal puncture. When the needle is in the desired position in the spinal column, the stylet is removed, and the syringe containing the medication or contrast agent is attached to the needle.

The physician who is performing the special procedure or an anesthesiologist administers intrathecal drugs. An open sterile tray containing the necessary equipment and drugs will be available. You assist by obtaining any extra articles that the physician needs and placing them on the sterile field and positioning the patient. For lumbar myelography, the patient is usually placed in a prone position with a pillow under the abdomen to raise the lumbar area slightly (Fig. 16–5).

Report any unusual symptoms or complaints that the patient has while the myelogram is in progress to the physician performing the procedure. Specimens of spinal fluid are often collected during this procedure and should be correctly labeled, bagged, and taken or sent to the laboratory immediately.

Patient Care and Education After Myelography

After a myelogram, the patient who receives a water-soluble contrast agent should be instructed to remain at bedrest for 8 to 10 hours with the head of the bed slightly elevated at a 35- to 45-degree angle. This prevents the contrast agent from being dispersed upward and possibly prevent headache after the examination. If air was injected into the subarachnoid space, the patient is positioned with the head lower that the trunk of the body for 48 hours to prevent headache. The air is usually absorbed within this time frame, and the patient can then resume a normal position.

Inform the patient that he or she may have increased lumbar pain after a lumbar myelogram. Also encourage the patient to increase fluid intake. You should inform the patient to notify the physician immediately if he or she is unable to urinate or develops a fever, drowsiness, stiff neck, seizures, or paralysis. Other complications of myelography are arachnoiditis (inflammation of the delicate spinal cord covering) and meningitis. Any unusual reactions that the patient had to the contrast agent or in general are recorded on

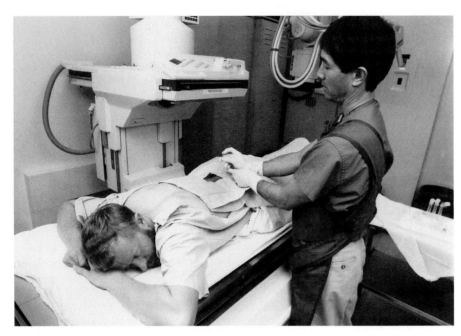

Figure 16–5. Patient receiving intrathecal drug administration.

the patient's chart. Also record the time that the procedure began and ended, specimens sent to the laboratory, and the patient's tolerance of the procedure. Instructions given to the patient for postmyelogram care are included on the chart.

CT scans are frequently used in combination with myelograms to improve visualization. They are described in the following section.

Contrast Agents

If you are the radiographer participating in special imaging procedures, you must learn the protocols for each procedure. You must also be certain that a health history and a drug history are taken for each patient to be examined. If a contrast agent is to be administered,

a history of allergic reactions as previously described must be taken. It is your responsibility to learn the intended action, the side effects, and the potential adverse effects of any drug that you administer. This includes contrast agents.

When the radiologist selects a contrast agent, he or she considers its viscosity, toxicity, iodine content, miscibility, and persistence. Contrast agents for intravascular use are either ionic or nonionic and are either of high or low osmolality. The positive intravascular contrast agents contain iodine to provide the contrast. You must become knowledgeable about the characteristics of the contrast agent selected. Table 16-1 lists some of the contrast agents and diagnostic imaging examinations for which they may be selected. The agents listed have been randomly selected and do not indicate authors' preferences or recommendations.

TABLE 16-1
Selected Contrast Agents and Examinations

EXAMINATION	AGENT	ROUTE OF ADMINISTRATION
Angiocardiography	Omnipaque 300 (iohexol)	Arterial catheter
	Visipaque (iodixanol)	
Arthrography	Hypaque Meglumine 60%	Injection
Computed tomography	Hypaque Meglumine 30%	Intravenous
	Omnipaque (iohexol)	
Cerebral angiography	Hexabrix (ioxaglate)	Arterial catheter
Magnetic resonance imaging	ProHance (gadoteridol)	Intravenous
	Magnavist (gadolinium)	
Myelography	Omnipaque 180 (iohexol)	Intrathecal

Summary

As a radiographer working in special procedures of diagnostic imaging, you are a member of a highly skilled technical team. As a member of this team, you must work with other team members to ensure positive patient outcomes from examinations and treatments. A successful outcome includes adequate patient preparation for the procedure and physical and emotional safety is it evolves.

Special procedures and radiographic imaging techniques in which you may participate as a radiographer involve specialized education. When working in these areas of patient care, you must be aware of the increased anxiety experienced by a patient who is about to undergo a complex procedure. You must not only be a highly skilled technologist but also have excellent therapeutic communication skills so that you are able to alleviate the patient's anxiety and fears.

Patients being examined by angiography, CT, ultrasonography, MRI, PET, radionuclide imaging, mammography, arthrography, lithotripsy, and myelography require special preparation and teaching. If you are the radiographer working in these areas of specialization, you must not neglect these aspects of patient care, since they are an important part of your professional practice.

One half of the patients who are diagnosed as having cancer receive external radiation therapy for treatment or control of symptoms. If you choose this area of specialization, you must understand that patients receiving this treatment are in varying stages of the grieving process and need extra time for communication. You must also realize that the cancer patient has an increased awareness of his or her body functions and focuses on physical symptoms that he or she would ignore at other times. You should make yourself available to discuss these problems with the patient whenever the patient desires. If you omit time for communication when caring for the patient receiving external radiation therapy, you are neglecting a vital professional obligation.

Patients receiving proton therapy have also been informed that they have a life-threatening disease. They will need the same thoughtful care as those receiving external radiation therapy.

If you are a radiographer working in a special procedures area, you must recognize your responsibility in drug administration. You must learn the protocols for each procedure and understand potential problems so that you are prepared to take the correct action should problems occur.

Chapter 16 Test

1. Discuss patient care responsibilities of the radiographer before and after cardiac catheterization.

2. Explain the patient teaching that must follow cardiac catheterization, angiography, and arteriography.

3. The patient teaching before CT should include the following: _____, _____, and _____.

4. A patient is to have a barium enema and an abdominal ultrasound examination. Explain how you as the radiographer will schedule these examinations.

5. Describe the common causes of anxiety before MRI. Explain how you may alleviate these fears?

6. Explain the potential problems that may occur if an elderly demented patient is to have PET.

7. Describe the patient teaching needs of a patient who has had radionuclide imaging.

8. Explain the generalized systemic reactions that may occur when a patient is receiving radiation therapy for cancer treatment.

9. Describe the special care considerations necessary for a patient receiving radiation therapy or proton therapy.

10. Define lithotripsy, and explain the medical indications for this treatment.

11. List the American Cancer Society guidelines for mammograms for women 40 years of age and older.

12. What are the common fears of women before mammography?

13. Explain the postarthrography teaching needs of a patient who has had a knee arthrogram.

14. Ms. Mary Misfeed is an 80-year-old white woman who has come to the diagnostic imaging department for a lumbar myelogram. She has come alone on the bus and plans to return home after the procedure. Discuss the problems, potential problems, and teaching needs of this patient.

Bibliography

Academy 2000: *IV Therapy and Phlebotomy Practicum*. Long Beach, California: Healthcare Education Academy, 2001.

Acello, B: Meeting HCAHO standards for pain control. *Nursing*, 30(3): 52–54, 2000.

Acello, B: Controlling pain, facing fears about opioid addiction. *Nursing*, 30(5): 72, 2000.

Agins, Alan P: *Pharmacology for Advanced Practice Clinicians*. Sponsored by Contemporary Forums, Los Angeles, 1995.

Andrews, TA: Radiology: Vitalt o child abuse detection. *Advance for Radiologic Science Professionals*, 13 (9): 13–25, 2000.

Asselin, M, and Cullen, HA: What you need to know about the new BLS Guidelines. *Nursing*, 31(3): 48–50, 2001.

Ballinger, Phillip W: *Radiographic Positions and Radiologic Procedures*, 9th ed. vol. 1. St. Louis: CV Mosby, 1999.

Ballinger, Philip, and Frank, Eugene: *Merrill's Atlas of Radiographic Positions and Radiologic Procedures*, 9th ed, vol. 2. St. Louis: CV Mosby, 1999.

Barcham, N, Egan, I, and Dowd, S: Gonadal protection method in neonatal chest radiography. *Journal of the American Society of Radiologic Technologists*, 69(2): 157–161, 1977.

Burton, Gwendolyn RW, and Engelkirk PG. *Microbiology for the Health Sciences*, 6th ed. Philadelphia: Lippincott Williams & Wilkins, 2000.

Carpenter, DO, et al: *Reading ECG Rhythm Strips Workbook*. Expert Nurse Video Series. Springhouse, Pennsylvania: Springhouse Corporation, 2001.

Chin, James: *Control of Communicable Diseases Manual*, 7th edition. Washington, DC: American Public Health Association, 2000.

Chohan, Naina, et al, eds. *Nursing 2001 Drug Handbook*, 21st ed. Springhouse, Pennsylvania: Springhouse Corporation, 2001.

Cohen, Mark: *Legislative Update*. Sutter Health Risk Management Department. AB 891, Health Care Decision Law, California, February 2000.

Coleman, E, and Kearney, K: Anthrax. *American Journal of Nursing*, 101(12): 48–49, 2001.

Collins, P, et al: Educating staff about pain management. *American Journal of Nursing*, 100(1): 59, 2000.

Connor, Barry C: *A Complete Course Practical Electrocardiography*. Bonita, California: Healthcare Education Academy, 2001.

Corwin, EJ: *Handbook of Pathophysiology*, 2nd ed. Philadelphia: Lippincott Williams & Wilkins, 2000.

Dansak, RL: Portable procedures: What RT's should know *RT Image*, 14(8): 41–43, 2001.

Dansak, RL: The power of poise and chitchat. *RT Image*, 13(35): 35–38, 2000.

Dillehunt, David B: Advance for administrators in radiology. *PACS Beyond Radiology*, 10(11): 54, 2000.

Dowd, SB, and Durick D: Addressing the needs of elderly radiology patients. *Journal of the American Society of Radiologic Technologists*, 66(5): 299–306, 1995.

Dowd SB, and Durick, D: Elder abuse: The R.T.'s role in diagnosis and prevention. *Journal of the American Society of Radiologic Technologists*, 68(1): 23–28, 1996.

Durbin, D: *Rapid Interpretation of EKG's*, 6th ed. Tampa: Cover Publishing Company, 2000.

Eastman, TR: Portable radiography. *Journal of the American Society of Radiologic Technologists*, 69(5): 475–478, 1998.

Eisenber, Roland, and Dennis, Cynthia: *Comprehensive Radiographic Pathology*, 2nd ed. St. Louis: CV Mosby, 1995.

Furlow, B: Bone fracture fixation.*Journal of the American Society of Radiologic Technologists*, 71(6): 543–562.

Galasko, Gail T: *Pharmacology for Advanced Practice Clinicians*. Sponsored by Contemporary Forums, Denver, New Orleans, Philadelphia, 2001.

Gilman, M: Transcultural care for the elderly. *RT Image*, 13(6): 30–32, 2000.

Gladwin, Mark, and Trattler, Bill: *Clinical Microbiology Made Ridiculously Simple*, 2nd ed. Miami: Med Master, Inc, 1999.

Goldman, Lee: Advance for administrators in radiology: Implementing. *PACS*, 20(11): 62, 2000.

Graham, MC, and Dellinger, RW: Emergency department patients within the scope of nurse practitioner practice. *American Journal of Nurse Practitioners*, 5(3): 29–42, 2001.

Hallstrom, A, et al: Taking the P out of CPR. *Clinician Reviews*, 10(7): 48, 2000.

Ingraham, JL, and Ingraham, CA: *Introduction to Microbiology*, 2nd ed. Pacific Grove, California: Brooks/Cole Thomson Learning, 2000.

Jensen, Steven C, and Peppers, Michael P: *Pharmacology and Drug Administration*. St. Louis: CV Mosby, 1998.

Karch, Amy M: *Focus on Nursing Pharmacology*. Philadelphia: Lippincott Williams & Wilkins, 2000.

Langford, Rae W, and Thompson, June D: *Handbook of Diseases*, 2nd ed. St. Louis: CV Mosby, 2000.

Laskowski-Jones, L: Responding to pediatric trauma. *Nursing 2001 Journal of Clinical Excellence*, 31(9): 37–41, 2001.

Linn-Watson, TerriAnn: *Radiographic Pathology*. Philadelphia: WB Saunders, 1996.

McCaffery, M: Understanding your patient's pain tolerance. *Nursing*, 29(12):17, 1999.

McCann, Judith, ed: *Diagnostics: An A–to–Z Nursing Guide to Laboratory Tests and Diagnostic Procedures*. Springhouse, Pennsylvania: Springhouse, Corporation, 2001.

Meeker, Margaret H, and Rothrock, Jane C: *Alexander's Care of the Patient in Surgery*, 11th ed. St. Louis: CV Mosby, 1999.

Motto, KP: Detecting and preventing elder abuse. *RT Image*, 13(21): 27–28, 2000.

Motto, KP: The role of radiology in diagnosing child abuse. *RT Image*, 13(44): 32–34, 2000.

Myeek, MJ, Harvey, RA, and Champe, PC: *Pharmacology: Lippincott's Illustrated Reviews*, 2nd ed. Philadelphia: Lippincott Williams & Wilkins, 2000.

National Center on Elder Abuse (1996–1999). Elder Abuse Information Series (On-Line). http//www.elderabusecenter.org.htm.

Norris, TG: Pediatric skeletal trauma. *Journal of the American Society of Radiologic Technologists*, 72(4): 245–264, 2001.

O'Brien, NM: Putting children at ease in radiology. *Advances for Radiologic Science Professionals*, 13(9): 10–11, 2000.

Pagana, D, and Pagana, T: *Mosby's Diagnostic and Laboratory Text Reference*. St. Louis: CV Mosby, 1997.

Pasero, C: Oral Patient-controlled analgesia. *American Journal of Nursing*, 1000(3): 24–25, 2000.

Paul, Richard: *Critical Thinking: How to Prepare Students for a Rapidly Changing World*. Edited by Jane Willsen and AJA Binker Foundation for Critical Thinking, Santa Rosa, California, 1995.

Peart, O: Pediatric imaging. *RT Image*, 12(21): 20–23, 2001.

Potter, Patricia A, and Perry, Anne Griffin: *Basic Nursing: A Critical Thinking Approach*, 4th ed. St. Louis: CV Mosby, 1999.

Ramsden, Elsa: *The Person as Patient*. Philadelphia: WB Saunders, 1999.

Rarey, LK: Radiologic Technologist Responses to Elderly Patients. *Journal of the American Society of Radiologic Technologists*, 69(6): 56–572, 1998.

Rosdahl, Caroline Bunker: *Textbook of Basic Nursing*, 7th ed. Philadelphia: Lippincott Williams & Wilkins, 1999.

Safran, Jeremy, and Nuran, J. Christopher: *Negotiating the Therapeutic Alliance: A Relational Treatment Guide*. New York, London: The Guilford Press, 2000.

Saia, DA: *Prep Program Review and Examination Preparation*, 2nd ed. Stamford, Connecticut: Appleton & Lange, 1999.

Salerno, Evelyn: *Pharmacology for Health Professionals*. St. Louis: CV Mosby, 1999.

Schoofs, Mark: The AIDS race: Can new drugs keep up with the wily virus? *The Village Voice*, New York, April 10, 2000.

Semb, S: Diabetes care: Competencies for patient teaching. *Continuing Medical Education Resource*. Sacramento, California, 2000, pp. 49–86.

Sisk, J: Are Hospital EDs kidfFriendly? *Radiology Today*, 2(18): 6, 2001.

Smeltzer, SC, and Bare, BG: *Brunner and Suddarth's Textbook of Medical-Surgical Nursing*, 8th ed. Philadelphia, Lippincott-Raven, 1996.

Smeltzer, SC, and Bare, BG: *Brunner and Suddarth's Textbook of Medical-Surgical Nursing*, 9th ed. Philadelphia, Lippincott-Raven, 1999.

Smeltzer, SC, and Bare, BG: *Brunner and Suddarth's Textbook of Medical-Surgical Nursing*. Philadelphia: Lippincott Williams & Wilkins, 2000.

Snopek, A: *Fundamentals of Special Radiographic Procedures*, 4th ed. Philadelphia: WB Saunders, 1999.

Stanley, Karen: *Making Appropriate End-of-Life Decisions*. Claremont, California, 2001.

Stapelton, ER, et al, eds: *BLS for Healthcare Providers*. Dallas: American Heart Association, 2001.

Tamparo, C, and Lewis, M: *Diseases of the Human Body*, 3rd ed. Philadelphia: FA Davis, 2000.

Weinstock, D, et al: *Nursing Procedures*, 3rd ed. Springhouse, Pennsylvania: Springhouse Corporation, 1999.

Wells, J, Salyer, S: Diagnosing pulmonary embolism: A medical masquerade. *Clinician Reviews*, 11(2): 67–70, 2000.

Whaley, Lynne, and Rue Mearns, Stephanie: *Critical Thinking*. Milbrea, California: California Academic Press, 1999.

Williams, Erica: *Patient Care*. New York: McGraw-Hill, 1999.

Index

Page numbers in italics denote figures; those followed by a t *denote tables; those followed by a* d *denote displays.*